OBSTETRICS AND GYNECOLOGY RECALL
SECOND EDITION

OBSTETRICS AND GYNECOLOGY RECALL
SECOND EDITION

EDITOR

F. JOHN BOURGEOIS, M.D., F.A.C.O.G., F.A.C.P.
Associate Professor
Department of Obstetrics and Gynecology
University of Virginia
Charlottesville, Virginia

ASSOCIATE EDITORS

PAOLA A. GEHRIG, M.D.
Assistant Professor
Division of Gynecologic Oncology
University of North Carolina at Chapel Hill
Chapel Hill, North Carolina

DAN S. VELJOVICH, M.D.
Gynecologic Oncology
Pacific Gynecology Specialists and
University of Washington
Seattle, Washington

 LIPPINCOTT WILLIAMS & WILKINS
A **Wolters Kluwer** Company
Philadelphia · Baltimore · New York · London
Buenos Aires · Hong Kong · Sydney · Tokyo

Acquisitions Editor: Neil Marquardt
Managing Editors: Daniel Pepper, Crystal Taylor
Development Editors: Elena Coler, Emilie Linkins
Marketing Manager: Scott Lavine
Production Editor: Jennifer Glazer
Compositor: Maryland Composition, Inc.
Printer: RR Donnelley

Printed in the United States of America

First Edition, 1997

Library of Congress Cataloging-in-Publication Data

Bourgeois, F. John.
    Obstetrics and gynecology recall / editor F. John Bourgeois; associate editors, Paola A. Gehrig, Daniel S. Veljovich.– 2nd ed.
        p. cm.—(Recall series)
    Includes index.
    ISBN 0-7817-4879-8
    1. Obstetrics—Examinations, questions, etc. 2. Gynecology—Examinations, questions, etc. I. Gehrig, Paola A. II. Veljovich, Daniel S. III. Title. IV. Series.
        [DNLM: 1. Obstetrics—examination questions. 2. Genital Diseases, Female—examination questions. WQ 18.2 B772o 2004]
    RG111.O38 2004
    618'.076—dc22
                                                                        2004044198
                                                                        CIP

The publishers have made every effort to trace the copyright holders for borrowed material. If they have inadvertently overlooked any, they will be pleased to make the necessary arrangements at the first opportunity.

To purchase additional copies of this book, call our customer service department at **(800) 638-3030** or fax orders to **(301) 824-7390**. International customers should call **(301) 714-2324**.

Visit Lippincott Williams & Wilkins on the Internet: **http://www.lww.com**. Lippincott Williams & Wilkins customer service representatives are available from 8:30 am to 6:00 pm, EST, Monday through Friday, for telephone access.

04 05 06 07 08
1 2 3 4 5 6 7 8 9 10

Dedication

This book recognizes Annie Bourgeois, who valued veracity and education, and did not care to compromise either. It is further an acknowledgment of the scholarship of W. Norman Thornton, Jr., M.D., who understood that the framework of knowledge and understanding does not require large volumes of words, but does require prioritization. I hope it reflects the philosophy of Joe Covelli, M.D., who understood that in clinical medicine compassion without accuracy doesn't do much good. However, it is dedicated to you.

RECALL SERIES EDITOR

LORNE H. BLACKBOURNE, M.D., F.A.C.S.
Fellow, Trauma/Critical Care
Department of Surgery
University of Miami
Jackson Memorial Hospital
Miami, Florida

Contents

CONTRIBUTORS TO THE FIRST EDITION

Gina Adrales, M.D.

Terry Allen, M.D.

Jessica Biesecker, M.D.

Susan Bliss, M.D.

Megan Bray, M.D.

Amy Erdman, M.D.

Maria Gluch, M.D.

Kathie Hullfish, M.D.

Amir Jazaeri, M.D.

Elizabeth Kane, M.D.

Sunita Kulshrestha, M.D.

Kelly MacMillan, M.D.

Niel Mason, M.D., Pharm.D.

Helen Malone, M.D.

Tanya Paul, M.D.

John Schnorr, M.D.

Amy Timmons, M.D.

Charrell Washington, M.D.

CONTRIBUTORS TO THE SECOND EDITION

Elizabeth Baker, M.D.

Christina Chandler, M.D.

Lisa Christianson, M.D.

Wendy Closshey, M.D.

Stephanie Flora, M.D.

Kimberly Galgano, M.D.

Jennifer Horton, M.D.

Daniel Kaelberer, M.D.

Lillian Mihm, M.D.

Erin Mullins, M.D.

Michelle Spears, M.D.

Preface

It's no accident that it's called "Recall." The questions and answers contained in this book review the fundamentals of obstetrics and gynecology, absent lengthy explanations and literature citations. *Obstetrics and Gynecology Recall* is designed to complement, not replace, more weighty sources. It is intended as a touchstone for testing students' mastery of already-gained knowledge—a good use for this book during both the clerkship and while preparing for the inevitable final exam.

But that's not all. What if you are just beginning your clerkship, and you are assigned a patient with a condition that you have barely heard of? Your guidebook to the essentials is *Obstetrics and Gynecology Recall*. By evening rounds you can be conversant regarding the condition, and well-prepared to consult a more comprehensive reference—a good way to generate knowledge and a great way to guarantee good evaluation.

Whether you need a rapid way to begin learning the fundamentals, or require a concise review of the key elements of obstetrics and gynecology to efficiently test your knowledge base, *Obstetrics and Gynecology Recall* is the place to start *and* to finish.

Section I

Obstetrics

1   Obstetric Glossary

Abortion

Pregnancy termination prior to 20 weeks' gestation with fetus weighing less than 500 grams

Complete—all products of conception are evacuated

Incomplete—some products of conception remain in the uterus

Inevitable—vaginal bleeding with an open cervix

Threatened—vaginal bleeding with a closed cervix

Abruption

Complete or partial separation of the placenta prior to the delivery of the fetus

AFP

Alpha-fetoprotein; produced primarily by the fetal liver, used as a screening test for congenital birth defects and chromosomal anomalies

Amniocentesis

Removal of amniotic fluid, usually by transabdominal aspiration; used either for therapeutic or diagnostic purposes

Amniotic fluid

During the first trimester, an ultrafiltrate of maternal plasma

Later in gestation, transudation of fetal plasma across the fetal skin

At 12 to 24 weeks, fetal urine begins to contribute.

Other sources include the fetal gastrointestinal and respiratory tracts, as well as transudate across the umbilical cord.

Apgar score

Assessment of the newborn, primarily at 1, 5, and 10 minutes by evaluating tone, heart rate, irritability, color, and respirations

β-HCG

Beta subunit of human chorionic gonadotropin
Produced by the syncytiotrophoblast
Maintains the corpus luteum in early pregnancy
Used to detect pregnancy

Battledore placenta

Umbilical cord attachment to the edge of the placenta

Betamethasone

Steroid given when preterm delivery is suspected, decreases incidence & severity of respiratory distress on the newborn.

Biophysical profile

Intrauterine evaluation of the fetus using nonstress test (NST), fetal breathing movements, fetal movement, fetal tone, and amniotic fluid index (AFI)

Bishop score

A scoring system used to assess the likelihood of success of induction of labor using factors such as dilatation, effacement, station, consistency, and position of the cervix

Breech

Complete (5%–10%)—flexed thighs and knees, feet above the buttocks
Frank (50%–75%)—flexed thighs, extended knees
Footling or incomplete (20%)—leg(s) extended below the umbilicus

Cervical incompetence

Cervical dilation without contractions

Chadwick's sign

A clinical sign consisting of a bluish discoloration to the cervix and vaginal walls that may suggest pregnancy

Chloasma

"Mask of pregnancy" brownish patches of facial skin that may occur during pregnancy or with oral contraceptive use (also known as melasma)

Chorioamnionitis

Acute or chronic infection/inflammation of the fetal membranes

Circumvallate placenta

Circumvallate caused by inappropriate placentation

CVS

Chorionic villi sampling—placental tissue is removed between 9 and 12 weeks by either transabdominal or transvaginal means and used for genetic evaluation

Coombs

Used to detect maternal red blood cell antibodies

Corpus luteum

Physiologic ovarian cyst; maintains progesterone production during early pregnancy until the placenta begins to function

CST

Contraction stress test

Crown rump length

In early pregnancy, used to estimate gestational age; add 6.5 weeks to the measurement obtained on ultrasound to estimate gestational age

DES

Diethylstilbestrol; fetal exposure to this drug may result in genital-tract anomalies, including incompetent cervix, cervical adenosis, vaginal adenosis, increased risk for clear-cell adenocarcinoma of the cervix and vagina, and other uterine structural anomalies in women.
Used archaically to prevent abortion

DIC

Disseminated intravascular coagulopathy

"Double setup"

Pelvic exam performed in the operating room with the means to perform an emergent cesarean section if there is significant bleeding or fetal distress;

	previously performed in women with suspected placenta previa
EASI	Extra ammiotic saline infusion - used for cervical ripening
Eclampsia	Seizures during pregnancy; the most severe manifestation of pregnancy-induced hypertension
EDC	Estimated date of confinement ("due date"); 280 days from the first day of the last menstrual period
Endometritis	Infection of endometrium (and myometrium) most commonly occurring after delivery
FHR	Fetal heart rate (normal is between 120 and 160 bpm, fetal bradycardia is < 120 bpm, and fetal tachycardia is > 160 bpm)
FHT	Fetal heart tone—refers to auditory detection of FHR
Episiotomy	Surgical procedure performed at the time of vaginal delivery in an attempt to minimize stretching of the perineum The most common form is a midline episiotomy extending from the posterior aspect of the vaginal introitus through the superficial perineal muscles and down through the vaginal mucosa.
FSE	Fetal scalp electrode—used to monitor fetal heart rate after rupture of the fetal membranes has occurred
Forceps	Mechanism to assist vaginal deliveries by shortening the second stage of labor

	Indications include maternal exhaustion, fetal distress, and fetal malposition. Several different types (e.g., Keilland, Piper, Tucker-McLean) are available, depending on the indication.
$G_a\ P_{bcde}$	a = number of pregnancies b = full-term deliveries c = pre-term deliveries d = abortions; (spont, elective, ectopic, etc) e = living children
GDM	Gestational diabetes mellitus
GTD	Gestational trophoblastic disease
Gravida	The number of times a woman has been pregnant or a pregnant woman
hCG	Human chorionic gonadotropin
HELLP	Subset of preeclampsia characterized by Hemolysis, Elevated Liver enzymes, and Low Platelets
hPL	Human placental lactogen or human placental somatomammotropin
Hydrops	Anasarca of the fetus associated with ascites, generalized edema, pleural effusions, etc; most commonly ascribed to anemia as a consequence of hemolysis
Hyperemesis gravidarum	Occurs in approximately 5/1000 pregnancies Associated with nausea and vomiting causing dehydration, electrolyte imbalance and weight loss Etiologic factors include psychosocial, thyroid disease, and trophoblastic disease.

IUGR   Intrauterine growth restriction
                                  Asymmetric—Head growth remains
                                  near normal.
                                  Symmetric—The entire fetus is small.

IUI   Intrauterine insemenation

IUPC   Intrauterine pressure cathether—allows
                                  for monitoring of frequency, duration
                                  and strength of uterine contractions

IVF   In vitro fertilization

Kell antigen   Major red blood cell antigen, may cause
                                  hydrops if present

Labor   Uterine contractions leading to cervical
                                  dilatation and effacement

Leopold maneuvers   Examination of maternal abdomen that
                                  allows fetal weight, position, and lie to
                                  be estimated

Lie   Relation of fetal spine to maternal spine;
                                  vertical or longitudinal is normal.

Macrosomia   Fetal weight greater than 4,000 grams;
                                  complicates approximately 5% of
                                  births
                                  Risk factors include maternal obesity,
                                  postdate pregnancy, maternal diabetes
                                  including GDM, and multiparity.

Magnesium sulfate   Used in the treatment of preterm labor
                                  and the prevention and treatment of
                                  eclamptic seizures

Mastitis   Infection of the breast, most commonly
                                  secondary to infections with S. *aureus*
                                  or *Streptococcus* as a result of breast-
                                  feeding
                                  Feeding from the affected breast may be
                                  continued, in contrast to a breast

abscess, in which feeding must be discontinued until treated.

Meconium   Infant's first bowel movement, composed of sloughed cells from intestinal mucosa May occur in utero as a result of stress and may lead to respiratory compromise if aspiration occurs

Molar pregnancy   Please refer to the chapter on gestational trophoblastic disease (see Chapter 41).

MSAFP   Maternal serum alpha-fetoprotein

Nifedipine   Calcium channel blocker used to treat preterm labor

Naegele's Rule   Formula to calculate Estimated Date of Confinement (EDC)

Nitabuch's layer   Layer between the uterus and the invading trophoblasts; absence will lead to abnormal placental implantation (i.e., accreta, increta, and percreta)

LMP   add 7 days
                             subract 3 months
                             add 1 year

NST   Nonstress test

NSVD   Normal spontaneous vaginal delivery

Nuchal cord   Umbilical cord around the fetal neck; may lead to distress during labor and delivery
                             Frequent cause of variable decelerations during childbirth
                             Often innocuous

Oxytocin   Hormone released by the pituitary that stimulates labor onset

Parturition	Process of labor and delivery
Pfannenstiel	Low transverse abdominal incisions
Pitocin	Synthetic form of oxytocin used in the induction of labor
Placenta accreta	Attachment of the placenta in the uterine musculature (myometrium) secondary to absence of Nitabuch's layer
Placenta increta	Invasion of the placenta into the myometrium
Placenta percreta	Penetration of the placenta through the myometrium to the serosa
Placenta previa	Placenta covering various degrees of cervical os
Postdates	Gestational age greater than 42 weeks - indication for induction
Postpartum hemorrhage	Greater than 500 cc blood loss at the time of vaginal delivery. Most common causes include uterine atony (inability to contract), retained products of conception (POC), obstetrical lacerations, abnormal placental implantation, and bleeding dyscrasia.
Preeclampsia	Pregnancy-induced hypertension; please refer to Chapter 15, Hypertensive Disorders in Pregnancy.
Preterm	Gestational age less than 37 weeks
PROM	Rupture of fetal membranes prior to the onset of labor
PPROM	Preterm premature rupture of

	membranes: Rupture of fetal membranes prior to 37 weeks' gestation
PUPPPs	Pruritic urticaria, pustules, and plaques of pregnancy
Pseudocyesis	The belief that one is pregnant without being pregnant
Puerperium	The period of time surrounding birth—commonly defined up to 6 weeks after delivery.
Quadruple screen	Offered between 8 and 18 weeks' gestation Involves four tests performed on maternal serum AFP, estriol, hCG, and inhibin Used to detect birth defects of chromosomal anomalies and neural tube defects.
Rh	Major blood group antigen of importance during pregnancy Incompatibility between mother (-) and fetus (+) may lead to hemolytic disease of the newborn.
RhoGAM	Rh immune globulin given to gravidas who are Rh negative if there is suspicion of fetal–maternal bleeding; for example, is given if there is bleeding during any trimester, after delivery, and prophylactically at 28 weeks
Scanzoni	Maneuver describing rotation of the fetal head through an arc of 180° to facilitate delivery from OP to OA
Sheehan syndrome	Pituitary ablation as a result of hypotension after delivery May result in amenorrhea, inability to breast-feed, etc.

Shoulder dystocia	Inability to deliver the fetus through the maternal pelvic outlet because of either macrosomic infant or relatively contracted pelvis
***Streptococcus* group B**	Found in approximately 30% to 40% of healthy women; may be a risk factor for preterm labor or premature rupture of membranes
Terbutaline	Betamimetic medication used in the treatment of preterm labor
Tocolysis	Therapy initiated to stop preterm labor
Tocomoter	External uterine contraction monitor—allows for monitoring of frequency and duration of contractions.
TOL	Trial of labor
Vasa previa	Placental vessels crossing the cervical os
VBAC	Vaginal birth after cesarean
Velamentous cord	Umbilical cord vessel attachment to the placenta by thin membranes; may lead to vasa previa
White's classification	Used to classify diabetes in pregnancy; please refer to the chapter on gestational diabetes.
Wood's maneuver	Used during a shoulder dystocia to rotate the anterior shoulder counterclockwise to an oblique position in an attempt to facilitate delivery
Zavanelli maneuver	Replacement of the fetal head through the vagina followed by a cesarean section; used in rare cases of **severe** shoulder dystocia

2

Maternal Physiology

What are hPL and hCG?

hPL = Human placental lactogen hormone

hCG = Human chorionic gonadotropin hormone

Where are they produced?

hPL and hCG are produced in the syncytiotrophoblasts of the placenta.

What are their functions?

hPL antagonizes effects of insulin and enhances lipolysis to ensure adequate blood glucose for the fetus; hCG stimulates the corpus luteum to produce progesterone and estradiol until the placenta is capable of autonomous steroidogenesis.

SKIN

What changes occur in the skin during pregnancy?

Striae gravidarum ("stretch marks"); vascular spiders (telangiectasias) and palmar erythema caused by increased estrogen levels; hirsutism and acne secondary to increased progesterone levels; hyperpigmentation of nipples, areolae, axillae, umbilicus, midline abdomen ("linea nigra"); and melasma or chloasma of the face ("mask of pregnancy") due to increased levels of melanocyte-stimulating hormone

BREASTS

What changes occur in the breast during pregnancy?

Enlargement, increased cystic consistency, dilatation of superficial venous patterns, darkening of areolae, sebaceous gland hypertrophy, colostrum production in late pregnancy

GENITAL TRACT

What is the Chadwick sign?	Bluish discoloration of the upper vaginal vault and cervix secondary to increased vascularity and hyperemia.
Other vaginal changes in pregnancy?	Increase in thickness of the mucosa, loosening of the connective tissue, and hypertrophy of the smooth-muscle cells.
What is the Hegar sign?	Softening of the lower uterine segment; often occurs in early pregnancy
How is this sign appreciated during examination?	Cervix is distinctly separate from the lower uterus; a soft isthmus is located between the cervix and uterus.
What is the leukorrhea of pregnancy?	Increased vaginal discharge of pregnancy secondary to increased vaginal capillary permeability and desquamation of vaginal epithelial cells
What changes occur within the cervix?	Increased eversion of cervical columnar epithelium onto the exocervix, making it more friable. Rearrangement of collagen-rich connective tissue reducing its mechanical strength by term.
What causes growth of the pregnant uterus?	During the first 8-10 weeks, uterine hypertrophy. Afterwards, it is mainly caused by the enlarging fetus and sac.
When does the uterus exceed the boundary of the pelvis?	12 weeks.

CARDIOVASCULAR

What percentage of cardiac output is devoted to uterine blood flow in pregnancy?	20% (approximately 500 ml/min) at term

In the nonpregnant state?	Less than 1%
What percentages of uterine blood flow are devoted to perfusing the different parts of theuterus?	5% perfuses the myometrium. 10%–15% perfuses the endometrium. 80%–85% perfuses the placenta.
What happens to the blood flow to the kidneys, breasts, and skin in pregnancy?	Increases
What changes in blood volume, red cell mass (RCM), and plasma mass occur in pregnancy?	Blood volume increases by 30%–50%. RCM increases by 35%. Plasma volume increases by 50%.
What is a consequence of the increase in plasma volume in pregnancy?	Physiologic "anemia" of pregnancy due to the relatively greater increase in plasma volume compared to RCM; hematocrit decreases approximately 5%, but the RBC count does not decrease.
When does this effect peak during pregnancy?	At approximately 28 weeks.
What causes true anemia in pregnancy?	Iron deficiency, folate deficiency, hemoglobinopathies
What changes in heart rate, stroke volume, and cardiac output occur during pregnancy?	Heart rate: increases 5%–15%, maximizing at term Stroke volume: increases 20%–35%, maximizing during the second trimester Cardiac output: increases 35%–45%, maximizing at 20–24 weeks' gestation; further increases of up to 40% during the second stage of labor
What are the consequences of these changes?	Rotation and elevation of the heart on the longitudinal axis, which manifests as slight left axis deviation on EKG and the appearance of cardiomegaly on chest x-ray

What heart murmurs are normal in pregnancy?

Late systolic or ejection murmurs

What effect does pregnancy have on blood pressure?

Blood pressure: falls from the first trimester to the middle of the second trimester; increases to prepregnancy levels by term

Systolic pressure: decreases approximately 4 mm Hg

Diastolic pressure: decreases approximately 10–15 mm Hg

What is the baseline blood pressure in pregnancy?

Early first-trimester blood pressures

What are the consequences of vena cava compression caused by the enlarging uterus in pregnancy?

Decreased cardiac output (secondary to decreased venous return) can cause nausea, dizziness, and syncope ("supine hypotensive syndrome") if not compensated for by increased peripheral resistance.

Increased venous pressure proximal to the area of compression can lead to worsening varicose veins in the legs and vulva, increased lower extremity edema, and decreased venous flow, which contributes to the increased risk of thrombosis in pregnancy.

RESPIRATORY

What changes in respiratory rate, tidal volume, total lung capacity, and vital capacity occur during pregnancy?

Respiratory rate: unchanged or slightly increased

Tidal volume: increased up to 40%

Total lung capacity: decreased from about 4200 to 4000 ml secondary to increased pressure from the enlarging uterus on the diaphragm

Residual volume: decreased from 1000 to 800 ml

Vital capacity: unchanged

Why is vital capacity unchanged during pregnancy?

Increased tidal volume is negated by decreased expiratory reserve volume.

What blood gas changes occur in pregnancy?

Increased pH and decreased PCO_2 secondary to hyperventilation (increased minute ventilation secondary to 40% increase in tidal volume at term)

Decreased serum HCO_3 due to increased renal excretion to compensate for mild respiratory alkalosis

Net pH between 7.40 and 7.45

What is physiological dyspnea?

Increased awareness of the desire to breathe

Why does it occur?

Increase in tidal volume slightly decreases PCO_2, which paradoxically causes dyspnea.

HEMATOLOGIC

How do WBC and platelet counts change in pregnancy?

WBC counts: increase slightly in pregnancy (10,000 to 14,000/mm^3); minimal left shift

Platelet counts: decrease slightly in later pregnancy, which may be related to increased platelet aggregation

What is the significance of thrombocytopenia during pregnancy?

It is not physiologic and should be investigated.

What are normal WBC count values during labor?

WBC count can reach 25,000–30,000/mm^3 without infection (average during labor and early puerperium is 14,000–16,000/mm^3).

How is the coagulation system affected by pregnancy?

Pregnancy is a hypercoagulable state. Coagulation factors I, II, VII, VIII, IX, and X are increased as a result of increased hepatic synthesis.
Fibrinogen is increased by 50%
D-dimer levels are also elevated.

What are the consequences of the coagulation system changes during pregnancy?

Increased risk of thromboembolism (especially in the late third trimester and puerperium); pulmonary embolism ranks second in causes of maternal mortality after hemorrhage.

MUSCULOSKELETAL

What causes lower back pain in late pregnancy?

Increased mobility in sacroiliac, sacrococcygeal pubic joints; along with a changing center of gravity caused by the enlarging uterus cause a progressive lordosis.

How does progesterone affect smooth muscle in pregnancy?

Inhibits smooth muscle peristalsis in GI, urinary, and biliary tracts

What are the consequences of smooth muscle inhibition?

GI tract: delayed gastric emptying, reflux esophagitis, and constipation
Urinary tract: ureteral dilatation, urinary stasis, and predisposition to pyelonephritis
Biliary tract: stasis plus changes in serum bile salt concentrations; may predispose to cholelithiasis and cholecystitis

GASTROINTESTINAL

What are the effects of pregnancy related to appendicitis?

Diagnosis may be delayed (and mortality is thus higher) because of the altered position of the appendix in the upper RLQ secondary to enlarging uterus.

What are the effects of pregnancy related to pancreatitis?

Increased frequency of cholelithiasis and perhaps hyperlipidemia lead to increased frequency of pancreatitis in pregnant women.

RENAL

How are renal blood flow and glomerular filtration rate (GFR) altered in pregnancy?

Both increase approximately 40%–50%.

What effects do these changes have on serum creatinine, BUN, and uric acid concentrations?

Serum concentrations decrease because of increased excretion secondary to the increased GFR.

What accounts for the increased incidence of pyelonephritis in pregnancy?

Progesterone-mediated laxity of ureteral smooth muscle leads to inhibition of peristalsis in the ureter.

Pressure of the enlarging uterus on the ureter (right greater than left due to the tendency of the pregnant uterus to lie to the right) leads to ureteral dilatation and urostasis.

High incidence of cystitis in pregnancy predisposes to upper urinary tract infection (UTI).

What is the major risk associated with pyelonephritis in pregnancy?

Preterm labor

What are the common UTI organisms in pregnancy?

Gram negatives: *Escherichia coli* (70%–80%), *Klebsiella pneumoniae* (5%–10%), *Proteus species* (5%–10%)

Gram positives: Group B streptococci (3%–5%), enterococci (3%–5%), staphylococci (1%–3%)

What is the serious complication associated with untreated pyelonephritis in pregnancy?	Adult respiratory distress syndrome.

ENDOCRINE

Does pregnancy affect thyroid function?	No, but results of thyroid function tests can be affected.
How are thyroid function tests affected in pregnancy?	Thyroid-binding globulin (TBG): increased secondary to estrogen-stimulated hepatic synthesis; reflected in low thyroid uptake [triiodothyronine (T_3) resin uptake] values Total thyroxine (T_4) and total T_3: elevated, because a significant percentage of each bind TBG Free T_4 and free T_3: normal Thyroid-stimulating hormone (TSH): normal
What lab values suggest true hyperthyroidism and hypothyroidism in pregnancy?	True hyperthyroidism: elevated free T_4 True hypothyroidism: elevated TSH
Can T_3, T_4, or TSH diffuse across the placental membrane?	Yes; transfer is negligible.
What about thyroid-stimulating immunoglobin and propylthiouracil?	Yes

3

Female Pelvic Anatomy

What are the layers of the abdominal wall?

From external to internal: skin, subcutaneous fat, superficial fascia (Scarpa's), anterior rectus sheath, muscle, posterior rectus sheath, preperitoneal fat, and peritoneum

What is the arcuate line?

Also known as the linea semicircularis
Superior to the arcuate line, the posterior aponeurosis of the internal oblique and aponeurosis of the transversalis lie posterior to the rectus abdominis.
Inferior to the arcuate line, these aponeuroses lie anterior to the rectus abdominis.

Which bones compose the bony pelvis?

Ilium, ischium, pubis, sacrum, and coccyx
The pubis, ilium, and ischium join to form the innominate bone (Figures 3-1 and 3-2).

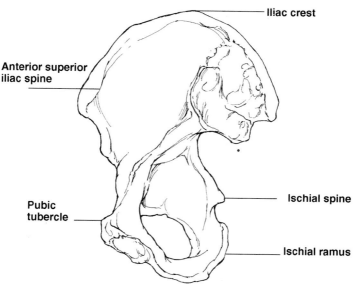

Figure 3–1

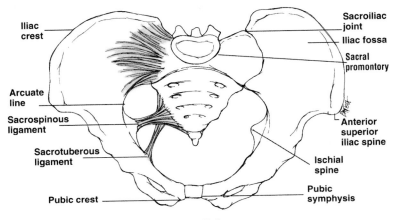

Figure 3-2

What are the four female pelvic configurations?	Gynecoid Android Anthropoid Platypelloid
What is a gynecoid pelvis?	"Typical" female pelvis shape found in approximately 50% of women. The anteroposterior and the transverse diameters are relatively equal, with straight pelvic sidewalls. The ischial spines are not usually prominent. The pubic arch is wide.
What is an android pelvis?	"Typical" male pelvis shape found in one-third of white women and one-sixth of nonwhite women Convergent sidewalls, prominent ischial spines, and a narrow pubic arch
What is an anthropoid pelvis?	This pelvic shape is found in 25% of white women and in approximately 50% of nonwhite women. The anteroposterior diameter is greater than the transverse diameter, giving this pelvis a "heart" shape.
What is a platypelloid pelvis?	Rarest pelvic type, found in 3% of women The transverse diameter is greater than the anteroposterior diameter, with wide sidewalls.

What is the pelvic inlet?

Its boundaries are the sacral promontory posteriorly, the pubic ramus and symphysis pubis anteriorly, and the linea terminalis laterally.

What is the fetal head "engaged"?

When the biparietal diameter of the fetal head passes through the inlet, the head is "Engaged."

What is the obstetric conjugate?

The shortest anteroposterior diameter between the sacral promontory and the symphysis pubis

Can only be measured radiographically

Normal measurement for the obstetric conjugate is > 10 centimeters (cm).

What is the true conjugate?

The anteroposterior diameter between the promontory of the sacrum and the superior margin of the symphysis pubis

What is the diagonal conjugate?

The distance between the sacral promontory and the inferior margin of the symphysis pubis; measured clinically

What is the midpelvis?

Measured at the level of the ischial spines

The interspinous diameter (the transverse of the midpelvis) should be at least 10 cm.

What are the organs of the external female genitalia?

Mons pubis, labia majora, labia minora, clitoris, vestibule, urethral opening, vagina, perineum, and perineal body

What is the composition of the labia majora?

Embryologically homologous to the male scrotum

Point of termination for the round ligaments

Composed primarily of subcutaneous fat with a prominent venous plexus and sebaceous glands

What is the composition of the labia minora?

Primarily composed of connective tissue and smooth muscle with dense nerve innervation

Fuse superiorly to form the frenulum and prepuce of the clitoris

What is the composition of the clitoris?

Homologous to the penis

Composed of a glans and two crura

Glans contains two corpora cavernosa, which are generously supplied with nerve fibers.

What are the Bartholin glands?

Homologous to the bulbourethral (Cowper's) gland in the male

Located beneath the vestibule on either side of the vagina, and open at the lateral border of the vagina

What and where is the urethral opening?

Located on the anterior edge of the vestibule and surrounded by Skene's or the paraurethral ducts, which are homologous to the prostate in the male

What is the composition of the perineum?

The area between the mons pubis, the buttocks, and the thighs laterally

Support for the perineum is provided by the pelvic and urogenital diaphragms.

The urogenital diaphragm is the area between the pubis symphysis and the ischial tuberosities.

The muscles of the perineum are the bulbocavernous, ischiocavernous, "sphincter" of the urethra, superficial and deep transverse perineal muscles, and the external sphincter of the anus (Figure 3-3).

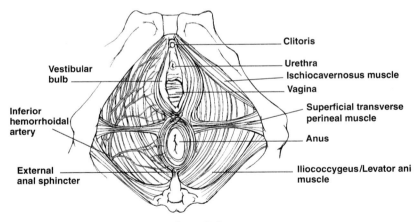

Figure 3–3

What is the blood supply to the perineum?

The internal pudendal artery (off anterior branch of internal iliac)

What is the innervation to the perineum?

Primarily from the pudendal nerve, which consists of the labial branch off the ilioinguinal, the perineal branch from the femoral cutaneous, and a branch from the genitofemoral nerve

What is the lymphatic drainage of the perineum?

Through the inguinal nodes

What structures comprise the pelvic diaphragm?

The levator ani and coccygeal muscles

What is the composition of the vagina?

The vagina is a muscular organ that extends from the vulva to the uterine cervix.

Anterior to the vagina lies the bladder, which is separated from the vagina by the vesicovaginal septum.

Posterior to the vagina lies the rectum, which is separated from the vagina by the rectovaginal septum.

The upper portion of the vagina is separated by the cervix into the anterior and posterior and lateral fornices.

The lateral fornices lie 1.0–1.5 cm from the point at which the uterine artery crosses the ureter.

The epithelium of the vagina is rugated stratified squamous epithelium.

What is the blood supply to the vagina?

Upper third: cervicovaginal branch of the uterine artery

Middle third: inferior vesical arteries

Lower third: internal pudendal artery and middle rectal artery

Venous drainage: through an interconnected venous plexus that drains into the internal pudendal vein

What is the innervation to the vagina?

No specific innervation; occasional free nerve endings are found in the papillas.

Parasympathetic innervation is supplied by S2–S4.

What is the lymphatic drainage of the vagina?

Lower third: through the inguinal nodes

Upper two-thirds: through the internal and external iliac nodes

What are the organs of the female internal genitalia?

The uterus and its supporting structures, the fallopian tubes and ovaries

What is the relationship of the uterus to the other pelvic organs?

Sits between the bladder and the rectum

The posterior wall of the uterus is covered by peritoneum; the peritoneal reflection forms the pouch of Douglas, or posterior cul de sac, between the uterus and the rectum.

Anteriorly, the vesicouterine peritoneum covers the uterus.

The bladder is in direct contact with the uterus (Figure 3–4).

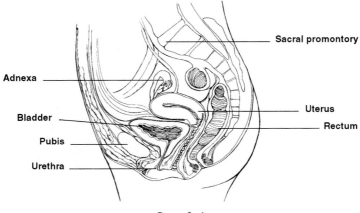

Figure 3–4

What are the parts of the uterus?

Uterine cervix, isthmus, corpus, and fundus (Figure 3–5)

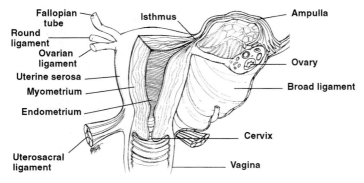

Figure 3–5

What is the uterine cervix?

Extends from the isthmus (constricted) portion of the uterus into the vagina

Portio: portion of the cervix visible from the vagina

Internal os: opening of the cervix into the isthmus

External os: opening of the cervix into the vagina

Cervical canal:

Area between the internal and external os
Measures approximately 4 cm
Lined by columnar epithelium, which
    forms the endocervical glands

What is the blood supply to the uterine cervix?

Cervical branch of the uterine artery,
which enters the cervix after coursing
through the cardinal ligament

What is the innervation to the uterine cervix?

Autonomic nerves that course with the
pudendal artery; the sympathetic nerves
from T12 to L3

What is the lymphatic drainage from the uterine cervix?

Through the external and internal iliacs
    to the common iliacs
The para-aortic nodes may also be
    involved.

What is the uterine corpus?

The "body" of the uterus
Composed of serosal, muscular, and
    mucosal layers
Mucosal layer is the endometrium,
    which is composed of a ciliated
    columnar surface epithelium; glands;
    and blood vessels known as the spiral
    arteries.
The muscular layer is called the
    myometrium.
Composed of smooth muscle and
    connective tissue.
The smooth muscle of the myometrium
    is arranged in a complex fashion of
    criss-crossing muscle fibers.

What are the ligaments of the uterus and cervix?

The broad, round, and uterosacral
    ligaments extend from both sides of
    the uterus.
The cardinal (Mackenrodt's) ligaments
    or the transverse ligaments of the
    cervix extend from either side of the
    cervix (Figures 3-6 and 3–7).

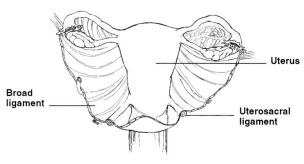

Uterus

**Broad
ligament**

**Uterosacral
ligament**

Figure 3–6

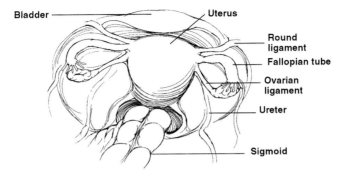

Bladder — Uterus

Round ligament

Fallopian tube

Ovarian ligament

Ureter

Sigmoid

Figure 3–7

What are the broad ligaments?

Composed of a reflection of the peritoneum

Extend from the lateral margin of the uterus to the pelvic sidewall

Comprise the mesosalpinx medially, and laterally form the infundibulopelvic ligament

The uterine vessels and the ureters are contained within the base of the broad ligaments.

What are the round ligaments?

Dense bands of connective tissue that extend from the lateral uterine fundus to the upper portion of the labia majora

Homologous to the gubernaculum in the male

Contains Sampson's artery

What are the uterosacral ligaments?

Dense bands of connective tissue that extend from the inferior and posterior portion of the uterus and attach to the fascia over the sacrum

What are the cardinal ligaments?

Dense bands of connective tissue located at the base of the broad ligament

Provide most of the support to the uterus

What is the blood supply to the uterus?

Primarily the uterine and ovarian arteries

Uterine artery:

Usually arises as a branch of the internal iliac artery (hypogastric)

Courses along the base of the broad ligament toward the lateral uterine wall

Divides into the cervicovaginal and uterine branches; uterine branch further divides into the fundal, ovarian, and tubal arteries

Also provides multiple perforating branches, called radial arteries, into the uterus

Crosses over the ureter ("water under the bridge") approximately 2 cm lateral to the cervix

Ovarian arteries branch directly off the aorta and anastomose with the uterine arteries.

Further anastomoses in the pelvis include that between the inferior mesenteric artery and the internal iliac (hypogastric) and internal pudendal arteries; that between the middle sacral artery and the lumbar sacral artery; and that between the deep circumflex artery (off the external iliac) and branches of the internal iliac.

Venous drainage of the uterus is through the uterine vein and the pampiniform plexus.

Why is the collateral circulation to the pelvic viscera important?

In profuse uterine or pelvic hemorrhage, the uterine or even the internal iliac (hypogastric) artery can be ligated to decrease bleeding by decreasing the pulse pressure. The collateral circulation ensures that the pelvic viscera are adequately supplied with blood.

What is the lymphatic drainage of the uterus?

Through the internal and external iliac nodes

The fundus of the uterus may drain to the para-aortic lymph nodes.

What is the composition of the fallopian tubes?

Eight- to 14-cm muscular tubes that extend laterally from the cornua of the uterus

Segments: interstitial, isthmic, ampullary, and infundibular

Similar to the uterus, composed of serosal, muscular, and mucosal layers

Muscular layer contains an external longitudinal layer and an internal circular layer of muscle.

The mucosa is composed of columnar epithelium.

The epithelial layer contains ciliated cells, which promote ova transport toward the uterus.

What is the blood supply to the fallopian tubes?

Primarily from the uterine and ovarian arteries, as well as from the previously mentioned anastomoses

The venous drainage is through the pampiniform plexus and the ovarian veins.

What is the lymphatic drainage of the fallopian tubes?

Through the aortic nodes

What is the relationship of the ovaries to other pelvic structures?

The ovaries are lateral to the uterus and are normally located in the ovarian fossae, which lie in the pelvic sidewall at the bifurcation of the common iliac artery.

The ovary is attached to the broad ligament by the mesovarium.

The suspensory ligament (infundibulopelvic ligament) is the lateral continuation of the broad ligament and contains the ovarian artery, vein, and nerves.

The ovarian ligament connects the ovary with the lateral wall of the uterus; this ligament runs within the broad ligament (mesovarium ligament).

On pelvic ultrasound, the ovaries usually lie above or near the iliac vessels.

What is the composition of the ovary?

Consists of cortex and medulla

Cortex (outer layer):Contains the ova in various stages of maturity

Outermost layer of the cortex is the tunica albuginea.

Medulla (central region) of the ovary contains connective tissue and the blood supply to the ovary.

What is the blood supply to the ovary?

Through branches from the uterine artery, ovarian vessels, and numerous anastomoses

The venous drainage is through the pampiniform plexus to the ovarian veins.

The right ovarian vein drains into the inferior vena cava.

The left ovarian vein drains into the left renal vein.

What is the lymphatic drainage of the ovaries?	Primarily through the aortic nodes Rarely, they may drain through the iliac node group.
What is the innervation to the ovaries?	Sympathetic and parasympathetic nerves that course along the ovarian and infundibulopelvic ligaments
What are the branches of the internal iliac (hypogastric) artery?	Anterior (visceral): Uterine Superior vesical Middle vesical Inferior vesical Middle hemorrhoidal Inferior hemorrhoidal Vaginal Anterior (parietal): Obturator Inferior gluteal Internal pudendal Posterior: Iliolumbar Lateral sacral Superior gluteal (Figure 3–8)

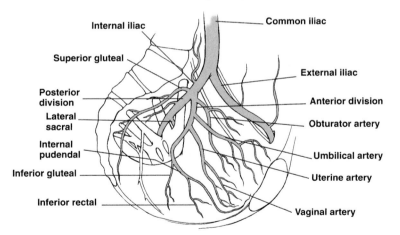

Figure 3–8

What is the innervation of the pelvis?	The hypogastric plexus supplies the sympathetic innervation; parasympathetic innervation is by S2–S4. As stated earlier, the perineum is also innervated by L1 (ilioinguinal), S1–S3

(femoral cutaneous), and L1–L2 (genitofemoral).

What is the relationship of the bladder to the other pelvic organs?

Anteriorly, the bladder rests against the lower abdominal wall and the pubic bones.
Posteriorly, the bladder abuts the vagina and cervix.

What is the composition of the bladder?

Consists of a dome and base
The muscle of the dome of the bladder becomes thin with distention of the bladder.
The base consists of the trigones (ureteral orifices and outflow to urethra) and the detrusor of the bladder; these muscles vary less with distention.

What is the blood supply to the bladder?

Superior and inferior vesical arteries and the middle hemorrhoidal artery
The superior vesical artery arises from the anterior branch of the internal iliac (hypogastric) artery; the inferior branch arises from the anterior branch of the internal iliac, the internal pudendal, or the vaginal artery.

What is the innervation to the bladder?

Sympathetic and parasympathetic nerves
The external urethral sphincter is innervated by the pudendal nerve.

What is the lymphatic drainage of the bladder?

Through the internal iliac nodes
The distal urethra drains to the inguinal nodes.

What is the composition of the ureters?

Measure approximately 25 cm from the renal pelvis to the trigone of the bladder
Segments: abdominal and pelvic
Composed of an inner longitudinal layer of muscle and an outer circular layer. Besides the muscular layer, the ureter has an outer serosal layer and an inner mucosal layer.

What is the course of the ureters?

With regard to the abdominal ureter, both the right and left ureters follow a similar course.
They run retroperitoneally down the anterior surface of the psoas major, then follow the common iliac artery

and cross the iliac vessels before entering the pelvis.

The right ureter crosses the common iliac artery at the bifurcation, whereas the left ureter crosses 1–2 cm above the bifurcation.

Both then follow the lateral pelvic wall and down the medial leaf of the broad ligament where it crosses under the uterine artery.

Both then continue medially and enter the cardinal ligaments. At this point, the ureter is approximately 1.5 cm lateral to the cervix.

Both continue medially to enter the bladder at the trigone of the bladder.

What is the blood supply to the ureters?

Several anastomoses from many vessels, including the renal, common iliac, internal iliac (hypogastric), ovarian, uterine, vaginal, vesical, and superior gluteal arteries

What are the most common points of injury to the ureter during gynecologic surgery?

The pelvic brim and the point at which the ureter crosses under the uterine artery and at the trigone of the bladder

How can the ureters be differentiated from vessels during surgery?

Two ways: watch for ureteral peristalsis, and identify Auerbach's plexus.

Auerbach's plexus is the area of anastomoses of the vessels supplying the ureter and is visualized on the anterior surface of the ureter

What intra-operative procedure can be used to assess ureteral injury?

IV infusion of Indigo Carmine and direct visualization of ureteral orifices in the bladder via cystoscopy

What is the relationship of the rectum to the other pelvic organs?

The rectum is the continuation of the sigmoid colon and begins at the point on the sigmoid colon where the mesentery ends (usually at the curvature of the sacrum).

The rectum does not have teniae coli or appendices epiploicae.

The distal third of the rectum is below the peritoneal reflection and lies posterior to the vagina.

The rectum continues into the anal canal.

What is the blood supply to the rectum?

Superior hemorrhoidal artery, which is a branch of the inferior mesenteric, and the middle and inferior hemorrhoidal arteries

What is the innervation to the rectum?

The sympathetic innervation follows the vasculature.
The parasympathetic innervation is from S2–S4.

What is the lymphatic drainage from the rectum?

Rectum: through the iliac nodes
Anus: through the inguinal nodes

During what kind of gynecologic surgery is the rectum most commonly injured?

Vaginal surgery, primarily vaginal hysterectomy, because the rectum lies only millimeters from the posterior vaginal wall

What are the most common points of injury to nerves during gynecologic surgery?

During radical gynecologic surgery, such as a radical hysterectomy, or during iliac and obturator node dissection, the genitofemoral or obturator nerves can be severed.
Injury to the obturator nerve interferes with adduction of the thigh and hip and with sensory function on the medial aspect of the thigh.
Injury to the genitofemoral nerve leads to anesthesia in the perineum.
During inguinal lymph node dissection, the anterior branches of the femoral nerve can be injured, which can interfere with sensory function on the anterior aspect of the thigh.
During abdominal surgery with the placement of a self-retaining retractor, the femoral nerve may be injured.
May cause temporary or permanent injury
   Prohibits flexion of the hip; patient is not able to lift leg off the bed.
If there is improper placement of a patient's leg in stirrups during surgery, the peroneal nerve may be injured.
   Causes sensory and motor loss over the lateral lower leg
   The patient will have footdrop.

4 ___ Prenatal Care

What are the goals of prenatal care?

Ensure mother's health.
Ensure delivery of a healthy infant.
Anticipate problems.
Diagnose problems early.

What should the initial visit consist of?

Confirmation of pregnancy with urine or blood test
History
Physical examination
Laboratory screening

What medical history is especially relevant?

STDs, Diabetes mellitus, hypertension, heart disease, autoimmune disorders, kidney disease, urinary tract infections, seizure or other neurologic disorder, psychiatric disorders, hepatitis, phlebitis, varicose veins, thyroid dysfunction, trauma, blood transfusions, pulmonary disease (tuberculosis or asthma), breast disease, and any previous surgery (specifically abdominal and cervical surgery)

What social history is particularly pertinent?

Cigarette use
Occupation/Exposure
Alcohol use
Illegal drug use
Domestic violence

What family history is pertinent?

Family history (both sides) of inherited disorders, birth defects, or mental retardation, including thalassemias, neural tube defects, Down syndrome, Tay-Sachs disease, sickle cell disease, hemophilia, muscular dystrophy, cystic fibrosis, and hereditary (Huntington) chorea

How is menstrual history obtained?

Pertinent questions include:
When was the last menstrual period?

Are the patient's periods regular?

What is the usual interval between periods?

Did the last period conform to the usual pattern in terms of timing, volume, and appearance?

Is the patient taking oral contraceptive pills?

Is the patient nursing?

What obstetric history is pertinent?

Pertinent questions include:

What were the patient's previous pregnancy outcomes?

Is there a history of infertility, which might suggest an anatomic or hormonal abnormality?

Were previous deliveries by cesarean section and how was the section done?

If deliveries were vaginal, how were they done?

What gynecologic history is pertinent?

Pertinent questions include:

Has the patient had any sexually transmitted diseases, including gonorrhea, chlamydia, herpes, warts, syphilis, hepatitis B, and human immunodeficiency virus (HIV) infection?

Has the patient had abnormal Pap smears?

Has the patient had gynecologic surgery?

Does the patient have any known uterine or other gynecologic anomalies?

Has the patient had previous first-trimester spontaneous abortions?

What are the normal findings from physical examination particular to pregnancy (depending on gestational age)?

Vital signs: Blood pressure decreases during second trimester; pulse increases.

Head, eyes, ears, nose, and throat: None

Neck: Diffuse mild enlargement of the thyroid

Skin:
- Increased pigmentation of the face (chloasma), abdomen (linea nigra), and vulva
- Stretch marks on the abdomen, thighs, or breasts

Lungs: Elevation of the diaphragm late in pregnancy

Heart:
- Systolic ejection murmur due to increased maternal cardiac output
- Heart rate is increased.
- S2 is loud.

Breasts: Increased nodularity

Abdomen:
- Fetal heart tones at approximately 12 weeks using Doppler
- Uterus grows out of pelvis at 12 weeks; at 20 weeks, uterus is at the umbilicus; after 20 weeks, the EGA equals the distance in centimeters from the pubic symphysis to the uterine fundus.

Upper abdomen tympany is heard late in pregnancy because of displacement of the small bowel and distention of the stomach.

What are the normal findings from pelvic examination particular to pregnancy (depending on gestational age)?

Vulva and perineum:
- Hyperpigmentation, varicose veins, or hemorrhoids
- Vagina: Increased secretions
- Cervix: Softer and pigmented
- Cervical mucus is more copious, often appearing thick and yellow.
- Bimanual: Uterine size is enlarged.

How is the shape of the pelvis assessed?

The diagonal conjugate is the distance from the pubic symphysis to the sacral promontory, which marks the pelvic inlet.

Check the ischial spines to determine if they are prominent, because they mark the midpelvis.

Assess the pelvic sidewalls to determine if they are parallel or convergent.

Assess the shape of the sacrum.

What laboratory evaluations are recommended at the initial visit?

Complete blood count to screen for anemia

Hepatitis B surface antigen test

Type and screen for maternal Rh status and antibodies to Rh or other blood antigens

Rubella titer

HIV, because the risk of transmission to the fetus can be reduced

Rapid plasma reagin (RPR) to screen for syphilis

Urine culture: Initial test for asymptomatic bacteriuria because pregnant women are more susceptible to urinary tract infections, leading to pyelonephritis

Cervical cultures for gonorrhea and chlamydia

Pap smear

What laboratory screens should be performed after the initial visit, and when should they be performed?

Quadruple screen at 15 to 20 weeks

Glucose screen to detect gestational diabetes mellitus at 24–28 weeks

Ultrasound to screen for fetal abnormalities is recommended by some experts at 20 weeks

Group B strep at 35–37 weeks

What is a quadruple screen?

Blood test that measures maternal serum α-fetoprotein (MSAFP), human chorionic gonadotropin (hCG), estriol (E3), and dimeric inhibin A

What is it used to determine?	The combination of measurements (with gestational age and maternal age and weight) assist in determining increased risk of neural tube defects or certain chromosomal anomalies, such as trisomy 21 and trisomy 18.
Abnormal results?	Trisomy 21: Elevated hCG and inhibin, and low MSAFP and E3 Trisomy 18: Low levels of all four Neural tube defects (spina bifida, myelomeningocele): Elevated MSAFP
Follow-up after abnormal result?	Detailed ultrasound and possibly amniocentesis
What is a 1-hour glucose screening test?	One hour after the patient drinks a 50-g oral glucose load, blood is drawn for glucose measurement.
Normal value?	< 135 mg/dl
Follow-up after abnormal result?	Three-hour glucose tolerance test
What is a 3-hour glucose tolerance test?	Patient prepares by consuming a high-carbohydrate diet for 3 days before the test. After the patient drinks a 100-g oral glucose load, blood is drawn for glucose measurement at time 0, and at 1, 2, and 3 hours.
Normal values?	Fasting < 95 mg/dl After 1 hour < 180 mg/dl After 2 hours < 155 mg/dl After 3 hours < 140 mg/dl
Abnormal values?	An abnormal fasting value >110 mg/dl alone or two other abnormal values indicate gestational diabetes.

What is examined during an ultrasound?

Fetal growth by measuring biparietal diameter, head circumference, femur length, and abdominal circumference

Limbs

Intracranial contents

Face (lip & palate)

Spine (neural tube defects)

Fetal organs, including diaphragm, kidneys, liver, heart, great vessels, stomach, and bladder

Placenta (location and grade)

Amniotic fluid volume

What general warning signs should the patient be aware of during pregnancy?

Vaginal bleeding:

In the first trimester, bleeding can indicate pending miscarriage or ectopic pregnancy.

In the second or third trimester, bleeding may indicate placenta previa, placental abruption, or labor.

Swelling of face or fingers, severe headache, or blurry vision may indicate preeclampsia (usually in late 2nd & 3rd trimester).

Dysuria, chills, or fever may indicate pyelonephritis or other infection.

Fluid leaking from the vagina could indicate premature rupture of the membranes.

Decreased fetal movement may indicate fetal compromise.

When should return visits be scheduled and what should each visit include?

Every 4 weeks until 28 weeks

Screening: Urinary tract infection, proteinuria, hypertension, preterm labor, gestational diabetes, and fetal well-being

Every 2 weeks until 36 weeks

Screening:

All of the above plus fetal growth

At 36 weeks, screening for chlamydia and gonorrhea

Every week until 41 weeks
Screening: All of the above
After 41 weeks, twice weekly until
  delivery
Screening: Fetal well-being by
  evaluation of amniotic fluid index
  and nonstress test

How is maternal condition evaluated at each visit?

Blood pressure: Actual and any change
  or trend
Weight: Actual and trend
Symptoms: Headache, vision, pain,
  nausea, vomiting, bleeding, dysuria,
  loss of fluid, contractions.
Vaginal examination if indicated

How is fetal condition evaluated at each visit?

Fundal height (to assess growth): Actual
  and trend
Fetal heart rate
Presenting part
Fetal activity
Amniotic fluid if indicated
Nonstress test at 41 weeks and later

What is the recommended total weight gain during pregnancy?

Approximately 12 kg
For underweight women, slightly more;
  for overweight women, less

What is the recommended weight gain throughout pregnancy?

1 kg in the first trimester; 0.5 kg per
week after 20 weeks

How is the weight gain accounted for during pregnancy?

9 kg is accounted for by the fetus,
placenta, amniotic fluid, uterine
hypertrophy, increase in maternal blood
volume, breast enlargement, and
maternal extracellular and extravascular
fluid. The remainder of the weight gain
is fat.

Can lack of weight gain be harmful in pregnancy?

Severe underweight (near-starvation) is
  required to establish clear differences
  in pregnancy outcome.

Starvation affects fetal birth weight, but does not cause central nervous system damage.

What are the recommended daily allowances in pregnancy?

Calories:

Increase daily caloric intake by approximately 300 calories per day depending on prepregnancy nutritional status.

Birth weight is influenced more significantly by the number of calories, not the form of calories.

Protein: Preferably from animal sources, such as meat, milk, eggs, cheese, poultry, and fish, to provide appropriate amino acids

Iron:

300 mg of iron is transferred to the fetus, and 800 mg is incorporated into maternal hemoglobin mass.

6 mg per day requirement in the second half of pregnancy

Very few women have sufficient iron stores, and diet seldom contains enough iron to meet the demand.

To ensure adequate iron intake, supplementation is recommended.

Another important aspect is the availability of the ingested iron; calcium and magnesium compounds can inhibit iron absorption.

Calcium:

30 g of calcium (or 2.5% of total maternal calcium) is needed for the fetus.

Most maternal calcium is in bone and can be easily mobilized to meet the needs of the fetus.

In addition, absorption by the intestine increases during pregnancy.

Iodine:
> Increased fetal requirement and theoretical increased maternal renal losses
>
> Use of iodized salt meets this requirement.

Copper:
> Pregnancy affects copper metabolism because it increases serum ceruloplasmin and plasma copper.
>
> However, copper deficiency in pregnancy has not been documented.

What elements do not need supplementation in pregnancy?

Chromium, manganese, potassium, sodium, fluorine, zinc, phosphorus, and magnesium

Which substances are potentially toxic in pregnancy?

Iron; zinc; selenium; and vitamins A, B_6, C, and D on high doses.

What vitamins are important in pregnancy?

Folic acid:
> Maternal folate requirements are slightly increased during pregnancy; thus, patients are more prone to folate deficiency, which rarely leads to hypersegmented neutrophils or megaloblastic anemia.
>
> Neural tube defects: Centers for Disease Control and Prevention recommends 0.4 mg daily for all women of childbearing age to prevent neural tube defects.

Vitamin B_{12}:
> Deficiency is usually seen only in strict vegetarians.
>
> In breast-fed infants of vegetarians, B_{12} deficiency may be pronounced.
>
> Excessive vitamin C ingestion can lead to deficiency of B_{12}.

Vitamin C:

Recommended requirement in pregnancy is 20% higher than for nonpregnant woman.

What are the current recommendations for exercise during pregnancy?

Women who exercise regularly may continue their prepregnant level of exercise, unless they have a hypertensive disorder of pregnancy, multifetal gestation, intrauterine growth restriction, or heart disease.

Women who did not previously exercise should slowly begin a low-impact exercise program.

Fetal reactivity is maintained even during vigorous exercise.

Employment?

Continue prepregnancy employment.

Travel?

No harmful effect on an otherwise healthy woman

Greatest risk is not being near an appropriate facility if a problem should arise.

Seat belts should be worn properly with three-point restraints; lap belt should be placed under abdomen and shoulder belt between breasts.

Air-travel is safe in the uncomplicated pregnancy up to 36 weeks' gestation.

Coitus?

If abortion or preterm labor threatens or if placenta previa has been diagnosed, coitus should be avoided.

Smoking?

Cessation should be emphasized because of increased risk of low birth weight.

Alcohol?

Should be avoided because prolonged exposure to alcohol can lead to fetal alcohol syndrome

Caffeine?

In 1980, the Food and Drug Administration advised pregnant women to limit caffeine intake, although it has not been shown to be teratogenic.

Illicit drugs?

Chronic use of cocaine and its derivatives is harmful to the fetus, causing intrauterine distress, low birth weight, placental abruption, and complications of drug withdrawal after birth.

Medications?

In general, any drug that exerts a systemic effect on the mother crosses the placenta.
The advantages to be gained by taking any medication must clearly outweigh any risks.

Provide an explanation and preventive measures (if applicable) for the following concerns expressed by pregnant women.

Bowel habits?

May become irregular owing to relaxation of smooth muscle and compression of the lower bowel by the enlarging uterus
Hemorrhoids are common because of impaired venous return.
Appropriate diet prevents this problem.

Nausea and vomiting?

The cause is not clear.
Small feedings at more frequent intervals help.
Increased lordosis from change in center of gravity with enlarging uterus.

Backache?

Mild backache can usually be alleviated with comfort measures and by avoiding strain.

Round ligament pain?

Usually occurs during the second

trimester as the uterus grows and stretches the round ligaments
Rest alleviates this pain.

Varicose veins?

Congenital predisposition to varicose veins
Can become more pronounced as pregnancy progresses
Management: Elevation and support stockings

Heartburn?

Caused by reflux due to upward displacement and compression of the stomach by the uterus, decreased gastrointestinal motility, and relaxation of the lower esophageal sphincter due to progesterone
Small, frequent meals help prevent heartburn.

Fatigue?

Common during the first trimester secondary to increased metabolic demand.

Leukorrhea?

Increased vaginal discharge is due to increased mucus formation by cervical glands in response to hyperestrogenemia.
Patients who complain of vaginal discharge must be evaluated for trichomoniasis, vaginitis, or bacterial vaginosis.

5

Labor and Delivery

What is labor?

Regular uterine contractions that cause progressive effacement and dilatation of the cervix and lead to expulsion of the fetus and placenta from the uterus

What are Braxton Hicks contractions?

"False labor"; contractions that occur with variable frequency and do not cause progressive cervical dilatation and effacement. Can begin as early as the 2nd trimester.

What is cervical dilatation?

The cervix being dilated or stretched beyond the normal dimensions

How is it measured?

In centimeters; measured at the width of the internal os of the cervix

What is effacement?

Shortening of the cervix and thinning of the cervical walls caused by the pressure of the fetus's head as it descends into the birth canal during labor

How is effacement expressed?

In terms of percentage of total effacement [i.e., 0% effacement (normal) to 100% effacement (completely thinned cervix)]

What is engagement?

Descent of the biparietal diameter of the fetal vertex below the level of the pelvic inlet

What is station?

Marks the descent of the fetal presenting part through the maternal pelvis

How is station measured?

In centimeters relative to the level of the maternal ischial spines
    0 station: presenting part at the ischial spines
    -1, -2, -3: above the ischial spines
    +1, +2, +3: below the ischial spines to the perineum. See Figure 5.1.

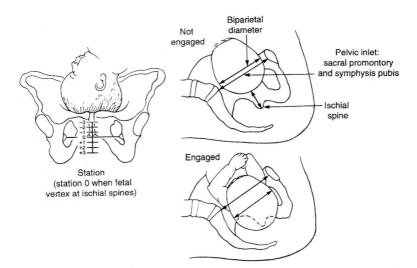

Figure 5.1. Station and engagement of the fetal head. Beckman CRB, Ling FW, Laube DW, Smith RP, Barzansky BM, Herbert WNP. Obstetrics and Gynecology, 4th Ed. Philadelphia: Lippincott Williams & Wilkins, 2002: 103.

UNCOMPLICATED LABOR

What are the stages of labor?	First stage: from the onset of contractions causing progressive cervical dilatation to complete dilatation of the cervix Second stage: from complete cervical dilatation to the birth of the fetus Third stage: from the birth of the fetus to the delivery of the placenta

FIRST STAGE OF LABOR

What are the two phases of the first stage of labor?	Latent: cervical effacement and early dilatation Active: slope of cervical dilatation increases; usually begins when the cervix is 3–4 cm dilated and contractions are regular

How long does the latent phase of labor last?	Primigravidas: up to 20 hours Multiparas: up to 14 hours
What is the normal progress of cervical dilatation during the active phase of labor?	Primigravidas: at least 1.2 cm/hr Multiparas: at least 1.5 cm/hr
What conditions may slow progress in the active phase of labor?	Uterine dysfunction, fetal malposition, cephalopelvic disproportion (CPD)
How should the mother be positioned during the first stage of labor?	Mother may ambulate (provided that intermittent monitoring is performed) or recline in the lateral recumbent position.
By what method and how often should the fetus be monitored in uncomplicated pregnancies?	Intermittent by auscultation
In complicated pregnancies?	Continuous fetal heart rate (FHR) monitoring
When should vaginal examinations be performed in the first stage?	On initial presentation of patient with contractions Latent phase: sparingly if membranes have ruptured Active phase: approximately every 2 hours If the patient reports the urge to push or FHR decelerates

SECOND STAGE OF LABOR

How long should the second stage of labor last?	Primigravidas: 30 minutes to 2 hours; with epidural analgesia, approximately 3 hours Multiparas: 45 minutes (average)
What are the cardinal movements of labor?	Engagement (usually occurs before the onset of true labor), descent, flexion, internal rotation, extension, external rotation. (Figure 5.2)

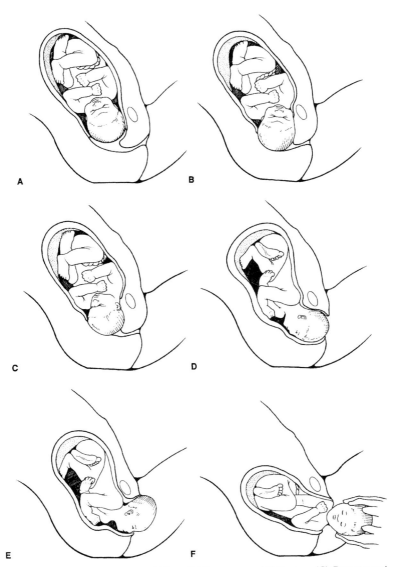

Figure 5.2. Cardinal movements of labor. (A) Engagement. (B) Flexion. (C) Descent and internal rotation. (D), (E) Extension. (F) External rotation. Beckman CRB, Ling FW, Laube DW, Smith RP, Barzansky BM, Herbert WNP. Obstetrics and Gynecology, 4th Ed. Philadelphia: Lippincott Williams & Wilkins, 2002: 105.

What forces bring about descent?	Combined forces of uterine contractions, maternal bearing-down efforts, and gravity
When does descent occur?	A variable degree of fetal descent occurs before the onset of labor and during the first and second stages.
When does the fastest rate of descent occur?	During the second stage of labor
How long does it last?	Until the fetus is delivered
What is flexion?	Flexion of fetal neck toward chest
When does flexion begin?	Partial flexion exists before labor as a result of the natural muscle tone of the fetus.
What causes flexion?	During descent, resistance from the cervix, the walls of the pelvis, and the pelvic floor results in further flexion of the cervical spine, causing the fetus's chin to approach its chest.
To what does "lie" refer?	The relationship between the long axis of the fetus and the long axis of the mother.

Identify the two types of lie.	Longitudinal
	   With either cephalic or breech
	      presentation
	Transverse
	   With shoulder/arm presentation

To what does "presentation" refer?	The part of the fetus arriving first in the birth canal.

Types of presentation?	Cephalic
	   Vertex (normal)
	   Face
	   Brow
	Breech
	   Frank
	   Complete
	   Incomplete
	Shoulder/Arm

What is meant by position?
The relationship between an anatomic feature of the presenting part and the maternal symphysis.

In normal labor, what are the lie, presentation, and position?
Longitudinal lie
Vertex presentation
Occiput anterior, occiput left anterior, or occiput right anterior

What determines the position of the fetus in vertex presentation?
The relationship of the fetal occiput to the maternal pelvis

What are the types of position in vertex presentation?
(LOA/Left Occipital Anterior)
(LOT/Left Occipital Transverse)
(LOP/Left Occipital Posterior)
[ROA-ROT-ROP same as above]

What landmarks are used to determine position?
Occipital, frontal & parietal sutures.

What is internal rotation?
Turning of the fetal head as the fetus descends through the pelvis.

When does it occur?
As the head descends through the pelvic cavity and meets the muscular sling of the pelvic floor

Why does it occur?
The presenting part of the fetus naturally seeks the most favorable position as it descends through the pelvis.

What type of presentation is most favorable at the pelvic brim?
Transverse

What type of presentation is most favorable at the outlet?
Because of the shape of the pelvic arch, the sagittal suture of the fetal head in the anteroposterior (AP) position relative to the pelvis

What is extension?
Extension of the fetal neck to negotiate under the pubic symphysis

What forces bring about extension?

Combined forces of descent, flexion, and internal rotation

What is the purpose of extension?

Because the vaginal outlet is directed upward and forward, extension must occur before the head can pass through.

What happens at crowning?

As the head continues to descend, the perineum bulges, followed by crowning; crowning occurs when the largest diameter of the fetal vertex is encircled by the vulvar ring.

What is the station at crowning?

+5

After crowning?

The vertex then extends as the occiput, nose, mouth, and chin pass over the perineum.

What is external rotation?

Return of the delivered head to its position at the time of engagement and return to its alignment with the fetal back and shoulders

What is expulsion?

Delivery of the anterior shoulder under the symphysis pubis, followed by delivery of the posterior shoulder and then the body

How should the mother be positioned during the second stage of labor?

In any comfortable position except supine

When should the mother be directed to bear down?

With each contraction

Why is this direction important for patients receiving regional anesthesia?

Reflex sensations may be impaired.

How often should the fetus be monitored during the second stage of labor?

Continuously or after each contraction

Why?

FHR decelerations secondary to head or cord compression often occur during this stage.

How often should vaginal examinations be performed during the second stage?

Every 30 minutes with particular attention to descent, extent of internal rotation, and development of molding or caput

What are the goals of assisted vaginal delivery?

Minimize maternal and fetal trauma.

What are the steps of an assisted vaginal delivery?

The patient is usually placed in the lithotomy position; the skin over the perineum and upper thighs is cleansed with antiseptic solution; appropriate sterile leggings and drapes may also be applied.

As the perineum bulges with the fetal vertex, an episiotomy is performed if necessary.

The fetal vertex delivers by extension; the Ritgen maneuver may facilitate delivery of the head.

The airway (oral cavity first, followed by nares) is cleared of blood and amniotic fluid using a suction bulb or suction catheter.

The operator checks for a nuchal cord (an umbilical cord that encircles the neck).

The shoulders then descend and rotate into the AP position relative to the maternal pelvis; delivery of the anterior shoulder is assisted by gentle downward traction on the head; delivery of the posterior shoulder is assisted by gentle elevation of the head.

The rest of the body is delivered without difficulty; the cord is clamped and cut.

What is the Ritgen maneuver?

The operator places a hand behind the rectum and applies upward pressure on the fetal chin and with the other hand applies gentle downward pressure on the fetal occiput to allow controlled delivery of the fetal head.

What is the procedure for a nuchal cord?

A nuchal cord can often be reduced over the head. If the cord is too tight, it can be clamped and cut on the perineum.

THIRD STAGE OF LABOR

How long does the third stage of labor last?

No more than 30 minutes

What are the stages of placental delivery?

Separation of the placenta from the uterine wall
Expulsion from the vagina

When does the placenta separate from the uterine wall?

Within 5 to 10 minutes of the end of the second stage

What are the signs of placental separation?

The uterus becomes firm and globular.
A gush of blood flows from the vagina.
The umbilical cord lengthens outside the vulva.
The uterine fundus rises in the abdomen.

What is the Brandt-Andrews maneuver?

Exertion of traction on the umbilical cord with one hand while the uterus is lifted out of the pelvis by suprapubic pressure on the uterus with the other hand; pressure on uterus is stopped as the placenta passes through the introitus.

Why must the operator be careful in performing this maneuver?

The membranes can tear and be left behind as the placenta is lifted away from the introitus.

Why is the placenta examined after delivery?

To ascertain its complete removal from the uterine cavity

How can the placenta present at the time of its delivery?

Duncan (**D**ull = Duncan): rough maternal edge presentation
Schultze (**S**hiny = Schultze): fetal membrane presentation

How is uterine hemostasis achieved after delivery of the placenta?

Vasoconstriction by myometria contraction

How can uterine contractions after delivery of the placenta be stimulated?

Agents such as oxytocin, methylergonovine, prostaglandin; uterine massage

What types of lacerations may require repair?

First-degree laceration involves the vaginal mucosa or perineal skin.
Second-degree laceration extends into the submucosal tissue of the vagina or perineum with or without involvement of the muscles of the perineal body.
Third-degree laceration involves the anal sphincter.
Fourth-degree laceration involves the rectal mucosa.

OPERATIVE DELIVERY

CESAREAN SECTION

What is a cesarean section (C/S)?

Delivery of the fetus through incisions in the anterior abdominal wall and the uterus

What are the indications for a C/S?

Maternal/fetal
 Dystocia
Maternal
  Maternal disease
    Eclampsia/severe preeclampsia
    Diabetes mellitus
    Cervical cancer
  Previous uterine surgery
    Previous classic cesarean section
    Previous uterine rupture
    Myomectomy
    More than one previous low
      transverse cesarean section
      (debatable)
  Obstruction in birth canal
  Fibroids
  Ovarian tumors
Fetal
  Fetal distress
  Cord prolapse
  Fetal malpresentation
    Breech
    Transverse
    Brow
Placental
  Placenta previa
  Abruptio placentae

What are the three types of C/S?

Low transverse, classic, and low vertical

C/S classifications refer to which incision: abdominal or uterine?

Uterine

What is the most common type of C/S?	Low transverse
What is a low transverse C/S?	The incision is made transversely in the lower uterine segment.
Advantage?	Decreased risk of scar rupture in subsequent pregnancies and generally less bleeding and adhesion formation
What is a classical C/S?	A vertical incision is made into the upper contractile portion of the uterus.
Indications?	Preterm breech fetus Fetus in a transverse lie with the back down Restricted access to the lower uterine segment secondary to fibroids or dense adhesions When a hysterectomy is to follow the delivery of the fetus Presence of an invasive cervical cancer Postmortem C/S to rescue a live fetus from a deceased mother
What is a low vertical C/S?	A vertical incision is made in the lower uterine segment.
Indications?	Preterm breech
What are the maternal morbidities for C/S?	Risk of maternal death is four to six times greater than for a vaginal delivery. Complications: hemorrhage; injury to surrounding structures such as the bowel, bladder, blood vessels, nerves and ureters; postoperative complications Postoperative complications: thromboembolic events; pain; prolonged hospitalization; postoperative infection involving the uterus, wound, bladder, lung, and IV site

How are subsequent pregnancies managed?

Decision to repeat C/S depends in part on the indications for the primary surgery.

Repeat C/S if any of the previously mentioned indications are present.

Previous classic C/S mandates a repeat C/S.

Patients with previous transverse C/S may labor in subsequent pregnancies unless contraindications exist.

OBSTETRIC FORCEPS DELIVERY

What are forceps?

An instrument used to provide traction, rotation, or both to the fetal head when the unaided expulsive efforts of the mother are insufficient to accomplish safe delivery

What do forceps used for traction (Simpson's and Tucker) look like?

They have a pelvic curve that corresponds to the axis of the birth canal.

What do forceps used for fetal rotation (Kielland's) look like?

They do not have a pelvic curve.

What are the indications for a forceps delivery?

Maternal
    Exhaustion: inability to expel the fetal head
    Medical conditions
    Cardiac disease (e.g., mitral stenosis)
    Pulmonary disease
Fetal
    Failure of the fetal head to rotate completely
    Control of the fetal head during a vaginal breech delivery
    Fetal heart rate decelerations with complete cervical dilatation and adequate station

How are forceps deliveries classified?	According to the station and position of the presenting part at the time the forceps are applied
Classifications?	Outlet forceps: applied when the scalp is visible at the introitus without separating the labia Low forceps: applied when the vertex is at +2 station or lower. Mid-forceps: applied when the head is engaged but the leading part is above +2 station or when the sagittal suture is not in the AP plane of the mother
Under what circumstances should forceps be applied to the unengaged fetal head?	Under **no** circumstances
What are the requirements for a forceps delivery?	The fetal vertex **must** be engaged. The position of the fetal vertex must be certain. Membranes must be ruptured. Uterine contractions must be present. The cervix must be fully dilated. The bladder should be emptied. Adequate anesthesia is optimal.
What are the complications of a forceps delivery?	Maternal Trauma to soft tissues Bleeding from lacerations Fetal Bruising or lacerations to the face Injury to the fetal scalp or cranium

VACUUM-ASSISTED DELIVERY

What is a vacuum?	An instrument that uses a suction cup applied to the fetal head to exert traction to aid the mother's expulsive efforts

What are the indications for a vacuum-assisted delivery?	Same as those for a forceps delivery, except for: Face or breech delivery Assisting fetal rotation Vacuum can also be used in multiparas in whom a small rim of cervix remains and the rim will displace easily over the fetal head.
What is an advantage of a vacuum-assisted delivery compared to a forceps delivery?	May require a smaller episiotomy than that for a forceps delivery and lower risk for vaginal lacerations
What are the contraindications to a vacuum-assisted delivery?	Preterm deliveries because of risk of fetal head and scalp injury from the suction cup
What are the complications of a vacuum-assisted delivery?	Vaginal laceration due to entrapment of vaginal mucosa between the suction cup and the fetal head Fetal scalp injuries Serious fetal eye injury if used in a face presentation

COMPLICATIONS AND ABNORMALITIES OF LABOR AND DELIVERY

What is dystocia?	Literally, "difficult labor"
What are the causes of dystocia?	Ineffective uterine expulsive forces Abnormal presentation, position, or fetal structure Disproportion between the size of the fetus and the maternal pelvis Obstruction of the birth canal
What are the three Ps?	Power: strength of the uterine contractions Passage: maternal pelvis Passenger: fetal size relative to the maternal pelvis

Significance?	Any abnormal progression during labor is likely caused by an abnormality in one of the three Ps.

ABNORMALITIES OF THE UTERINE EXPULSIVE FORCES

When is the latent phase of labor considered prolonged?	Primigravida: latent phase exceeds 20 hours Multipara: exceeds 14 hours
Causes?	Hypertonic uterine contractions that do not lead to effective contractions and cervical dilatation Hypotonic uterine contractions Premature or excessive use of sedatives or analgesics
What are the management options for a prolonged latent phase?	Hypertonic uterine activity: therapeutic rest with morphine sulfate or an equivalent drug Hypotonic contractions: IV oxytocin in a continuous infusion beginning with 0.5 mU to 1.0 mU per minute and increased incrementally; artificial rupture of membranes (AROM)
Why is AROM controversial?	Added risk of intrauterine infection when performed in the latent phase and labor does not improve Risk of cord prolapase if head not firm in pelvis.
What abnormalities can occur during the active phase of labor?	Protraction disorder: failure of the cervix to dilate greater than 1.2 cm/hr in a primigravida and 1.5 cm/hr in a multipara after the cervix has reached an accelerated slope of dilatation (usually at 3–4 cm) Arrest of dilatation: period of 2 or more hours without progress in cervical dilatation, usually at 3–4 cm

Arrest of descent: period of more than 1 hour without a change in station of the fetal presenting part with adequate contractions

What is failure to progress?

Failure of either cervical dilatation or descent of the fetal vertex during labor despite adequate uterine contractions

Etiologies?

CPD, uterine anomalies, uterine fibroids, cervical mass; often no definable etiology

How is adequacy of labor measured?

With an intrauterine pressure catheter (IUPC)

What measurement is considered adequate?

Greater than 200 Montevideo Units (MVU) in a 10-minute period

How are Montevideo Units Calculated?

Take maximum pressure of each contraction and subtract the base line & add them together over a 10-minute period.

What are the management options for a prolonged active phase?

Oxytocin infusion
IUPC to assess adequacy of labor

When is a C/S necessary for failure to progress?

No cervical change occurs for 3–4 hours despite adequate labor; the size of the fetus, adequacy of the pelvis, and the well-being of the fetus should also be assessed.

Second stage of labor exceeds 2 hours (3 hours if epidural analgesia is used), provided maternal expulsive effort has been sufficient; some patients can be delivered by forceps.

What other factors should be considered when assessing the need for a C/S?

Physician must balance the morbidity incurred by the mother from C/S against the benefit to the infant from avoiding prolonged labor and possible difficult delivery.

ABNORMAL PRESENTATIONS AND POSITIONS

What are the abnormal fetal presentations and positions?

Any presentation other than longitudinal lie, cephalic (vertex), and occiput anterior (OA)

What is a breech presentation?

Presentation of the fetal buttocks or lower extremities into the maternal pelvis

What are the types of breech presentation?

Complete (5%–10%): flexed thighs and flexed knees, feet above the buttocks
Frank (50%–75%): flexed thighs and extended knees
Footling or incomplete (20%): leg(s) extended

What is the effect of a breech presentation on the progress of labor?

Only a small effect on rate of dilatation and descent; however, likelihood of dysfunctional labor is greater

What are the criteria for a trial of labor in breech presentation?

Estimated fetal weight > 1500 or < 3800 g
Frank breech presentation
Nonextended fetal head (may be determined by ultrasound)
Adequate maternal pelvis
Absence of fetal anomaly that may impair vaginal delivery
No evidence of fetal distress
Ability to perform a rapid C/S

Why is vaginal delivery contraindicated for a footling breech presentation?

20% prolapse of the cord; entrapment of the aftercoming head on the cervix may occur because the fetal trunk does not adequately dilate the cervix.

When should a C/S be performed?	When the above criteria for a trial of labor are not met In some institutions: if a dysfunctional labor pattern develops
What is the perinatal morbidity for a breech?	Ranges from 9% to 25% in breech fetuses (three to five times higher than in a vertex infant at term)
What factors contribute to increased risk of morbidity and mortality in breech presentations?	Factors that may have caused the breech presentation, such as prematurity and congenital anomalies
What is a face presentation?	A variety of cephalic in which the head is extended & with the face at the introitus
Cause?	Complete extension of the fetal head results in a larger diameter of the fetal presenting part; does not include the normal extension of the fetal vertex that occurs as one of the cardinal movements of labor
How is a face presentation managed?	Mentum posterior: vaginal delivery of a term infant is impossible Spontaneous rotation of the fetus to mentum anterior occurs in most cases. Rotation with forceps should **not** be attempted. C/S if spontaneous rotation does not occur; sometimes required if it does occur
What is a brow presentation?	A variety of cephalic in which the head is extended & the brow at the introitus
Cause?	Incomplete extension of the fetal head results in a presentation midway between a vertex and a face presentation.

Effects on dilatation and descent?	Dilatation: usually none Descent: may be prolonged because this presentation provides a larger diameter to maneuver the maternal pelvis
How is a brow presentation managed?	May convert spontaneously to a vertex or face Observation to determine whether spontaneous conversion will occur C/S if conversion does not occur Vaginal delivery if the fetus is unusually small or the maternal pelvis large
What is an occiput transverse position?	Failure of the head to rotate to an OA or OP position
Causes?	CPD Altered pelvic architecture Relaxed pelvic floor that does not encourage rotation
Why does arrest of descent occur with this presentation?	The OT position leads to a larger diameter of the presenting part.
How is a persistent OT position managed?	Normal-size pelvis or small fetus: oxytocin augmentation if arrest is secondary to inadequate contractions Large pelvis or smaller fetus: no labor management necessary Manual or forceps rotation C/S if rotation fails or CPD exists
What is an OP position?	The occiput is in the posterior instead of the normal anterior position.
How is an OP position managed?	No fetal distress: observation with expectant management Delivery of the fetal head may occur spontaneously. Difficult delivery of head or maternal exhaustion: forceps delivery

What is a transverse lie?	The fetal spine lies transverse to the maternal vertical axis.
Causes?	Fetal prematurity, pelvic deformity, abnormal placental location
How is a transverse lie managed?	Before labor and rupture of membranes: expectant management because of possibility of spontaneous resolution Risk for cord prolapse if membranes rupture C/S: term infant with a transverse lie Low transverse C/S: if infant is "back up" Classic C/S: if infant is "back down"

ABNORMALITIES OF FETAL STRUCTURE

What is fetal macrosomia?	Fetal weight greater than 4000 g
Above what percentage of normal fetal weight constitutes macrosomia?	90% for a term pregnancy
Etiology of fetal macrosomia?	Genetic determinants, maternal diabetes, maternal weight gain during the pregnancy, or post-term gestation
What is a shoulder dystocia?	Inability to dislodge the anterior shoulder from under the pubic symphysis
Can traction on the fetal head help?	No
What is the risk of exerting traction on the fetal head in this condition?	May damage the brachial plexus and cause Erb's palsy

What is Erb's palsy?

Results from stretching or tearing of the upper branches of the brachial plexus

Paralysis of the deltoid and flexor muscles

Paralysis is transient and resolves within 3 to 6 months after delivery.

How is a shoulder dystocia managed?

The following maneuvers in the following order:

Call for help.

McRoberts maneuver: flexing the maternal thighs to alter the angle between the sacrum and the spine

Downward pressure with the hand over the maternal suprapubic region to guide the anterior shoulder under the symphysis

Pushing the anterior shoulder into an oblique position

Pushing the posterior shoulder forward; may lead to rotation and delivery (woods screw)

Moving the posterior shoulder across the fetal chest to facilitate delivery; may lead to rotation of the fetus and delivery

Fracture of one or both of the fetal clavicles

What if none of the above maneuvers work?

The fetal head is manually replaced into the vagina and delivery is accomplished by C/S (Zavanelli maneuver); this technique is rarely performed, and is considered a last resort.

What fetal anomalies can affect delivery?

Fetal hydrocephalus, fetal ascites, gastroschisis, omphalocele, spina bifida, sacral teratomas

Management?

Depends on prenatal diagnosis of the fetal anomaly and the severity of the defect

FETAL DISTRESS

What is the etiology of fetal distress?

Hypoxia caused by the temporary interruption of blood flow that supplies the fetus with oxygen through the placental exchange of respiratory gases during a contraction

What is the role of fetal health in fetal distress?

In a normal fetus, sufficient oxygen exchange occurs during the interval between contractions; a fetus whose oxygen supply is marginal cannot tolerate the stress of contractions and becomes hypoxic.

What are the results of hypoxia?

Contraction-related FHR changes and fetal acidosis

How is fetal acidosis assessed?

Blood is sampled from the presenting part.

How is baseline FHR determined?

Determination of the rate in beats per minute (BPM) and the variability

What is a normal FHR?

Between 120 to 160 BPM

What is short-term variability?

Also known as beat-to-beat variability; reflects electrical events of the cardiac cycle. Can only be assessed with a fetal scalp electrode.

How is short-term variability calculated?

The standard deviation calculated from the baseline interval between beats

What is normal short-term variability?

Fluctuates between 5 and 25 BPM

What is long-term variability?

Fluctuations of FHR that occur in cycles, usually three to five cycles per minute

What are the types of FHR decelerations?	Early, late, and variable (Figure 5.3)

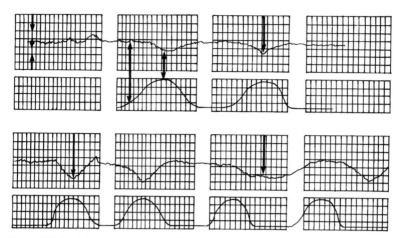

Figure 5.3. Fetal heart rate patterns. Beckman CRB, Ling FW, Laube DW, Smith RP, Barzansky BM, Herbert WNP. Obstetrics and Gynecology, 4th Ed. Philadelphia: Lippincott Williams & Wilkins, 2002: 135.

What is an early deceleration?	A deceleration, the radii of which occur prior to the peak of contraction.
Cause?	Fetal head compression leads to an increase in intracranial pressure, which elicits a vagal response with subsequent decrease in FHR.
Description?	Onset, maximal fall, and recovery coincide with the onset, peak, and end of the uterine contraction; nadir of the deceleration coincides with the peak of the contraction. Usually occur with fetal descent.
What is a late deceleration?	Deceleration in which the onset & nadir occur after the peak of contraction.
What does it indicate?	Uteroplacental insufficiency
Description?	Onset, maximum decrease, and recovery

are shifted to the right in relation to the contraction.

How is severity measured?

By the magnitude of the decrease in FHR at the nadir of the deceleration

Grades of severity?

Mild: FHR drops < 15 BPM
Moderate: FHR drops 15–45 BPM
Severe: FHR drops > 45 BPM

What are the management options for late decelerations?

Left or right lateral maternal position
Oxygen by face mask
Stop oxytocin infusion if uterine hyperstimulation is suspected of causing the decelerations.
A tocolytic drug may be necessary to stop uterine contractions.
Monitor maternal blood pressure to exclude maternal hypotension as the etiology (especially if an epidural has been administered).
Fetal blood sampling if late decelerations persist for > 30 minutes (some institutions)

When is operative delivery for fetal distress indicated?

Fetal acidosis
Persistent late decelerations in early labor
Deterioration of fetal status and vaginal delivery cannot be accomplished promptly

What is a variable deceleration?

A deceleration, the radii of which may occur before, during, or after the peak of contraction

Cause?

Secondary to cord compression; causes a sudden increase in blood pressure in the central circulation of the fetus with a subsequent decrease in FHR

Description?

Onset and forms vary; may be nonrepetitive.

How is severity measured?	By the duration of the deceleration and the decrease in FHR
Grades of severity?	Mild: lasts < 30 sec, or > 80 BPM Moderate: 30–60 sec Late: > 60 sec, or < 70 BPM
What are the management options for variable decelerations?	Change maternal position to the right or left side (may relieve fetal pressure on the cord). Temporarily stop oxytocin. Amnioinfusion to alleviate pressure on the cord If deceleration occurs during the second stage of labor, delivery of the fetus with low or outlet forceps C/S if progressive acidosis or deterioration of variability occurs and vaginal delivery is not imminent
What is an amnioinfusion?	Instillation of sterile saline into the uterine cavity through a catheter

MECONIUM

What is meconium?	Fetal colonic contents
What is the significance of meconium before delivery?	May indicate current or past fetal distress, but usually does not
Classification?	Light or heavy
Outcome of light staining?	**Not** necessarily associated with poor outcome
Management of an infant with meconium-stained fluid?	At delivery: fetus needs vigorous suction, usually with De-lee suction catheter, on the perineum. Intubation may be necessary. Check with laryngoscope for meconium below the vocal cords; indicates aspiration, which can lead to pneumonia.

Remove meconium from the oropharynx and trachea with suction through an endotracheal tube.

What is terminal meconium?

Usually occurs during the second stage of labor, after clear amniotic fluid has been noted earlier; usually heavy and thick

Significance?

Associated with some event late in labor causing fetal distress (e.g., umbilical cord compression or uterine hyperstimulation)

6

The Postpartum Period (Puerperium)

What is the puerperium?

Time period from delivery of the infant and placenta to 6 weeks postpartum, during which maternal reproductive organs and physiology return to the prepregnancy state

ANATOMIC AND PHYSIOLOGIC CHANGES

What are the anatomic and physiologic changes in the reproductive tract during the puerperium?

Uterus: Weight decreases from about 1000 g at delivery to approximately 50 g 3 weeks postpartum

Cervix: Cervical opening contracts; cervix itself thickens; canal reforms. At 1 week postpartum, it is difficult to introduce a finger into the os.

Lochia:

    Days 1–3 after delivery, contains blood and appears red (lochia rubra)

    Days 3–4, becomes paler (lochia serosa)

    Day 10, is white or yellow-white (lochia alba)

Vagina: Rapidly regains tone but does not return to the prepregnancy state

Supportive tissues of the pelvic floor: Gradually regain tone

Menstruation: Resumes 6–8 weeks postpartum in nonnursing women; resumes in 70% of women by 10 weeks postpartum

Ovulation: May not occur for several months, especially in nursing women; contraceptive counseling still should be provided.

What are the physiologic changes in the cardiovascular system?

Peripheral vascular resistance: Markedly decreases immediately after delivery

Plasma volume: Rapidly decreases to prepregnancy level

Cardiac output: Returns to its prepregnancy state by 8–10 weeks

Hematocrit: Returns to prepregnancy level by 8 weeks

What are the anatomic and physiologic changes in the urinary tract?

Hydronephrosis: No evidence by 6–12 weeks in most patients; one study showed that 50% of patients continue to have mild urinary stasis at 12 weeks, suggesting long-standing changes secondary to pregnancy.

Glomerular filtration rate and creatinine clearance: Normal by 8 weeks

What changes lead to lactation?

Levels of placental hormones drop (especially estrogen).

Suckling leads to release of prolactin and oxytocin, which cause contraction of myoepithelial cells in the alveoli and milk ducts.

When is colostrum secreted?

Approximately 2 days postpartum

When is mature milk secreted?

Approximately 3–6 days postpartum

What are the major components of mature milk?

Proteins, lactose, water, and fat

How do the nutrients in colostrum and milk compare?

Colostrum contains more protein (globulin) and minerals than mature milk, but less sugar and fats.

What are the psychological changes during the puerperium?

Mild "maternity blues" occur in 50%–70% of women during the first week after delivery; not associated with hormonal changes.

Postpartum depression occurs in 10%–15% of women.

Postpartum psychosis occurs in 0.1%–0.3% of women.

What medications are effective for postpartum depression?	Selective serotonin re-uptake inhibitors, tricyclic antidepressants
What are the signs, symptoms, and duration of postpartum psychosis?	Similar to those of acute psychosis; usually lasts 2–3 months. Several authors have not found an association between postpartum depression and prenatal depression, social class, parity, and marital status.

POSTPARTUM CARE OF THE MOTHER

How is the postpartum uterus evaluated?	The uterus should be firm, with its upper margin just below the umbilicus after delivery of the placenta.
What is standard care for the perineum?	Application of an ice pack immediately postpartum to minimize swelling and discomfort. Witch hazel-impregnated pads are helpful "Sitz baths" to minimize discomfort and keep the area clean Evaluation for a hematoma wound breakdown or infection if a woman complains of increasing pain
When is RhoGAM indicated?	When the mother is Rh- and the infant is Rh+
When and how much RhoGAM is given?	300 g of RhoGAM within the first 72 hours after delivery

COMPLICATIONS OF THE POSTPARTUM PERIOD

POSTPARTUM HEMORRHAGE

What is a postpartum hemorrhage?	Vaginal delivery: Blood loss > 500 ml Cesarean section: Blood loss > 1000 ml
When does it usually occur?	In the immediate postpartum period, but can occur in the first 24 hours after delivery

What is the term for hemorrhage after the first 24 hours?	Late postpartum hemorrhage
Usual cause?	Subinvolution of the uterus or retention of placental fragments
What is the incidence of postpartum hemorrhage?	Occurs in approximately 8% of vaginal deliveries
Etiologic factors?	Uterine atony Genital tract trauma (lacerations of perineum, vagina, cervix) Retained placental tissue or blood clots Coagulation disorders Ruptured uterus Uterine inversion Abnormal placental adherence (accreta, percreta, increta)
What is uterine atony?	Inability of the uterus to contract; causes 75%–80% of postpartum hemorrhages
Etiologic factors?	Overdistention of the uterus secondary to multiple gestations, fetal macrosomia, or polyhydramnios Grand multiparity (parity > 5) Prolonged use of oxytocin for the induction or augmentation of labor Use of magnesium sulfate for the treatment of preeclampsia Uterine infection
Treatment?	Identification of at-risk patients Adequate IV access Fluid resuscitation Frequent vital signs Manual exploration of the uterine cavity for evidence of retained placenta Medications (use in the following order): 　1. Oxytocin 20 U in a liter of crystalloid given rapidly plus 10 U of oxytocin IM

2. Methylergonovine (Methergine) 0.2 mg IM (contraindicated in hypertension and heart disease)
3. 15-Methyl prostaglandin $F_{2\alpha}$ (Hemabate) 250 IM (contraindicated in asthma)
4. Prostaglandin E_1 (Misoprostil) 1000 mg PR

Evaluation for possible abnormal placentation or uterine rupture if above measures fail

Last resort: Surgery

What are the surgical options for uterine atony?

1. O'Leary sutures (ligation of uterine arteries and uterine and parametrial tissue bilaterally)
2. B-Lynch suture (formation of "net" with absorbable suture to keep uterus manually contracted)
3. Ligation of hypogastric arteries bilaterally (after superior gluteal branch)
4. Hysterectomy
5. Uterine artery embolization

How are genital lacerations managed?

Place first suture well above the apex of the laceration (or episiotomy) to incorporate any bleeding retracted arterioles.

Vaginal lacerations: Reapproximate the tissue without dead space; a running locked suture is the most hemostatic.

Cervical lacerations: These do not require suturing unless actively bleeding.

Expanding vaginal or vulvar hematomas: May require surgical evacuation of the clot; locate and ligate bleeding vessels.

What kind of hematoma can develop from a large dissecting perineal hematoma?

Retroperitoneal hematoma

What is the management of retained placental fragments?	Manual exploration of the uterus with manual removal of the placental fragments Curettage of the uterus (with adequate anesthesia) if hemorrhage continues Hysterectomy or uterine repair (if possible) if evidence of abnormal placentation (placenta accreta) is present
What is an inverted uterus?	The uterine fundus inverts into the uterine cavity.
Cause?	Excessive traction applied during the delivery of the placenta (can be associated with abnormal placentation)
Management?	Rapid intervention to prevent cardiovascular shock Immediate intravascular volume replacement **Without** removing the placenta, replacement of the uterus by placing a cupped hand around the fundus and elevating it into the long axis of the vagina Sublingual nitroglycerine or general anesthesia (halothane) may be needed to allow uterine relaxation Oxytocin after uterine replacement
How are coagulopathies managed?	Postpartum hemorrhage associated with a coagulopathy: Infusion of blood products or necessary factors to correct specific defect Significant thrombocytopenia: May require platelet transfusions Von Willebrand disease: Fresh frozen plasma or DDAVP (a synthetic vasopressin analog)

POSTPARTUM FEVERS

What is included in the differential diagnosis of postpartum fevers?

Endometritis
Pelvic thrombophlebitis
Breast engorgement
Mastitis
IV site phlebitis
Atelectasis
Pneumonia
DVT
Wound infection
Urinary tract infection
Drug fever

What is endometritis? (Endomyometritis)

Inflammation most commonly caused by polymicrobial infection
Primarily involves the endometrium (specifically the decidua and the myometrium)
The most common cause of postpartum fever

Signs and symptoms?

Body temperature > 38.0°C, on 2 occasions 6 hours apart, or once > 38.5°C
Increasing fundal tenderness
Change in lochia: More profuse, foul smelling or purulent
Leukocytosis, which may be difficult to interpret due to physiologic leukocytosis often seen postpartum

Etiologic factors?

Gram-positive cocci (group A streptococci, group B streptococci)
Gram-positive anaerobic cocci (*Peptostreptococcus*, *Peptococcus*, *Streptococcus*, *Bacteroides*) in up to 90% of cultures
Gram-positive bacilli (*Clostridium* and *Listeria*)
Gram-negative cocci (*Neisseria gonorrhoeae*)
Gram-negative bacilli (*Escherichia*, *Klebsiella*, and *Proteus*)

What are the risk factors for postpartum endometritis?

Prolonged rupture of membranes, cesarean section after labor and ruptured membranes, retained fetal membranes or placental fragments

What is the management for postpartum endometritis?

Initial close observation for patients without significant symptoms and body temperature < 38.0°C

Clindamycin plus gentamicin (most tested and effective treatment); second- or third-generation cephalosporins; ampicillin/sulbactam sodium; extended-spectrum penicillins

Other penicillin-betalactamase inhibitor combinations

What is the management of the patient who remains febrile after several days of antibiotic treatment?

Search for other sites of infection (e.g., hematoma, pelvic abscess, septic pelvic thrombophlebitis, or a wound infection)

Reassess antibiotic coverage

What is pelvic thrombophlebitis?

Extension of endometritis along the veins that drain the uterus; sometimes involves the ovarian veins (often including veins of the placental site) because they drain the upper part of the uterus

Usually a right unilateral process

Tests (e.g., Doppler ultrasound and computed tomography scan) usually not diagnostic

Often a diagnosis of exclusion when a patient does not respond to antibiotics for suspected endometritis but responds to addition of heparin

Management?

Treatment of phlebitis with continued use of antibiotics

Heparin therapy to increase partial thromboplastin time to two times above normal

What is breast engagement?

Lymphatic obstruction resulting in bilaterally tender breasts, often with mild temperature elevation; onset usually over the first days after delivery

Management?

Binding breasts with an Ace bandage or tight-fitting bra, placement of ice packs on the breasts, and avoidance of nipple stimulation if not breast-feeding

Continue breast-feeding if desired

Parlodel (bromocriptine) therapy no longer recommended because of increased risk of cerebrovascular accident

What is mastitis?

Unilateral or bilateral infection of the breast; usually caused by *Staphylococcus aureus* and *Streptococcus* species; transmitted to the mother from the child's oropharynx

Management?

Continue breast-feeding or pumping from the affected breast

Antibiotic therapy with dicloxicillin

Formation of breast abscess:
Discontinuation of breast-feeding from the affected breast; may require surgical drainage and intravenous antibiotic therapy

7

Spontaneous Abortion

What is an abortion?

Termination of a pregnancy before 20 weeks' gestational age

Can also be defined as the expulsion of fetal tissue < 500 g

Can be spontaneous or induced by medical or surgical means

What is preterm birth?

Expulsion of a fetus after 20 weeks' gestational age and before 37 completed weeks' gestation

What is intrauterine fetal demise?

Death of the fetus after 20 weeks' gestational age

What is a stillbirth?

Expulsion of a dead fetus after 20 weeks' gestational age

What are the categories of abortion?

Induced abortion: Pregnancy termination by medical or surgical means for therapeutic or elective reasons

Spontaneous abortion ("miscarriage"): Pregnancy loss before 20 weeks' gestational age

Complete abortion: Abortion with complete expulsion of all products of conception (POC)

Incomplete abortion: Abortion without complete expulsion of all POC; fetal or placental components remain in the uterus.

Threatened abortion: Bleeding from the uterus (as seen on visualization of cervical os) without cervical dilatation and with or without contractions before 20 weeks' gestational age; no expulsion of POC

Inevitable abortion: Bleeding from the uterus with cervical dilatation with or without perceived contractions before 20 weeks' gestational age; no expulsion of POC

Missed abortion: Fetal death before 20 weeks' gestational age without expulsion of POC

Septic abortion: Induced or spontaneous abortion with uterine and systemic infection

Recurrent abortion: Three or more consecutive spontaneous abortions

How is spontaneous abortion evaluated?

Confirm pregnancy by history, physical examination, and possibly ultrasound or human chorionic gonadotropin (hCG) assay.

Establish location of the pregnancy (intrauterine vs. ectopic) by history, physical examination, ultrasound, and hCG trends.

Establish whether expulsion of POC is partial, complete, or absent by history and pelvic examination.

May rule out retained POC with ultrasound if patient passes tissue.

May confirm fetal loss by laboratory tests (static or declining hCG values) or ultrasound (lack of fetal cardiac activity or movement, or the absence of POC); histologic evaluation of passed tissue can also help in diagnosing spontaneous abortion.

What are the common pathologic findings in spontaneous abortion?

Hemorrhage into the decidua basalis

Necrotic changes in tissue adjacent to bleeding

Edematous, thickened villi

Blood (carneous) mole: Ovum encapsulated in clotted blood

Fetal maceration: Skull collapse, hemorrhagic abdominal distention, red appearance, skin softening and peeling, organ necrosis

What are the differential diagnoses of spontaneous abortion?

Bleeding and pain are common gynecologic complaints and, without a β-hCG, the differential diagnosis includes:

Ectopic pregnancy
Placental separation
Trauma
Hydatidiform mole
Bleeding submucous fibroid
Bleeding pedunculated fibroid
Cancer (cervical or uterine)
Dysfunctional uterine bleeding

What is the incidence of spontaneous abortion?

Occurs in 15%–20% of clinically diagnosed pregnancies

One study found a 50%–75% spontaneous abortion rate in chemically diagnosed pregnancies (positive hCG assay in women followed with sequential hCG assays).

Subclinical spontaneous abortion (early losses not diagnosed for lack of symptoms) rate is about 10%.

During what trimester do most spontaneous abortions occur?

First trimester

In approximately how many early pregnancies do the common signs and symptoms of spontaneous abortion (pain and vaginal bleeding) occur?

Approximately one in four

How many of these pregnancies will be spontaneously aborted?

Fifty percent

What is the incidence of recurrent abortion?

Estimates vary from 0.5% to 1% of pregnant women.

What is the risk of recurrence of spontaneous abortion?

Women who have had a single early spontaneous abortion have a 10%–20% chance of recurrence.

Women who have had two consecutive spontaneous abortions have a 25%–45% risk of recurrence.

At what gestational age do most abortions occur?

Eighty percent of pregnancy losses occur before 14 weeks' gestational age.

Fifteen percent are lost before implantation (undetectable clinically).

Two percent are lost during implantation.

What are the etiologic factors of spontaneous abortion?

Genetic

Over 50% of first trimester losses demonstrate abnormal karyotypes (30% at 16–19 weeks).

Half of the abnormal karyotypes are aneuploid (abnormal chromosomal number, e.g., trisomy, monosomy, triploidy, tetraploidy).

Half are euploid (single gene mutation or polygenic with a normal number of chromosomes).

Fetal: Abnormal morphologic embryonic growth and development [e.g., blighted ovum, in which the embryo is degenerated or absent (anembryonic)]

Maternal endocrinologic or metabolic disorders: Diabetes mellitus, thyroid dysfunction

Maternal autoimmune disorders: Antiphospholipid syndrome, lupus erythematosus

Infection: Implicated organisms include *Mycoplasma hominis, Ureaplasma urealyticum,Treponema pallidum, Borrelia burgdorferi, Chlamydia trachomatis, Neisseria gonorrhoeae,* and *Listeria monocytogenes.*

Uterine abnormalities: Müllerian defects, fibroids, adhesions

Incompetent cervix: Reduced ability of
cervix to support pregnancy in uterus

Progesterone deficiency: Failure of
corpus luteum or placenta to
synthesize normal levels of
progesterone (luteal phase defect) to
maintain pregnancy

Trauma: Penetrating or blunt wounds or
surgical trauma (e.g., corpus luteum
cystectomy or appendectomy)

Drugs: Substances that may play a role
include tobacco, alcohol, aminopterin,
methotrexate, chloroquine, and
anesthetic gases.

Radiation: Lethal dose of approximately
ten radiation absorbed dose (rad)
during implantation

Severe malnutrition

**What laboratory values can
be helpful in managing
spontaneous abortion?**

hCG assay

Confirms pregnant status

Serial values can be followed when the
diagnosis is uncertain (e.g., in early
pregnancy, in which falling or stable
values suggest abortion).

Blood type and screen

Blood type should be determined in all
patients with bleeding in pregnancy.

Rh immunoglobulin should be given
within 72 hours if patient is Rh-
negative.

Complete blood count: Determines
extent of hemorrhage (if any) and
likelihood of infection

Progesterone levels: Some authorities
recommend this assay. This test
determines whether the progesterone
level is adequate to support the
pregnancy.

**How is ultrasound useful
in the evaluation of
spontaneous abortion?**

Ultrasound (usually transvaginal in early
pregnancy) is helpful in differentiating
intrauterine pregnancy from extrauterine

(ectopic) pregnancy when evaluating first-trimester bleeding without prior evidence of an intrauterine pregnancy.

For each of the following hCG values, give the findings that should be seen on transvaginal ultrasound:

hCG > 1500 MIU?
Gestational sac

hCG > 5000 MIU?
Fetal pole

hCG > 17,000 MIU?
Fetal heart motion

What is the discriminatory zone?
The hCG value above which the gestational sac should be seen in the uterus

How should a patient with threatened abortion be managed when the β-hCG is below the threshold for visualization of a sac and no intrauterine pregnancy is seen?
This clinical scenario (early pregnancy with inability to rule in an intrauterine pregnancy or rule out an ectopic pregnancy) is frequently encountered. The principal management is close follow up, but the following measures are commonly accepted in stable patients (no pain or hemodynamic instability):

Serial β-hCG measurements to determine trend (intrauterine pregnancies generally have a doubling of β-hCG values every 48 hours, whereas ectopic pregnancies generally have an abnormally low increase in β-hCG values)

Serial ultrasound examinations to determine whether there is a gestational sac once the discriminatory zone is reached

Ectopic precautions: The patient should be told to return with heavy bleeding, abdominal or pelvic pain, dizziness, syncopal episodes, or any symptom that might suggest ectopic pregnancy.

Suction curettage remains an option for patients who do not desire the pregnancy and are either noncompliant or otherwise poor candidates for follow-up

How is threatened abortion diagnosed?

Bleeding or cramping in early pregnancy
Closed cervix

How is threatened abortion treated?

Intravenous fluids for stabilization if needed
No known proven "treatment" exists that prevents miscarriage, although pelvic rest (avoiding intercourse) may be beneficial.

What is the follow-up if spontaneous abortion occurs after threatened abortion?

Follow-up with repeat physical examinations is justified if the patient is stable and without pain.
Blood type and Rh screen followed by administration of Rh immunoglobulin to Rh-negative women
Suction curettage may be needed in cases where there is heavy bleeding or the patient is having pain not responsive to NSAIDS

On what is the diagnosis of inevitable abortion based?

Bleeding or cramps with a dilated cervical os

What is the treatment of inevitable abortion?

Intravenous fluids for stabilization if needed
No treatment can prevent miscarriage once the cervix has dilated; therefore, options include (if bleeding is minimal and the patient is stable and compliant) dilation and curettage or spontaneous abortion at home with close follow-up to ensure that all POC has been passed.
Blood type and Rh screen followed by administration of Rh immunoglobulin to Rh-negative women

What are the treatment options for women who do not want to pass tissue at home?	Suction curettage or inpatient observation while aborting
What are the risks of passing tissue at home?	It is safe at the usual 6 to 8 weeks' gestational age and does not require hospitalization or intervention.
On what is the diagnosis of incomplete abortion based?	Continued bleeding after passage of tissue
What is the treatment of incomplete abortion?	Intravenous fluids for stabilization if needed Removal of tissue protruding from os with ring forceps Ultrasound to evaluate for intrauterine POC D&C; treatment of choice to evacuate the uterine cavity definitively Oxytocin or methylergonovine, or both, to stimulate uterine contractions to decrease blood loss Blood type and Rh screen followed by administration of Rh immunoglobulin to Rh-negative women Antibiotics after D&C Histologic evaluation of any available tissue
What is a side effect of methylergonovine?	It is an ergot and can therefore exacerbate chronic hypertension, or rarely lead to thromboembolic events.
On what is the diagnosis of complete abortion based?	Tissue is passed after bleeding and cramping. Cramps and bleeding cease after tissue passage.
What is the treatment of complete abortion?	Histologic confirmation that tissue is POC and not a mole

hCG values may be followed if tissue is unavailable.

Blood type and Rh screen followed by administration of Rh immunoglobulin to Rh-negative women

On what is the diagnosis of missed abortion based?

Fetal demise is confirmed, signs and symptoms of spontaneous abortion are absent, and the cervix is closed.

How can fetal demise be confirmed?

Laboratory: Static or abnormally slow increases in hCG values

Ultrasound: Absence of fetal cardiac activity in a fetus with prior cardiac activity or at a gestational age in which fetal cardiac activity should be demonstrated

What is the treatment of missed abortion?

Options include:

Outpatient follow-up

D&C

Vaginal suppository or intra-amniotic prostaglandin administration to effect uterine contractions and delivery in the second trimester

Blood type and Rh screen followed by administration of Rh immunoglobulin to Rh-negative women

Why do most authorities opt for intervention (D&C or prostaglandin administration) over observation?

Intervention decreases the risk of infection or coagulopathy, depending on the estimated time since fetal death and estimated gestational age.

What are the etiologic factors of coagulopathy after a missed abortion?

Rarely develops after a missed abortion (after several weeks) as a result of trophoblastic tissue (thromboplastin) entering the maternal circulation and triggering the intrinsic coagulation pathway

On what is the diagnosis of coagulopathy in a missed abortion based?

Diagnosis is made with laboratory and clinical evidence of altered coagulation.

Platelet values
  Simple screening test
  Usually low in the coagulopathic patient

Low fibrinogen and increased fibrin degradation products also suggest coagulopathy.

Very rarely, full-blown disseminated intravascular coagulation can develop.

On what is the diagnosis of septic abortion based?

Evidence of localized infection:
  Suprapubic, uterine, pelvic, or cervical motion tenderness; foul-smelling cervicovaginal discharge; peritonitis)
  and
Systemic evidence of infection: Fever, shock, leukocytosis after an induced or spontaneous abortion

What is the treatment for septic abortion?

Intravenous antibiotic administration
Evacuation of the infected uterine contents
Hospitalization

When is intensive care required for a patient with a septic abortion?

If systemic sepsis occurs, to allow proper hemodynamic monitoring and respiratory care

What factors should guide the choice of intravenous antibiotics?

Initial antibiotic therapy should be broad spectrum and cover anaerobic and aerobic bacteria.
After results of culture, antibiotics should be chosen according to organism antibiotic sensitivities.

When during the course of treatment of septic abortion should D&C be performed?

Only after initiation of antibiotic therapy

When is hysterectomy a treatment option for septic abortion?

In cases unresponsive to antibiotics, particularly with abscess formation

What is the differential diagnosis for recurrent pregnancy loss?

Uterine anomalies
Intrauterine lesions (fibroids, polyps, synechiae)
Luteal phase defect
Thrombophilia
Mycoplasma infection
Chromosome abnormalities
Maternal disease

What questions should be asked when taking a history for recurrent abortion?

Has the patient been exposed to environmental toxins or drugs?
Does the patient have known gynecologic or obstetric infection?
Does the patient have antiphospholipid syndrome-associated historical factors (thrombosis, autoimmune thrombocytopenia, or false-positive syphilis tests)?
Is the patient related to the father of the child?
Does the patient have a family history of recurrent pregnancy loss?

What tests can be included in the work-up of recurrent abortion?

Thyroid function evaluation
Hysterosalpingography
Parental karyotypes to determine parental chromosome abnormalities
Endometrial biopsy to determine the presence of a luteal phase defect (histologic dating of the endometrium lags behind menstrual dating by 3 days), serum progesterone d 21-24
Hypercoagulability studies:
Anticardiolipin Ab
Factor V leiden
Factor II, III
PT, PTT
ANA
Fasting homocysteine
Protein S, C

Lupus anticoag (modified RVVP, Staclot)
Methyltetra-hydrofolate reductase
Coagulation Studies:
Factor V deficiency
Protein S deficiency
Protein C deficiency
Factor II level
Factor III level
PT
PTT
ANA
Homocysteine
Lupus anticoagulant (RVVT)
Hydrofolate reductase

What are potential treatments for recurrent pregnancy loss?

Supplemental progesterone or clomiphene citrate for luteal phase defect
Surgery to correct uterine abnormalities
Treatment of infection, if present
Empiric treatment of couple with erythromycin & doxycycline to eradicate *Mycoplasma* has been proposed.
Aspirin or subcutaneous heparin for antiphospholipid syndrome
Prenatal genetic studies if warranted by parental karyotypes

What is the major threat to future reproductive potential when performing a D&C for septic abortion?

Asherman syndrome (the development of extensive intrauterine synechiae)
Risk is increased if a D&C is performed in the presence of infection.
Can also result from overzealous uterine curettage in the absence of infection

Prevention?

Treatment with antibiotics before the D&C

Treatment?

Hysteroscopic lysis of adhesions

What are the complications of D&C for inevitable,

Uterine perforation: Can result from dilation, curettage, forceps probing, or

incomplete, missed, or septic abortion?

an overly soft uterine wall that permits easy instrument penetration

Bladder or bowel injury: Results from uterine perforation and occasionally the suction of bowel into the suction curette

Fistula formation secondary to perforation

Infection

Amenorrhea and infertility (Asherman syndrome)

Why is it important to send tissue, if available, for histologic confirmation?

Histologic evaluation can confirm:

Intrauterine pregnancy when chorionic villi are present

Passage of POC

Ectopic pregnancy in the absence of chorionic villi

Gestational trophoblastic disease

For each of the following structural or mechanical causes of pregnancy loss before 20 weeks' gestational age that are amenable to treatment, give the diagnosis and treatment.

Cervical incompetence (premature cervical dilatation)

Diagnosis: Painless (no contractions) dilatation of the cervix and passage of POC

Treatment: Placement of a cervical cerclage to reinforce the structural integrity of the cervix; usually treated in the second trimester vs. bedrest

Leiomyomas

Diagnosis: Hysterosalpingogram, ultrasonography, or hysteroscopy

Treatment: Removal (myomectomy) at laparotomy, laparoscopy, or hysteroscopy; hysteroscopy is usually used now in treating submucosal fibroids in infertility patients.

Müllerian anomalies, such as a "double uterus" (bicornuate, septate, or didelphic)

Diagnosis: Hysterosalpingogram, hysteroscopy, and laparoscopy
Treatment: Surgery

Uterine synechiae (intrauterine adhesions seen in Asherman syndrome)

Diagnosis: Hysterosalpingogram, hysteroscopy, or both
Treatment: Hysteroscopic lysis of adhesions

When are causes of early pregnancy loss usually treated?

With the exception of premature cervical dilatation, which is a clinical diagnosis, extensive workup and subsequent treatment of causes of early pregnancy loss is not undertaken until the patient has experienced three consecutive losses (recurrent pregnancy loss).

8

Ectopic Pregnancy

What is it?

Extrauterine pregnancy

Most commonly occurs in the fallopian tubes (97%)

78% occur in ampullary portion of tube

Can also occur in the abdomen 1–2%, ovary 1%, and cervix < 0.5%

Life-threatening condition for the mother due to hemorrhage in the case of rupture through implantation site

Successful completion of the pregnancy is not usually a consideration.

Incidence?

Complicates ~2% of pregnancies

Has risen steadily since 1970

What is its mortality rate?

~3.5/10,000 cases (12% of all maternal deaths)

Highest risk of mortality for interstitial and abdominal gestations

What are the major risk factors?

Salpingitis/PID: Risk increases sixfold; chlamydial infection is more important than *Neisseria gonorrhoeae*.

Previous tubal pregnancy: 10%–25% will have another tubal pregnancy (10-fold increased risk).

Age: age greater than 35 increases risk threefold

Race: increased risk in Black & Hispanic women

Previous sterilization, hormonal birth control, & IUD do not increase risk of ectopic pregnancy.

This is because these are effective means of preventing prenancies.

If pregnancy occurs, however, the relative risk is higher if these factors are present.

–Surgical sterilization: 15% are ectopic

–IUD: 5% are ectopic

What are the symptoms?
Classic triad: **Abdominal pain** (generalized in nature 50% of the time), **abnormal uterine bleeding**, and **history of amenorrhea**

Other: Dizziness or lightheadedness; gastrointestinal symptoms (e.g., nausea, vomiting, and diarrhea), referred pain (to back or shoulder)

Common for pain to worsen acutely around the time of rupture, or for syncope to occur after rupture

What are the signs?
Abdominal tenderness

Adnexal tenderness (unilateral or bilateral)

Cervical motion tenderness in > 50% of patients

A tender adnexal mass may be palpable in approximately 50% of patients.

Fever: unusual occurs in <10% of patients and could suggest infectious etiology

Other: Depends on the presence and extent of rupture and hemorrhage; includes peritoneal signs, tachycardia, tachypnea, and orthostatic changes

What are the laboratory findings?
Quantitative serum β-human chorionic gonadotropin (β-hCG): Urine pregnancy test is enough in emergent clinical setting.

Serial quantitative values show a blunted rate of increase; in a normal pregnancy, β-hCG doubles every 2 days.

Complete blood count

Hematocrit—usually normal or slightly decreased; more valuable when measured serially to indicate blood loss

Type & Screen: to assess Rh status and to have blood ready if needed

Serum progesterone: can be used as an adjunct.

Levels < 5.0 ng/ml indicate a nonviable pregnancy. Only 2.5% of abnormal pregnancies have levels > 5.0 ng/ml.

What are other useful studies?

Pelvic ultrasound

Intrauterine and extrauterine pregnancies rarely occur simultaneously (1 in 30,000 pregnancies); evidence of intrauterine pregnancy excludes an ectopic.

Abdominal sonography can identify an intrauterine sac only when pregnancy is advanced enough for β-hCG levels to reach 5000–6000 mIU/ml (~7 weeks after last menstrual period).

Vaginal ultrasound: Detects an intrauterine sac at β-hCG levels between 1500 and 2000 mIU/ml (~6 weeks after last menstrual period).

Culdocentesis

Presence of nonclotting blood is diagnostic of free blood in the peritoneal cavity; supports diagnosis of ectopic pregnancy.

Useful for surgical intervention along with other findings; not very sensitive or specific for ectopic pregnancy

Dilation and Curettage: presence of chorionic villi excludes diagnosis of ectopic. Do not perform if early desired pregnancy in the differential.

Laparoscopy or laparotomy: indicated when peritoneal signs present.

What are the differential diagnoses?

Acute appendicitis

Adnexal torsion

Aborting intrauterine pregnancy

Corpus luteum or follicular cyst rupture

Pelvic inflammatory disease
Degenerating fibroids (in pregnancy)
Endometriosis
Urinary tract infection
Kidney stone
Gastroenteritis
Diverticulitis
Meckel's diverticulum

What are the treatment options?

Laparoscopy, laparotomy, medical treatment, expectant management with serial β-hCGs.

What does laparoscopic treatment entail?

1. **Linear salpingostomy:** Linear incision over the antimesenteric aspect of fallopian tube; the ectopic is exposed and evacuated. Incision closes by secondary intention and tubes reepithelialize, or may be sutured.
2. **Segmental resection:** Removal of the affected portion of the tube, with reanastomosis of tubal ends
3. **Salpingectomy removal of the tube:** Performed when the tube is severely damaged or persistently bleeding;
4. **Abdominal pregnancies:** Placenta often implants in vital organs (bowel) or over blood vessels. Therefore, fetus is removed but placenta sometimes left intact to avoid life-threatening hemorrhage. Patient often treated with methotrexate after surgery.

What are the indications for laparotomy?

Profuse hemorrhage
Certain locations of the pregnancy (cornual, interstitial, abdominal, ovarian)
Inadequate visualization, exposure, or treatment of adnexa during laparoscopy

What does medical management of ectopic pregnancy involve?

Methotrexate (folic acid antagonist):
Single intramuscular injection, with repeat dose 7 days later if β-hCG not adequately falling

What are the absolute contraindications to using methotrexate?

Active liver disease
Active renal disease

What are the relative contraindications to methotrexate?

Gestational sac > 3.5 cm
Fetal cardiac activity present
β-hCG > 5000
Questionable patient compliance with follow-up

What are the side effects of methotrexate?

Abdominal pain
Neutropenia

What are the complications of an ectopic pregnancy?

Intra-abdominal hemorrhage
Persistent trophoblastic tissue (5%); requires subsequent surgery or methotrexate
Rh sensitization secondary to fetomaternal hemorrhage: Rare; however, all Rh− patients should receive dose of RhoGAM.

What is the long-term prognosis for patients treated for an unruptured ectopic pregnancy?

Subsequent intrauterine pregnancy : ~70%
Recurrence of ectopic pregnancy: 8%
Infertility, probably secondary to tubal dysfunction and adhesion formation after treatment: 20%

9   Preterm Labor

What is preterm labor?

Contractions and progressive cervical change between 20 and 37 completed weeks' gestational age

What is cervical incompetence?

Also called premature cervical dilation; cervical dilation in the absence of contractions before term; should not be confused with preterm labor

What is the incidence of preterm labor?

Occurs in 5%–15% of all pregnancies; rates have remained unchanged for decades despite efforts to intervene.

What is the percentage of neonatal deaths caused by preterm birth?

Seventy-five percent of neonatal deaths not caused by congenital anomalies

What are the risk factors for preterm labor?

Preterm rupture of the membranes
Polyhydramnios
Multiple gestation
Maternal systemic disease
Low socioeconomic status
Nonwhite race
Maternal age: < 18 or > 40
Low prepregnancy weight
Multiple gestation (10% of all preterm births)
Fetal death
History of preterm births (17%–37% risk after one preterm birth)
Repeated second-trimester spontaneous abortion
Uterine infection/vaginal infection/colonization [group B streptococcus (GBS), gonorrhea, *Chlamydia*, *Ureaplasma*, syphilis, trichomoniasis, *Gardnerella*]

Uterine anomalies (unicornuate uterus,
  bicornuate uterus, uterine
  leiomyomata)
Pyelonephritis
Smoking
Cocaine use
Use of IUD
Lack of prenatal care
Fetal anomalies
Placental anomalies

What is the percent of all preterm births caused by preterm labor?

Approximately 30%

What are other causes of preterm birth?

Preterm premature rupture of the
  membranes (30%–35% of all preterm
  births)
Placental abruption
Placenta previa
Maternal indication for delivery
Isoimmunication
Multiple gestation
Hypertensive disorders
Diabetes mellitus
Congenital malformations

What constitutes "labor"?

Regular uterine contractions with:
Contractions lasting at least 30 seconds
At least two contractions in a 10-minute
  period
Persistence of contraction pattern for at
  least 30 minutes
Progressive cervical change

What questions should be asked in the history of the preterm labor patient?

Does the patient have:
A history of preterm birth?
A history of cystitis or pyelonephritis?
A known multiple gestation?
A known placenta previa?
A known fetal anomaly?
A known uterine anomaly?
Good fetal movement?

Untreated infections?
Cigarette or cocaine use?
An accurate last menstrual period (LMP) or dating ultrasound?

What conditions should be ruled out in preterm labor?

Preterm premature rupture of the membranes
Placental abruption
Placenta previa
Fetal death
Infection
Multiple gestation
Fetal anomalies

Why is gestational age important in preterm labor?

It determines the risks to the fetus in the extrauterine environment and guides aggressiveness of treatment.

How is gestational age calculated?

By determining the estimated date of confinement (EDC, "due date") using Naegele's rule:
EDC = (**LMP** + 7 days) − 3 months

How is gestational age calculated when LMP is not precisely known and early ultrasonographic dating is not available?

Use best estimate of the LMP and the earliest possible ultrasound to estimate gestational age.

What form of preterm birth can be prevented?

Iatrogenic preterm birth due to elective induction of labor or elective cesarean section when the maturity of the fetus is not precisely known

What are preventive measures for preterm labor?

Home uterine monitoring for women with a history of preterm labor
Prophylactic tocolytic agents for women at high risk for preterm labor
Reduced activity
Bed rest
Frequent cervical examinations to detect early cervical change

What are general treatment options?	Hydration Bed rest Tocolytic therapy Glucocorticoid administration Transfer of patient to a high-risk facility
How do hydration and bed rest stop preterm labor?	Hydration: Mechanism is unknown. Bed rest: Little evidence supports its use. Both continue to be used liberally because their use entails almost no risk and may benefit the patient.
What are tocolytic drugs?	Agents that decrease uterine contractions by a variety of mechanisms; used to stop the progression of labor when continued uterine contractions or labor could have negative consequences
What are the short- and long-term goals of tocolysis?	Short-term goal: Prevent delivery for at least 48 hours to allow administration of glucocorticoids to the mother (fetal lung benefits optimized at least 48 hours after institution of therapy) Long-term goal: Allow fetus to gain lung maturity in utero to increase the chances of a good outcome after delivery
Contraindications?	Intrauterine fetal demise Oligohydramnios Intrauterine growth retardation Fetal distress Chorioamnionitis PPROM Fatal congenital anomalies
What are β-mimetic agents?	β-Adrenergic agonists that act through smooth muscle relaxation
Specific β-adrenergic agents used?	Only ritodrine is FDA-approved for tocolysis, but terbutaline is commonly used.

Side effects?

Tachycardia
Palpitations
Tremors
Nervousness
Restlessness
Pulmonary edema
Decreased K^+
Insulin release
Increased glucose
Lactic acidosis

Contraindications?

Maternal heart disease
Hyperthyroidism
Uncontrolled hypertension
Pulmonary hypertension
Drug-dependent asthma
Possibly diabetes

How do calcium channel blockers (nifedipine) act in tocolysis?

They reduce smooth muscle activity and myometrial contractions by reducing cytoplasmic free calcium.

Side effects?

Minimal; animal experiments suggest fetal hypoxemia and decreased uteroplacental blood flow, but these effects are not found in humans.
Headache
Hypotension
Dizziness

What are indomethacin (Indocin) and sulindac?

Prostaglandin inhibitors that prevent prostaglandin-induced myometrial contractions by blocking prostaglandin synthetase activity; possibly more effective than ritodrine in delaying delivery and increasing birth weight

What primary concerns limit the use of prostaglandin inhibitors as tocolytics?

Premature closure of ductus arteriosus and fetal nephrotoxicity

What is the mechanism of action of magnesium sulfate in tocolysis?

Exerts stabilizing effects on smooth muscle by calcium antagonism

Side effects?

Decreased deep tendon reflexes, pulmonary edema, heart block, respiratory and cardiac depression, and drowsiness; not usually seen if renal function is normal and administration rates are acceptable (2 g/hour)

Indications?

First-line drug in obviously progressive labor, especially at an early gestational age
Second-line drug with failed oral tocolysis
When other tocolytics are contraindicated

What is the therapy for magnesium toxicity?

1 g calcium gluconate intravenously

What are the beneficial effects of corticosteroids in preterm labor?

Betamethasone or dexamethasone aids fetal lung maturity and decreases the incidence of neonatal respiratory distress syndrome (RDS), neonatal intraventricular hemorrhage, and neonatal mortality.

At what gestational age should they be used?

At 24–34 weeks' gestational age in women at risk for preterm delivery, before 30–32 weeks' gestation in women with preterm premature rupture of membranes in the absence of clinical chorioamnionitis

Neonatal risks?

No evidence of increased neonatal infection risk or adrenal suppression

Maternal risks?

Generally low; include pulmonary edema (increased risk with tocolytics, fluid overload, or multiple gestation), slight increase in infection with preterm premature rupture of the membranes (controversial), and glucose/insulin control effects

What common organism poses a threat to fetus and mother in preterm labor?

Group B *Streptococcus* (GBS)

Incidence of colonization?

Fifteen percent to forty percent of pregnant women are colonized with GBS.

Fifty percent of these women colonize their infants during delivery.

Maternal complications related to GBS?

Chorioamnionitis, endomyometritis, cystitis, and pyelonephritis

Prophylaxis and treatment?

Culture of women in preterm labor and a penicillin (erythromycin or clindamycin in penicillin-allergic patients) until culture proves negative

Full course of antibiotics for women with positive GBS cultures to prevent maternal/sexual transmission of ODS, neonatal sepsis, chorioamnionitis, and postpartum endomyometritis.

Treatment of all women with GBS in their urine

Should patients at risk for delivery of a preterm neonate be transferred to high-risk centers before or after delivery?

Historically, concern for potential delivery en route to perinatal centers prevented routine transfer of patients with risk of preterm delivery.

Current practice mandates transfer to a perinatal center of all stable women at risk of delivery if the fetus weighs less than 1500 g (~32–34 weeks).

Should preterm neonates be delivered by cesarean section (C/S)?

Cephalic presentation: Vaginal delivery has same outcome as C/S despite the theoretical risk of head trauma and intraventricular hemorrhage.

Breech: C/S is indicated because of the risk of head entrapment by the incompletely dilated cervix (infrequent but potentially devastating).

What underlying fetal deficiency leads to neonatal respiratory distress syndrome (RDS)?

Deficient surfactant biosynthesis in neonatal lung type II pneumocytes leads to RDS because of alveolar collapse from increased alveolar surface tension.

Treatment?

Surfactant administration for neonates at high risk for RDS

What determines outcome in preterm neonates?

Level of neonatal care
Gestational age
Birth weight
Presence of asphyxia
Presence of intracranial hemorrhage
Presence of periventricular leukomalacia
Presence of retinopathy of prematurity
Parental socioeconomic factors/education
Presence of necrotizing enterocolitis
Presence of congenital anomalies

What are the generally accepted values for low–birth-weight neonates?

$\geq$ 2500 g = "normal"
< 2500 g = low birth weight
$\leq$ 1500 g = very low birth weight
$\leq$ 1000 g = extremely low birth weight

What is the difference in risk of neonatal death between normal and very low–birth-weight infants?

Very low–birth-weight infants have a 200-fold increased risk of death compared with neonates weighing > 2500 g (Table 9-1).

What is the incidence of RDS from 33 to 38 weeks' gestation?

Decreases with increasing gestational age:
Thirty-one percent at 33 weeks' gestation
Thirteen percent at 34 weeks' gestation
Six percent from 35 to 38 weeks' gestation

Table 9–1. Mortality rates by gestational age and birth weight

Gestational Age (wk)	Mortality Rate (%)	Birth Weight (g)	Mortality Rate (%)
23	82	500–600	80–90
24	42	600–700	53–85
25	20	700–800	41–65
26–27	6	800–900	29–42
28–29	9	900–1000	17–25
<26	44	1000–1250	13

Courtesy R. J. Boyle, MD, University of Virginia.

What are the early and late problems associated with preterm birth?

Early: Developmental delay, cerebral palsy, visual impairment, hearing loss, chronic lung disease, rehospitalization

Late: Mental retardation, learning disabilities, attention deficit disorder, language impairment, school problems

What is the incidence of problems?

Twenty-six percent of survivors weighing < 800 g have major handicaps.

Seventeen percent to twenty percent of survivors weighing 750–1000 g have major handicaps.

10

Premature Rupture of the Membranes

What is premature rupture of the membranes (PROM)?

Disruption of the integrity of fetal membranes before the onset of labor at any gestational age

What is preterm PROM?

PROM before term (before 38 weeks' gestation)

What is prolonged PROM?

More than 24 hours elapsed between rupture of membranes and the onset of labor (latent period).

What is the incidence of PROM?

Complicates 10% of all pregnancies
Associated with 30% of preterm births
Most common diagnosis on admission to neonatal intensive care units

Does PROM occur more frequently at term or preterm?

Ninety-four percent of all cases occur at term.
Five percent occur in pregnancies with fetuses weighing 1000–2500 g.
One percent of all cases occurs in fetuses weighing less than 1000 g.

How do term and preterm patients differ in their propensity to go into labor after PROM?

Ninety percent of term patients will be in labor 24 hours after PROM.
Fifty percent of preterm patients will be in labor 24 hours after PROM.
75 percent of preterm patients will be in labor within 1 week after PROM.
Earlier gestational age is associated with greater potential for prolongation of pregnancy

What are the causes of PROM?

Not definitively known, but linked to:
Membrane infection
Hydramnios
Incompetent cervix

cerclage placement
Abruptio placentae
Amniocentesis
Lower socioeconomic status
History of STDs
Prior preterm delivery
Cigarette smoking

What organisms have been linked to PROM?

Ureaplasma urealyticum, Trichomonas vaginalis, Bacteroides species, Chlamydia trachomatis, group B streptococcus (GBS), *Gardnerella vaginalis*, and others

How do they cause PROM?

Production of various factors may weaken fetal membranes and render them susceptible to rupture
It is unknown whether positive vaginal or amniotic fluid cultures are the result of (1) infection causing PROM through weakening of the membranes, or (2) PROM leading to colonization with microorganisms.

What is a common symptom in PROM?

Sudden "gush" of fluid or a steady "trickle" of fluid per vaginum that may or may not be associated with the passage of a small amount of blood or mucus. **Note:** Patients frequently confuse loss of urine, vaginal discharge, or bloody show with loss of amniotic fluid.

How is PROM diagnosed?

With a "sterile" speculum vaginal examination

What are the three signs of PROM?

1. Pooling of vaginal fluid in the posterior fornix
2. Positive nitrazine test—i.e., nitrazine paper reveals pH >6.0–6.5 (normal vaginal pH 4.5–6.0)
3. "Ferning" on a slide prepared with a thin layer of fluid obtained from the vaginal wall and allowed to dry

How can false-positive diagnoses of membrane rupture be avoided?

Nitrazine test: False positives can occur if discharge is obtained from the cervical os because the cervical mucus, like amniotic fluid, has a pH higher than that of the vagina; blood, semen, or vaginitis can also raise pH.

Ferning: Cervical mucus can also cause "ferning" (a distinct arborization pattern seen under microscopy) in the absence of ruptured membranes.

Collection of fluid: Collect fluid *only* from the vaginal wall to avoid cervical mucus unless fluid can be seen flowing from the os into the posterior fornix with the Valsalva maneuver, cough, or fundal pressure.

How is cervical dilatation evaluated in preterm PROM?

No digital cervical examination if rupture of the membranes is confirmed or suspected in preterm patients due to the risk of introducing infection into the amnionic sac

Visualization with a "sterile" speculum for cervical assessment

How is potential infection evaluated?

Assess for symptoms clinically—fever, fundal tenderness, etc.

Cultures for genital tract organisms, including GBS as well as gonorrhea and chlamydia

Amniocentesis in women with preterm PROM for Gram stain and culture to evaluate for infection

Benefit: also allows evaluation of fetal lung maturity

Risk: procedure carries some risk; questionable whether this practice results in improved pregnancy outcomes

How is ultrasound useful in the evaluation of PROM?

Evaluation of fetal biometry [in the absence of a known last menstrual period (LMP) or prior ultrasound] to determine gestational age of the fetus

Evaluation of amniotic fluid volume for oligohydramnios, which may help to confirm the rupture

Determination of fetal presentation (vertex, breech, or transverse) when vaginal examination is inappropriate and abdominal examination is inconclusive

Evaluation for a fetal anomaly if PROM occurs preterm

What is a dye test?

Injection of dye into the amniotic sac followed by evaluation of the presence of dye on a tampon placed intravaginally

How can a dye test be used to evaluate PROM?

To confirm diagnosis if equivocal

To determine if membranes have "sealed over" in a woman who has stopped leaking

How is the fetus evaluated before initiating treatment in PROM?

Rule out fetal stress (from cord compression in oligohydramnios or cord prolapse) with fetal heart monitoring in preterm or term PROM.

Why is knowing the gestational age important in PROM?

The risks to the fetus from preterm delivery vary with gestational age.

How is gestational age determined?

With the patient's LMP, or ultrasound if LMP is uncertain

What are the risks of PROM to the fetus and the mother?

Infection of the fetus (fetal/neonatal sepsis or death), the fetal membranes (chorioamnionitis), or the uterus (endomyometritis)

Differences in risks between preterm and term PROM?

Preterm PROM: The risks are primarily related to prematurity (RDS, IVH, NEC) and secondarily related to infection.

Term PROM: No risk of prematurity; primary risk is infection.

What is expectant management of PROM?

Preterm patient: patient observation for evidence of chorioamnionitis without active attempts at tocolysis

Term patient: patient observation without active attempts at induction

What is active management of PROM?

Preterm patient: active attempts at halting the progression or preventing the onset of labor (to increase fetal maturation in utero) with or without the use of steroids or antibiotics

Term patient: active attempts at delivery of the infant (induction or augmentation of labor)

What are the primary risks of expectant management versus active management in *preterm* PROM?

Principal risks of preterm PROM are related to prematurity, not infection; delivery of the preterm fetus is undesirable.

Expectant management risk: chorioamnionitis

Active management risks: risks involved with tocolysis, risks of antibiotics, and risks of corticosteroids

The debate of expectant management versus active interventions is ongoing, but the benefits of close observation for evidence of fetal or maternal infection and induction of labor if chorioamnionitis is diagnosed are established.

What are the primary risks of expectant management versus active management in PROM *at term*?

Principal risk is chorioamnionitis (with potential neonatal sepsis and maternal endomyometritis), not prematurity; delivery is desirable.

Expectant management risks: risks of infection—significant if delivery does not occur within 24 hours

Active management risks: risks of labor induction (uterine hyperstimulation, fetal distress, and uterine rupture, all relatively small risks)

Because the risks of induction are relatively low and the morbidity of chorioamnionitis relatively high, most practitioners induce labor or augment labor 8–24 hours after membranes have ruptured.

What maternal and fetal signs and symptoms suggest chorioamnionitis in PROM?

Uterine tenderness on abdominal examination
Maternal white blood cell count ≥ 16,000—difficult to interpret
Maternal temperature ≥ 38♂C
Maternal and fetal tachycardia
Flu-like symptoms, back pains, or a subtle change in vaginal discharge
Foul-smelling or purulent vaginal fluid on speculum examination

Why is tocolysis in preterm PROM controversial?

Tocolytics may mask an important sign of infection (uterine irritability with resultant contractions). Alternatively, some feel tocolytics do not delay diagnosis because other reliable signs (fever ≥ 38°C, uterine tenderness, leukocytosis, purulent amniotic fluid, fetal or maternal tachycardia) can be used to diagnose chorioamnionitis.
Also, most studies have failed to show a benefit of tocolysis in preterm PROM in terms of neonatal outcome.

What role do antibiotics play in the treatment of PROM at term?

Depends on GBS status. If GBS, or with risk factors for GBS, prophylactic penicillin is given to decrease the risk of neonatal infection.

Of preterm PROM?

In the preterm PROM patient, a course of antibiotic therapy has been shown to prolong pregnancy and to reduce the incidence of chorioamnionitis, postpartum endomeritis, neonatal sepsis, RDS, IVH, and NEC.

What is the treatment of chorioamnionitis?

In both term and preterm PROM: antibiotic therapy and prompt delivery of the fetus (labor induction) to prevent neonatal sepsis

Cesarean section: reserved for usual obstetric indications; consequences of postoperative uterine infection are severe during chorioamnionitis.

What are the NIH recommendations for the use of corticosteroids in the treatment of PROM?

Controversial because of the theoretical risk of immunocompromise and infection

Antenatal corticosteroid use for women with preterm PROM at less than 30–32 weeks of gestation in the absence of clinical chorioamnionitis

Benefits of steroids in the treatment of PROM?

Neonatal benefits; reduced incidences of IVH, RDS, NEC (necrotizing enterocolitis) and neonatal death

What are the risks of PROM associated with gestational age less than 24 weeks?

Low odds of neonatal survival (< 30%) and a high risk of severe short- and long-term neonatal morbidity if fetus lives. At 24–26 weeks, 57% survival.

How is PROM managed in the nonviable gestation?

Because of risks, termination of the pregnancy and labor induction should be considered.

What are the complications of preterm PROM?

Fetus/Neonate:
Neonatal sepsis
RDS
 — IVH
Patent ductus arteriosus
Necrotizing enterocolitis
Pulmonary hypoplasia in fetuses < 24 weeks
Cord prolapse/intrauterine demise
Mother:
Chorioamnionitis/endomyometritis
Puerperal sepsis

11   Intrauterine Growth Restriction (IUGR)

What is intrauterine growth restriction (IUGR)?

Estimated fetal weight less than expected—often defined as (10th percentile)

What is a small for gestational age (SGA) infant?

An infant below the 10th percentile in birth-weight for its gestational age

What is the incidence of IUGR?

Occurs in 10% of all pregnancies

What are the potential risks to a fetus (or neonate) with IUGR?

Neonatal risks:
Sepsis
Hypoglycemia
Temperature instability
Asphyxia
Meconium aspiration
Metabolic derangements
Hematologic disorders
Malformations
Fetal risks:
Oligohydramnios
Increased risk of IUPD
Increased risk of abnormal FHR pattern in labor

What are the classifications of IUGR?

Symmetric and asymmetric. It is unclear at present whether this distination is important with regard to neonatal outcome.

What is symmetric IUGR?

Overall decrease in infant size
Affects both head and body
Usually secondary to an early gestational insult

What percentage of IUGR cases are symmetric?

Twenty percent

What is asymmetric IUGR?

Decrease in subcutaneous fat and abdominal circumference (AC)

Relative sparing of head circumference (HC) and femur length (FL)

Usually secondary to an insult later in gestation

Verified as increased HC/AC ratio or FL/AC ratio

What percentage of IUGR cases are asymmetric?

Eighty percent

What are the etiologic factors for IUGR?

Constituionally small mother

Poor maternal weight gain or nutrition

Lower socioeconomic status

Congenital or chromosomal anomalies

Teratogen exposure

Maternal disease (especially vascular disease)

Placental abnormalities

Multiple gestation

Infection

How does congenital infection affect fetal growth?

By interfering with cellular development; generally, the earlier the infant is infected, the more severe the outcome.

What percentage of IUGR cases are caused by congenital infection?

Up to 5%

What organisms are most commonly involved in IUGR?

Toxoplasmosis, Syphilis, **R**ubella, **C**ytomegalovirus

How do chromosomal anomalies and congenital anomalies affect fetal growth?

Overall decrease in cell number

What chromosomal anomalies are associated with IUGR?

Trisomies 13, 18, and 21

What congenital anomalies are associated with IUGR?

Cardiac and renal anomalies with or without an associated chromosomal anomaly. Generally, a more severe anomaly carries a higher risk for an SGA infant.

What percentage of IUGR cases are caused by chromosomal and congenital anomalies?

Ten percent

How does maternal drug use affect fetal growth?

Smoking: Decreases uteroplacental blood flow; risk of SGA infant is increased threefold over nonsmokers.

Alcohol abuse: may cause dysmorphic features and IUGR (fetal alcohol syndrome)

Cocaine use: causes vasospasm and decreased uteroplacental blood flow; 30% of pregnant women using cocaine will have an SGA infant.

How does maternal disease affect fetal growth?

Maternal vascular disease (e.g. lupus, hypertension, diabetes, renal disease): decreased uteroplacental blood flow→decreased fetal oxygenation→ IUGR.

Diseases that affect maternal oxygenation (e.g., hemoglobinopathies) also affect fetal growth.

What placental defects lead to fetal IUGR?

Decreased placental mass (decreases fetal oxygenation and transfer of nutrients)

Placental anomalies including placental abruption, circumvallate placenta, placental infarction, placenta accreta

Possibly abnormal placental implantation (may be a risk factor; placenta previa may limit oxygenation and nutrient transfer)

How do multiple gestations lead to fetal IUGR?

Decreased placental surface per fetus
Eighteen percent of twin gestations are associated with IUGR

What tests are used to diagnose IUGR?

Physical examination with measurement of maternal fundal height

Ultrasound evaluation of fetal size and interval growth

How is fundal height measured?

From the maternal pubis symphysis to the top of the uterine fundus in centimeters

How is fundal height measurement used in the diagnosis of IUGR?

As a screening test

What is fundal height lag?

A fundal height smaller than fetal gestational age

When should fundal height lag raise suspicion of IUGR?

A lag greater than 3–4 weeks

What fetal indices are evaluated with ultrasound?

Head circumference relative to abdominal circumference and femur length

Amniotic fluid volume (AFV)

Placental grade

Estimated fetal weight

Fetal gestational age: a MUST prior to assessing for IUGR; do not confuse a misdated fetus with a fetus with symmetric IUGR

Congenital anomalies: may indicate a chromosomal anomaly

How are head and abdominal circumference used to assess for IUGR?

Established head circumference to abdominal circumference ratios:

In normal fetuses: HC/AC > 1.0 before 32 weeks; HC/AC = 1.0 at 32 to 34 weeks; HC/AC < 1.0 after 34 weeks.

In fetuses with asymmetric IUGR: The head remains larger relative to the body; therefore, HC/AC is elevated.

In fetuses with symmetric IUGR: Both HC and AC are reduced; the ratio remains normal.

When is femur length used to assess for IUGR?

When fetal position prevents accurate measurement

Femur length is spared in asymmetrical IUGR, increasing the FL/AC ratio.

How is AFV used to assess for IUGR?

Decreased AFV may be an early sign of IUGR.

70–80% of IUGR fetuses are affected by oligohydramnios.

Why does decreased AFV occur in IUGR?

Decreased renal blood flow secondary to shunting to other organs leads to decreased fetal urine output and, thus, decreased AFV.

How is placental grading used to assess for IUGR?

A placenta of a higher grade than expected for a gestational age may indicate decreased placental function and subsequent IUGR.

What indices are evaluated in placental grading?

Placental calcium deposits and indentations in the chorionic plate.

What are the placental grades?

Grade 0: no calcifications and no indentations in the chorionic plate

Grade 1: few calcifications throughout the placenta

Grade 2: calcifications along the uterine wall and indentations in the chorionic plate

Grade 3: significant calcium deposits and indentations in the chorionic plate that appear to outline individual cotyledons

How is estimated fetal weight (EFW) determined with ultrasound?

Established charts and formulas determine EFW using biparietal diameter, head circumference, abdominal circumference, and femur length.

What are the most useful ultrasound criteria for determining IUGR?

EFW below the 10th percentile
Decreased AFW, elevated HC/AC

How are Doppler flow studies used to assess for IUGR?

Doppler ultrasound can be used to evaluate uterine umbilical or fetal middle cerebral artery blood flow.

What are normal results of Doppler flow studies?

Forward flow through the umbilical arteries throughout the cardiac cycle

What are results of Doppler flow studies that may indicate IUGR?

Decreased end diastolic flow with a corresponding increased systolic/diastolic ratio (S/D ratio > 2.6). Most reliable—no diastolic flow

What is the general goal of monitoring fetuses with suspected IUGR?

To balance the risks of delivering a premature infant against the risk of stillbirth

What are the general considerations in management of the constitutionally small and asymmetric and symmetric IUGR fetuses?

Constitutionally small fetuses: Majority of SGA infants are constitutionally small and do not require any intervention.
Symmetric IUGR: Due to possibility of early insult, therapy may not be available.
Asymmetric IUGR: It may be possible to alter the uterine environment or deliver the fetus early to minimize negative effects.

What is the management plan for fetuses with IUGR?

Serial examinations of the fetus
Maternal education about daily fetal activity (kick counts)
Ultrasound examinations every 3 to 4 weeks to evaluate the HC/AC ratio, EFW, possible congenital anomalies, AFV
Regular fetal monitoring:
Frequent nonstress tests (NST)
Contraction stress test (CST), biophysical profile (BPP), or Doppler

flow studies if a fetus has a nonreactive NST (especially if the fetus had a previously reactive NST); CST is positive (fetal heart rate [FHR] decelerations in > 50% of contractions) in 40% of IUGR fetuses
Possible amniocentesis to time the delivery of the fetus

What findings from amniocentesis indicate delivery?

Evidence of fetal lung maturity (either an L/S ratio > 2 or the presence of phosphatidylglycerol)

When should a preterm fetus with IUGR be delivered?

Worsening growth lag, development of oligohydramnios, nonreassuring fetal monitoring; Amniocentesis for evidence of fetal lung maturity can be helpful. Depends on degree of prematurity.

What is the recommended management of progressive growth lag, development of oligohydramnios, or nonreassuring fetal monitoring when amniocentesis indicates fetal lung immaturity?

Steroids to accelerate fetal lung maturity
Close fetal monitoring
Consideration of delivery if fetal condition worsens—depends also on degree of prematurity.

What is the intrapartum management of a fetus with IUGR?

Continuous fetal heart rate monitoring
If reassuring FHR: normal delivery
Persistent FHR decelerations: possible cesarean section

What are the etiologic factors of hypoglycemia in IUGR infants?

Two factors:
1. Decreased glycogen stores secondary to malnutrition
2. Decreased sensitivity of gluconeogenesis pathway to hypoglycemia

What are the etiologic factors of hypothermia in IUGR infants?

Decreased body fat stores

What are the etiologic factors of meconium aspiration in IUGR infants?

Passage of meconium is common and its concern is high when amniotic volume is low.

What metabolic derangements are common in IUGR infants?

Hypocalcemia
Hypokalemia
Hyponatremia
Hyperphosphatemia

What hematologic disorders are common in IUGR infants?

Polycythemia secondary to fetal hypoxia and an increased production of red blood cells (RBCs) to compensate for the decreased oxygenation
Hyperbilirubinemia secondary to increased RBC breakdown

What is the long-term follow-up for infants born with IUGR?

By 2 years of age, most otherwise normal SGA infants have caught up to normal birth weight infants.
Neurologic complications: The extent of persistent neurologic damage in IUGR infants remains unclear.
Overall, the degree of long-term sequelae is related to the degree of growth retardation, prematurity, and gestational age at which the insult occurs (the earlier the insult, the greater the level of neurologic damage).

12

Hematologic Diseases in Pregnancy

What normal hematologic changes occur in pregnancy?

Fifty percent increase in maternal plasma volume (1,000 ml) plus 25% increase in red blood cell (RBC) mass→decrease in hematocrit.

Decrease in hematocrit is greatest in the second trimester.

Late pregnancy: Plasma expansion ceases while RBC mass continues to increase.

How is the decreased hematocrit compensated for?

Iron absorption from the duodenum increases.

What defines anemia in pregnancy?

A hematocrit less than 30 or a hemoglobin less than 10

What are the etiologic factors of anemia in pregnancy?

Most common: secondary to iron deficiency anemia

Other causes: nutritional deficiencies, acute blood loss, anemia from chronic disease, drug-induced hemolytic anemia, hemoglobinopathies, malignancy

IRON DEFICIENCY ANEMIA

What is the daily iron requirement in pregnancy?

One gram of elemental iron needs to be absorbed into the bloodstream to maintain a steady state (over the course of the pregnancy).

How can this be accomplished?

By taking 150 mg ferrous sulfate/day (equivalent of 30 mg elemental iron)—or by diet

What are the symptoms of iron deficiency anemia?

Fatigue and lethargy; these symptoms are also common in pregnancy.

What are the associated lab findings?	Complete blood count (CBC): Hematocrit is decreased.
	Peripheral blood smear: May show hypochromic microcytic cells; however, if the patient is also folate-deficient, normochromic normocytic cells may be seen
	Decreased ferritin
	Other: decreased serum iron concentration, decreased saturation of transferrin
What is the effect of iron deficiency anemia on a developing fetus?	Causes no adverse effect on the fetus; the fetus maintains its iron stores by active transport mechanisms despite maternal deficiencies.
What is the effect of pregnancy on the hematocrit?	A decrease in the hematocrit that is most marked in the second trimester
What is the treatment?	Supplemental iron (PO or IV or dietary)
What is the dosage?	325 mg of simple iron compounds, such as ferrous sulfate or ferrous gluconate, each day; doses in excess of this standard dose do not result in more rapid RBC production because excess iron is excreted in the stool.
What are the instructions for maximum absorption?	Ingest 30 minutes before a meal.
What can increase or decrease absorption?	Vitamin C ingestion increases iron absorption; simultaneous antacid ingestion decreases absorption.
What are indicators of patient response to iron supplementation?	A reticulocytosis indicating a hematologic response should be seen within 2 weeks of beginning iron therapy.
	The hematocrit should increase by 1% to 2% each week.

FOLATE DEFICIENCY

What is folic acid?

Folic acid (folate) is a water-soluble vitamin usually found in green vegetables, peanuts, and liver. It is a member of the B-complex group of vitamins. In humans, the only source of folate is from the diet.

What is the recommended dose of folate/day for reproductive age women?

0.4 mg/day

What are folic acid requirements in pregnancy?

0.8 to 1 mg/day
Increased requirements with multiple gestations and patients with hemoglobinopathies

What effects does folate supplementation around the time of conception and in early pregnancy have on fetal development?

Supplemental folate (1 mg per day) around time of conception and in early pregnancy (organogenesis) may decrease the incidence of neural tube defects.

What is the incidence of folate deficiency in pregnancy?

Low serum folate levels occur in ~10% to 25% of pregnant women; second most common nutritional anemia in pregnancy

What is the relationship between folate deficiency in pregnancy and megaloblastic anemia?

Folate deficiency is the most common cause of megaloblastic anemia in pregnancy.
However, even without folate supplementation, less than 5% of patients with a folate deficiency will develop a megaloblastic anemia.

What are the symptoms of folate deficiency?

Fatigue and lethargy, which are related to the degree of anemia
Nausea, vomiting, anorexia, roughness of the skin, glossitis

What are the lab findings?

CBC: reveals normochromic macrocytic anemia or a normochromic normocytic anemia with hypersegmentation of neutrophils

Reticulocyte count: normal or low; elliptocytes may be seen.

WBC count: sometimes decreased

Platelet count: sometimes decreased

Concurrent iron deficiency may produce a mixed population of RBCs, detectable on smear, but not MCV.

Serum folate level: low (< 4)

How is folate deficiency distinguished from vitamin B_{12} deficiency?

Unlike folate deficiency, vitamin B_{12} deficiency may produce a peripheral neuropathy.

What is the effect of folate deficiency on a developing fetus?

Folate deficiency does not cause adverse effects on a developing fetus because the fetus preferentially obtains folate from the mother and maintains normal levels.

Although the incidence of congenital anomalies is not increased in folate-deficient mothers, folate supplementation around the time of conception may decrease the overall incidence of neural tube defects.

What is the effect of pregnancy on folate requirements?

Pregnancy increases the folate requirement by three- to fourfold.

Patients with multiple gestations, malabsorption syndromes, hemoglobinopathies, or those taking phenytoin are more likely to develop a folic acid deficiency.

What is the treatment of folate deficiency?

Folate supplementation with 1 to 3 mg folate daily

What are the indicators of patient response to folate supplementation?

Rapid increase in the reticulocyte count

After 1 week of treatment, the hematocrit may increase as much as 1% each day.

SICKLE CELL DISEASE

What is sickle cell disease?	Most common hemoglobinopathy Hemoglobin (Hb) S ("sickle") results from a single amino acid substitution of valine for glutamic acid in the beta chain of hemoglobin. RBCs with Hb S: Have reduced oxygen-carrying capacity and survival time (half-life of 5 to 10 days) Have an increased chance of sickling
How is sickle cell disease inherited?	Autosomal recessive disease
What is sickle cell trait?	Sickle cell trait (Hb AS) is the heterozygous form of disease.
Who should be screened?	All African Americans. Those with family history of sickle disease or trait
What other hemoglobinopathies result in sickling?	Hb C, Hb D, and Hb sickle cell-beta thalassemia
What is sickle cell-Hb C disease?	It is a double heterozygous condition in which patient carries one gene for Hb S and one gene for Hb C. It causes milder hemolytic anemia and fewer painful crises than sickle cell-Hb S disease. Pregnant women have an increased frequency of skeletal pain with respiratory and/or neurologic compromise in the third trimester, at term, and immediately postpartum. Pregnant women have an increased tendency for complicated pregnancy; management during pregnancy is the same as that of sickle cell anemia.

What is sickle cell-Hb D disease?	Patients may be asymptomatic or may have a mild hemolytic anemia. Pregnancy is usually uneventful.
What is the incidence of sickle cell trait?	Occurs in 1/12 of adult African Americans
What percentage of Hb is Hb S in people with sickle cell trait?	25–35%
What is the incidence of sickle cell disease?	Occurs in 1/625 of African-American children
What percentage of Hb is Hb S in people with sickle cell disease?	90%
Diagnostic tests?	Screening tests for the sickle cell gene (e.g., sickledex test) Hb electrophoresis: diagnostic Polymerase chain reaction and Southern blotting may be used for prenatal diagnosis in the fetus.
What screening test is used?	Hemoglobin electrophoresis
What laboratory findings are consistent with sickle cell disease?	Hematocrit: Low Bilirubin: Hyperbilirubinemia (bilirubin = 1–7 in sickle cell disease; 15–20 in a crisis)
What are the signs and symptoms?	Patients with sickle cell trait are asymptomatic. Patients with sickle cell disease: Have "crises," frequent painful vaso-occlusive episodes in the extremities, joints, and abdomen. Have symptoms of anemia and frequent infections.

What is the pathophysiology of sickle cell crisis?

Sickling of RBCs is triggered by hypoxia, acidosis, and dehydration.
Sludging in small vessels results in microinfarction of the affected organs.
Crises can lead to a rapid drop in hematocrit, deoxygenation, and pain; splenic sequestration may occur.

What is the effect of sickle cell disease on a developing fetus?

It has been hypothesized that sickling in the uterine vessels may lead to decreased fetal oxygenation.
Sickle cell trait has no adverse effect on a developing fetus.
Sickle cell disease may complicate pregnancy; associated with an increased incidence of spontaneous abortion, preterm birth, intrauterine growth retardation, perinatal mortality, stillbirth, pyelonephritis, and preeclampsia.

What is the effect of pregnancy on a person with sickle cell disease?

Increased incidence of severe anemia, vasoocclusive episodes, and painful crises

What are the complications of the disease?

Increased incidence of urinary tract infections
Osteomyelitis, jaundice, cholelithiasis, high-output cardiac failure secondary to chronic anemia, infections, and pulmonary and splenic infarctions

What is the management?

Pneumococcal vaccine to prevent infection early in or prior to pregnancy
Supplemental iron when iron deficiency exists
Folic acid supplementation (1 mg/day)
Avoidance of crises with prevention of infections and dehydration
Antenatal fetal surveillance with NSTs
Serial ultrasonography to assess fetal growth

Monitoring for preeclampsia (e.g., blood pressure checks)

Regular monitoring of reticulocyte count, bilirubin, and hematocrit

How is a crisis managed during pregnancy?

Search for an infection (up to one-third of crises are associated with infection).

If no infection is found, search for other possible causes of pain and/or anemia such as ectopic pregnancy, placental abruption, pyelonephritis, appendicitis, and cholecystitis.

Manage pain with acetaminophen and meperidine hydrochloride (Demerol®); avoid morphine sulfate because of its potential smooth muscle constrictive properties.

Replace fluid and electrolytes because of increased insensible fluid loss that occurs during a crisis.

Prophylactic exchange transfusions and simple transfusions significantly decrease the incidence and severity of painful crises. However, improvement in perinatal outcome is controversial.

In labor, provide supplemental oxygen and continuous fetal monitoring.

How can sickle cell disease be prevented?

Through carrier screening in populations at risk and prenatal screening when both parents have the sickle cell trait

When both parents have the trait, the risk of a child with disease is 25%.

Prenatal diagnosis of this condition is possible.

VON WILLEBRAND DISEASE

What is von Willebrand disease?

A lack of or abnormality in von Willebrand factor

What is the function of von Willebrand factor?

Von Willebrand factor is a glycoprotein complex that associates with and stabilizes factor VIII, enhances platelet aggregation, and contributes to the ability of platelets to attach to injured endothelium.

What are the components of factor VIII?

Factor VIII is a multimer composed of factor VIII-related cofactor, factor VIII-related antigen, and factor VIII-coagulant protein (VIIIc).

What is the incidence of von Willebrand disease?

Affects 1/10,000 individuals

How is the disease inherited?

As an autosomal dominant trait

What are the symptoms?

Easy bruising, easy bleeding, gingival bleeding, and epistaxis; abnormal menstrual bleeding

How is the disease diagnosed?

Bleeding time: prolonged
PTT: occasionally increased
Factor VIII levels: decreased
Platelet count: normal
Factor VIII cofactor: qualitatively or quantitatively deficient

What is the function of factor VIII-related cofactor?

Necessary for platelet adherence to the endothelium

How does von Willebrand disease affect pregnancy?

Patients have an increased incidence of postpartum hemorrhage related to concentration of factor VIIIc (problems arise if factor VIIIc value is < 50% of normal).

What is the effect of pregnancy on women with von Willebrand disease?

Clotting factors normally increase in pregnancy and thus bleeding time usually improves. Labor and delivery often proceed uneventfully because factor VIII levels usually increase to hemostatic levels beginning at 11 to 12 weeks.

What is the management?

Avoidance of episiotomies, deep injection of local anesthetic, and conduction anesthesia

Infusions of factor VIII–containing preparations if a patient has inadequate hemostasis

Transfusion with cryoprecipitate (rich in factor VIII) or fibrinogen if the concentration of factor VIIIc is below 50% at term

1-desamino-8-D-arginine vasopressin (ddavp) for patients with von Willebrand disease who have decreased levels of normal circulating factor (quantitative deficiency)

What are the considerations for caesarean section?

Factor VIIIc levels should be 80% of normal and the bleeding time should be in the normal range.

Why does the risk of delayed postpartum hemorrhage exist?

Postpartum, factor VIII levels fall to pre-pregnancy levels after 48 to 72 hours.

What are the considerations for the newborn?

Assume the newborn has von Willebrand disease; circumcisions should be performed only after exclusion of disease.

What are the risks associated with cryoprecipitate infusion?

Cryoprecipitate is pooled from several donors and therefore places the patient at a higher risk for transfusion-related infection.

THROMBOCYTOPENIA OF PREGNANCY

What is the definition of thrombocytopenia?

Platelet count less than 150,000

What is the incidence of thrombocytopenia during pregnancy?

Occurs in 7–8% of pregnancies

GESTATIONAL THROMBOCYTOPENIA

What is the most common cause?

Represents 2/3 cases of thrombocytopenia during pregnancy

Most women are asymptomatic, usually an incidental finding on CBC

Platelets rarely fall <70,000

Usually manifests during the 3rd trimester

What are the other causes of thrombocytopenia during pregnancy?

HELLP Syndrome

HIV infection

ITP

TTP

Lupus

Hemolytic uremic syndrome

Antiphospholipid syndrome

Congenital thrombocytopenia

Hypersplenism

Medications (heparin, quinine, zidovudine, sulfonamides)

DIC

Is there a risk to the fetus with gestational thrombocytopenia?

Extremely low risk of fetal or neonatal thrombocytopenia

What is the etiology of gestational thrombocytopenia?

May be due to accelerated platelet consumption

How is gestational thrombocytopenia differentiated from ITP?

Repeat platelet counts every 1–2 months to evaluate for falling levels

Platelet levels less than 70,000 should increase concern for ITP

With gestational thrombocytopenia, platelet levels will return to normal after delivery

ITP

What is ITP?	An autoimmune disease leading to thrombocytopenia
What is the pathophysiology?	Production of IgG antiplatelet antibodies leading to peripheral destruction and sequestration of platelets by the reticuloendothelial system
What are the symptoms?	Epistaxis, gingival bleeding, ecchymoses which precedes pregnancy Some females are completely asymptomatic Abnormal skin and mucous membrane bleeding usually occurs with platelet counts <100,000 Spontaneous bleeding occurs with platelet counts <20,000
How is the disease diagnosed?	Demonstration of IgG platelet associated antibody *Presence of anti-platelet antibodies is not diagnostic for ITP. They may be present with gestational thrombocytopenia* Platelet count usually between 75,000–150,000 Peripheral smear with megathrombocytes Coagulation tests normal Bleeding and MG increased if count is <50,000
What is the incidence?	1–2/1,000 pregnancies
What is the effect of ITP on pregnancy?	Increased incidence of spontaneous abortion Increased incidence of postpartum hemorrhage (usually associated with genital tract injury)

What is the effect of ITP on the infant?

Depression of fetal platelet count due to transplacental passage of anti platelet antibodies (IgG)

Rare incidence of intracranial hemorrhage which appears to be unrelated to mode of delivery

70% of infants born to mothers with ITP will develop thrombocytopenia—usually mild—peaks 4–6 weeks after delivery and gradually corrects within 2–3 months

How does maternal platelet count relate to fetal platelet count?

No reliable relationship

What is the effect of pregnancy on ITP?

No effect

What is the management?

Avoidance of trauma and salicylates (which impair platelet function)

Initiation of corticosteroids (Prednisone) when platelet counts <50,000

A favorable response is seen with a rise in platelet count in 7–21 days

Dose is tapered to minimum dose able to achieve a stable platelet count

Hospitalization and intravenous glucocorticoid therapy if patient has a bleeding diathesis or if platelet counts are <20,000

Consider plasma exchange for refractory or complicated cases

Platelet transfusions are of little benefit because the transfused platelets are destroyed 1–4 hours after infusion

Does therapy affect circulating antiplatelet antibodies that cross the placenta?

No, medications are poorly transmitted across the placenta

What is the benefit of splenectomy?

Produces remission in 70–80% of patients

If performed prior to pregnancy there is a decreased incidence and severity of complications during pregnancy

If performed during pregnancy (due to refractory case or hemorrhage), fetal mortality rate may be as high as 30%

Should fetal platelet counts be obtained?	No, due to low risk of intracranial hemorrhage (<1%) and lack of difference in outcome with vaginal delivery vs. cesarean delivery
Can patients with ITP breast feed?	It is not recommended due to possible transmission of antiplatelet antibodies through breast milk
What is the rationale for using steroids for management of ITP in pregnancy?	Steroids increase the platelet count by increasing production decreasing antiplatelet antibody production, binding and antibody-coated destruction

NEONATAL ALLOIMMUNE THROMBOCYTOPENIA

What is the etiology?	Maternal alloimmunization to fetal platelet antigens
What is the incidence?	1/1,000–2,000 live births
How does this differ from Rh disease?	It can occur during 1st pregnancy Almost one half of clinically evident cases are discovered in first live born infant Neonates are born with evidence of profound thrombocytopenia such as generalized petechiae or ecchymosis
What is a serious complication of this disease?	Intracranial hemorrhage Occurs in 10–20% of infants Can occur in utero and be diagnosed during fetal ultrasound
How does the management differ from ITP?	Recommend fetal platelet sampling If <50,000, cesarean delivery is preferred over vaginal delivery

What is the recurrence risk with future pregnancies?   Approaches 100%

What is the mother's platelet count?   Normal

13

Post-term Pregnancy

What is post-term pregnancy?

Gestation of 42 completed weeks (294 days) or more (from the first day of the LMP)

What is the incidence?

Occurs in 3% to 12% of all pregnancies

Why is correct dating of pregnancy important in evaluating for post-term pregnancy?

Incorrect determination of gestational age may lead to the misdiagnosis of a normal pregnancy as post-term.

What are common errors that are made in dating a pregnancy?

Inaccurate history of the last menstrual period (LMP)
Inaccurate estimation of ovulation (prolonged follicular phase)

What are the etiologic factors?

The cause of a post-term pregnancy usually cannot be found.
Rare conditions that may predispose patients to prolonged gestation include:
Anencephaly
Fetal adrenal hypoplasia
Absence of the fetal pituitary
Placental sulfatase deficiency
Extrauterine pregnancy
Obesity: Women who are obese at conception may have as much as a 50% increase in the frequency of post-term pregnancy over that of the general population.
Excessive weight gain during pregnancy: Weight gain has also been found to be an independent factor for post-term pregnancy that compounds the effect of pre-pregnancy obesity.

What are the maternal complications?

Consist mainly of maternal discomfort, anxiety, increased expense, and risk of antenatal testing

Increased induction and cesarean section rate, with the attendant risks

For what complication are most cesarean deliveries performed in post-term pregnancies?

Fetal distress

What is the increase in the rate of cesarean deliveries?

May be fourfold over non–post-term pregnancies

What is the increase in the rate of fetal complications?

Two- to threefold increase in neonatal/perinatal morbidity rate

Name the four main factors that contribute to neonatal/perinatal morbidity.

Oligohydramnios, macrosmia, passage of meconium, dysmaturity

What is oligohydramnios?

Loss of amniotic fluid volume (AFV)

May lead to cord compression, which can cause both acute and chronic fetal hypoxia and sudden death

Peak AFV (mean = 1000 [ml]) occurs at 37 weeks; AFV declines after 37 weeks.

The mean volume at term is 800 ml; at 42 weeks, 250 ml.

What is macrosomia?

Fetal weight in excess of 4,000 g (8 lbs, 13 oz)

Fetuses grow at a rate of 224 g (or about 0.5 lb) per week for the last 4 weeks at term.

Occurs due to prolonged gestation with continued nutrition and resultant increased fetal growth.

Associated with an increased risk of shoulder dystocia or other birth trauma and a high cesarean section rate

What is passage of meconium?

It is thought to occur with maturation of innervation of the gastrointestinal tract or the presence of a fetal stressor.

Increased incidence with increasing gestational age:

Rare prior to 32 weeks

Occurs in 10% to 15% of normal term pregnancies

Occurs in 25% to 30% of pregnancies at 42 weeks

The presence of meconium with oligohydramnios may result in meconium of increased viscosity, which increases the risk of aspiration pneumonia should aspiration occur.

What is dysmaturity?

Abnormal maturation in neonates associated with a characteristic appearance and increased morbidity and mortality rates

Classically described as a loss of vernix, peeling skin, loss of subcutaneous fat, long fingernails, thin abdominal girth, and an "old man" appearance, often with meconium staining of skin, nails, and placenta

Thought to result from placental insufficiency because area available for exchange of nutrients begins to decrease from a maximum of 11 m^2 at 37 weeks

What is the difference between macrosomia and dysmaturity?

Placental compromise does not occur in macrosomia; therefore, the fetus continues to grow.

What is the antepartum management?

Induction of labor between 42 and 44 weeks, regardless of cervical condition; most experts agree that at 42 weeks, if the patient is found to have a favorable cervix, induction should be recommended.

Trial of cervical ripening agents and/or antepartum testing if the cervix is unfavorable at 42 weeks

If at any time antepartum test results are abnormal, labor should be induced.

If the cervix ripens during this period, labor should be induced.

Some authorities begin screening earlier than 42 weeks.

What does antepartum testing involve?

Twice-weekly fetal surveillance by either nonstress test (NST) or contraction stress test (CST) combined with determination of AFV using the Amniotic fluid index (AFI)

May also include several other tests (e.g., fetal kick counts, biophysical profile, placental grade, Doppler flow studies)

Fetal kick count is a simple screening tool that can be instituted early and done at home on a daily basis. The mother is instructed to lie on her left side for 1 hour three times a day after meals. If she notices decreased fetal movement (usually described as fewer than 4–5 kicks per hour), further evaluation is necessary.

AFI uses ultrasound to measure the vertical height of the largest amniotic fluid pocket in each of four quadrants. A value of 5 to 20 cm is considered adequate.

Biophysical profile measures five indices, including AFV, fetal tone, fetal body and respiratory movement, and NST.

Placental grade (0, 1, 2, or 3) is an assessment of placental maturity based on ultrasonographic changes in the chorionic plate, placental substance, and basal layer.

Grading cannot predict the likelihood of postmaturity syndrome, but correlates generally with gestational age, and may be of some value in the management of delivery when combined with placental thickness and other clinical variables.

Doppler flow studies of the umbilical artery have not been shown to add any useful information in evaluating post-term pregnancy in the absence of other complicating factors, such as hypertension.

What are the risks associated with cervical ripening agents?

Prostaglandin E_2 and dilapan laminaria risks include rupture of membranes, infection, bleeding, and allergic reaction including anaphylaxis.

What is the intrapartum management?

Close monitoring of fetal heart rate (FHR) and uterine contractions to monitor for variable decelerations that indicate umbilical cord compression

Amnioinfusion (i.e., infusion of saline into the amniotic sac of a patient with oligohydramnios)

Placement of a fetal scalp electrode and intrauterine pressure catheter after rupture of membranes to allow more accurate measurement of uterine contractions and FHR

Evaluation of amniotic fluid for meconium following membrane rupture; if present, evaluation of meconium viscosity

Presence of meconium: suctioning of the infant's oropharynx when the head is delivered and before the thorax is delivered to reduce the risk of aspiration pneumonia should aspiration occur

Consideration of macrosomia (especially with a prolonged second stage of labor) and shoulder dystocia in vaginal delivery

Avoidance of oxytocin overstimulation, because umbilical cord compression may occur secondary to decreased AFV

What is the rationale for amnioinfusion for intrapartum management of a post-term pregnancy?

May reduce cesarean section rate for fetal distress

May improve infant outcome by increasing AFV and thereby decreasing the risk of umbilical cord compression and meconium aspiration syndrome

14

Multiple Gestation

What is the incidence of multiple gestation?	Occurs in 3% of all pregnancies
List, define, and state the incidence of the two types of twin pregnancies.	Dizygotic (also called fraternal) pregnancy results from the fertilization of two ova; comprises two-thirds of twin pregnancies. Monozygotic (also called identical) pregnancy results from the fertilization of one ovum and then cleavage; comprises one-third of twin pregnancies.
What factors influence the incidence of dizygotic twinning?	Race (African Americans > whites) Parity (increased incidence with increased parity) Age (increases with maternal age up to 37 years). Maternal size (increased incidence in larger women) Family history Fertility drugs including clomiphene citrate (Clomid®, 5%–10%) and menotropins (Pergonal®, 20%–40%)
What factors influence the incidence of monozygotic twinning?	Incidence is constant at 1/250. However, fertility drugs may increase the incidence. Largely independent of race, heredity, age, & parity. It is thought that delayed transport of the egg through the tube may increase M2 twinning. Progestational agents & combination OCPs decrease tubal motility & there is an increase in twinning if conception occurs in close proximity to OCP use.
What types of placentas exist in twin pregnancies and how is the type determined?	In dizygotic twins: The placental type is always dichorionic–diamniotic. In monozygotic twins: Type of placenta depends on the timing of embryo cleavage.

Table 14–1

Fertilization	4 days	8 days	13 days
Dichorionic Diamniotic (30%)	Monochorionic Diamniotic (70%)	Monochorionic Monoamniotic (1%)	Conjoined twins (1/600)

How are twins usually diagnosed?	Ninety-five percent of twin pregnancies are diagnosed prior to the onset of labor. History: Use of fertility drugs Family history (if mother herself is a twin, incidence is 1/60) Rapid weight gain Physical exam: Large uterine size for gestational age Identification of two fetal heart tones Visualization via ultrasound Laboratory data: Possibly elevated MSAFP
What are the complications?	Increased mortality rate: Perinatal mortality rate is 6% to 12%, five to ten times higher than singletons Prematurity is the largest contributor to mortality. Twins with a monochorionic placenta have two to three times higher mortality rate than dichorionic twins because of: 1. Twin–twin transfusion syndrome 2. Cord accidents (occur in up to 50% of monoamniotic twins) 3. Conjoined twins (occur in 1/60,000 live births) Single fetal death in utero occurs in approximately 1% to 5% of twin pregnancies. Preterm Delivery: It is the number one contributor to perinatal mortality.

Fifty percent of twins deliver before 36 weeks.

Ten percent of all preterm deliveries are multiple gestations.

Low birth weight: Fifty percent of twin infants have weights less than 2500 grams.

Prematurity

Intrauterine growth retardation (IUGR): may occur in up to 40% of twins

Discordant growth:

Estimated fetal weight (EFW) difference is 25%.

Discordant growth causes IUGR of one twin or macrosomia of the other twin.

Twin–twin transfusion syndrome (TTTS) results from the shunting of blood through arteriovenous communications within the placenta.

1. Occurs in monochorionic diamniotic twins, 5% to 10% overall

2. Donor twin is small, anemic, and may have oligohydramnios.

3. Recipient twin is large, polycythemic, and may have polyhydramnios.

4. Mortality rate is greater than 50%.

Pregnancy-induced hypertension:

Risk is twice as high as with singleton pregnancy, or 12% to 16%.

It may be more severe with earlier onset.

Malformations:

Risk is increased two to three times compared to singletons.

Both twins are affected in less than 20% of cases.

Anomalies associated with twinning include conjoined twins, TTTS.

Placenta previa/abruptio: slightly more common

Cord accidents: Entanglement may occur in 50% of monoamniotic twins.

Operative delivery:
Malpresentation occurs in almost 20% of twin pregnancies.
Cord prolapse
Postpartum hemorrhage

What is the mortality rate for triplets?

Fifteen to thirty percent

At what average gestational age are triplets delivered?

Thirty-three to thirty-five weeks

What is the management?

Early detection and frequent visits:
Ultrasound reduces missed diagnoses to less than 5%; visits should include education and screening for preterm labor.
Ultrasound:
To determine gestational age, evaluate anatomy, determine chorionicity
To assess serial growth and amniotic fluid volume (AFV) every 4 weeks
To confirm fetal presentations prior to delivery
Transvaginal U/S to evaluate shortening cervical length can help predict who is at increased risk for preterm delivery.
Bed rest/Hospitalization:
May help prevent preterm delivery; controversial
Hospitalization is not cost-effective.
Prophylactic cerclage: useful in cases of incompetent cervix only
Tocolysis:
Its use prophylactically is not generally supported.
Use is similar to preterm labor in singleton pregnancies.

How is the delivery of twins different from singleton deliveries?

Average gestational age for twins is 37 weeks.
Delivery must be performed when cesarean section can be expedited.

Continuous fetal heart surveillance is mandatory.

Mode of delivery depends on presentation of twins:

Vertex–vertex presentation (42%): Vaginal delivery

Nonvertex presentation (20%): Cesarean section

Breech–vertex presentation carries risk of heads interlocking.

Vertex–nonvertex presentation (35%): Controversial

1. Deliver vertex twin vaginally.
2. Turn nonvertex twin to vertex; then deliver vaginally.
3. Vaginal breech delivery of second twin when:

   • Standard criteria are met for vaginal delivery
   • Second twin is of similar size

4. Breech extraction
5. Cesarean section of both twins

15   Hypertensive Disorders in Pregnancy

PREGNANCY-INDUCED HYPERTENSION

How is hypertension categorized in pregnancy?

Gestational Hypertention:
Elevated BP without proteinuria developing after 20 weeks' gestation and returning to normal post partum
Preeclampsia:
Hypertension developing after 20 weeks' gestation (140/90) and associated with at least 0/3 q of proteinuria in a 24-hour collection
Chronic Hypertension:
Hypertension anteceding and succeeding pregnancy. It can be aggravated by pregnancy. It is usually essential hypertension

PREECLAMPSIA

What is preeclampsia?

An idiopathic disease exclusive to pregnancy, characterized by hypertension, proteinuria, and edema
Blood pressure > 140/90 mm Hg; this elevation must be present on two measurements at least 6 hours apart while patient is resting.
Proteinuria is defined as ≥ 300 mg or more of urinary protein per 24 hours, or ≥ 100 mg/dl.

What are the two classifications of preeclampsia?

Mild preeclampsia:
Blood pressure ranges from 140/90 to 160/110 mm Hg.
Proteinuria < 5 g/24 hrs
Edema of face, hands, and feet
Severe preeclampsia
Blood pressure > 160/110 mm Hg

Proteinuria > 5 g per 24 hours
Oliguria < 400 ml in 24 hours
Cerebral or visual disturbances
Epigastric pain or, more specifically,
    right upper quadrant (RUQ) pain
    that may indicate liver involvement
Pulmonary edema
Hepatocellular dysfunction
Thrombocytopenia
Intrauterine growth restriction
    (IUGR)
Elevated serum creatinine
Microangiopathic hemolysis

What is the epidemiology of preeclampsia?

Unique to human primates; does not
    occur in subhuman primates
Occurs in 6%–8% of pregnancies
Incidence is affected by parity.
    More common in nulliparous women
        (incidence of 14%–20% in
        primigravidas compared to 6%–7%
        in multiparas)
    Associated in multiparous women with
        multiple gestations, fetal hydrops,
        and coexisting vascular or renal
        disease such as diabetes mellitus, or
        when the paternity of current
        pregnancy is different from that of
        previous pregnancies
    Affects women at either end of
        reproductive age range
    Onset typically after 20 weeks'
        gestation
    Appears to be inherited and occurs
        more commonly in families with
        history of hypertension
    More common in patients with
        essential hypertension
    Occurs more frequently in
        pregnancies involving multiple
        gestations, in polyhydramnios, and
        with the occurrence of a
        hydatidiform mole

Second to embolism as most common cause of maternal mortality in the United States, accounting for 15% of maternal deaths

Major cause of perinatal morbidity and mortality in the United States

What are the possible etiologies of preeclampsia?

Possibilities include:
Immunologic phenomena
Genetic predisposition
Dietary deficiencies or excesses (specifically calcium)
Vascular reactivity changes
    Renin–angiotensin–aldosterone system
    Prostaglandins
    Autonomic nervous system
    Calcium
    Endothelial cell function
Abnormal trophoblast invasion
Cardiovascular maladaptation
Coagulation abnormalities

What is the pathophysiology of preeclampsia?

The major feature is the generalized occurrence of arteriolar constriction leading to significantly elevated systemic vascular resistance. Associated changes include:

Uterine vascular changes: Endothelial injury, ranging from swelling to erosion in placental and nonplacental sites

Hemodynamic changes:
    Myocardial contractility rarely impaired; ventricular function normal
    Changes that do occur include elevation of afterload, decreased cardiac output, increased vascular resistance, reduced ventricular preload, and reduced total blood volume.

Hematologic changes:

> The primary hematologic change is hemoconcentration; the plasma volume contracts during decreased regional perfusion.

> Other changes include thrombocytopenia; decreased clotting factors; and red blood cell destruction characterized by hemolysis.

Endocrine and metabolic changes:

> During pregnancy, plasma levels of renin, angiotensin II, and aldosterone increase. In preeclampsia, these levels often return toward prepregnancy range.

> Increase in levels of antidiuretic hormone and atrial natriuretic factor

Fluid and electrolyte changes:

> Extracellular volume increases as a result of increased capillary permeability.

> In eclampsia, bicarbonate levels decrease owing to lactic acidosis and compensatory respiratory alkalosis.

Renal changes:

> During pregnancy, renal blood flow and glomerular filtration rate (GFR) increase. In preeclampsia, these factors are reduced toward nonpregnant levels.

> Other changes include sodium retention, increased plasma creatinine, increased uric acid, decreased urinary excretion of calcium, increased permeability to large–molecular-weight proteins leading to proteinuria, and endothelial damage to renal vasculature.

Hepatic changes:
　　HELLP occurs in 10% of women with severe preeclampsia.
　　Serum transaminase levels increase.
　　Hepatic rupture is possible but rare, requires surgical intervention, and is associated with a high (70%) mortality rate.
Uteroplacental perfusion: Vasospasm causes compromised placental perfusion and can result in poor fetal growth or even death.
Central nervous system (CNS):
　　Headaches and visual disturbances (blurred vision and scotomata) occur because of retinal artery spasm. Retinal detachment occurs rarely.
　　Reflexes can become hyperactive.
　　CNS signs and symptoms may indicate a high risk of seizure.

What are the signs and symptoms of preeclampsia?

Elevation of blood pressure
Proteinuria, which may follow hypertension
Excessive weight gain from extravascular fluid accumulation and edema
Dyspnea: May result from pulmonary edema secondary to cardiac failure (rare) or volume overload (more common)
Abdominal pain/tenderness: RUQ or epigastric pain may indicate hepatic subcapsular swelling from edema (common) or hematoma (rare); hepatic rupture is rare but can occur.

On what is the diagnosis of preeclampsia based?

Demonstration of hypertension, proteinuria, and edema

What laboratory evaluations are appropriate after a diagnosis of preeclampsia?

Hematocrit
Platelets
Blood urea nitrogen
Creatinine

Carbon dioxide
Uric acid level
Transaminase levels to test for liver
    damage
Total protein
Albumin
24-Hour urine protein
Protime and bilirubin to test for liver
    function
Nonstress test (NST)
Ultrasonography to evaluate growth and
    amniotic fluid level

**What is important to
remember about the
alkaline phosphatase level?**

It is increased in pregnancy owing to
placental production.

**What are the sequelae of
preeclampsia?**

Pulmonary edema
Hepatic hemorrhage, infarction, or
    necrosis
Intracerebral hemorrhage
Abruptio placentae
HELLP syndrome (see p. 141)
Acute renal failure
Shock
Ventricular arrhythmias
IUGR/Intrauterine fetal demise (IUFD)

**How is preeclampsia
managed?**

The only definitive treatment is delivery.
Other objectives of therapy include
seizure prevention with anticonvulsant
agents, delivery of an infant that
subsequently thrives, and restoration of
maternal health.

**How is mild preeclampsia
managed?**

Hospitalization, including bed rest,
    frequent monitoring of vital signs and
    fetal monitoring by NST, as indicated
At less than 37 weeks, continued
    maternal and fetal observation with
    seizure prophylaxis
Past 37 weeks, begin seizure prophylaxis
    and induction of labor

How is severe preeclampsia managed?

Consideration of prompt delivery is warranted, regardless of fetal age. Some forms of severe illness may not indicate delivery when the fetus is very immature.

When immediate delivery is not performed, monitoring for organ system impairment, as previously outlined, must be continued.

Vaginal delivery is preferable. Labor induction using IV oxytocin can be attempted and cesarean section can be reserved for those patients in which it fails.

Seizure prophylaxis should be instituted immediately using anticonvulsant medication. Antihypertensive medications should be used if DBP rises above 110 mmHg. Intake and output should be closely monitored.

What is the appropriate pharmacologic management of preeclampsia?

Anticonvulsant medication:

Seizure prophylaxis should be instituted in all preeclamptics during labor and delivery and should be continued for 48 hours after delivery.

Magnesium sulfate is the agent of choice. It can be initiated at 8 g/hour for the first hour, reduced to 4 g/hour for the second hour, and then maintained at 2 g/hour with a controlled infusion device. In patients with normal urine output, the level of magnesium in this protocol is predictable and does not require checking.

Monitoring of deep tendon reflexes (DTR), which should be present, can be followed to prevent toxic levels of this medication.

Therapeutic levels = 8 mg/dl. The following occur at the indicated blood magnesium levels:

Loss of DTR: 10 mg/dl
Respiratory suppression: 15 mg/dl
Cardiac arrest: > 25 mg/dl
For overdose, treat with 1 g calcium gluconate IV push.

Antihypertensive medication:

Indicated for systolic blood pressure > 170 mm Hg or diastolic blood pressure > 110 mm Hg to decrease risk of intracranial or hepatic hemorrhage and abruptio placentae

Acute control of high blood pressure may be achieved with IV labetalol 5–15 mg slow push every 10 minutes, not to exceed a dose of 300 mg/day.

Alternative medications include hydralazine 5–10 mg every 20–30 minutes as needed, and nifedipine 10 mg sublingually repeated after 30 minutes.

For refractory hypertension, sodium nitroprusside 0.5–3 U/kg/minute in a controlled infusion may be given, but not to exceed 800 U/kg/minute.

HELLP SYNDROME

What is HELLP syndrome?

A syndrome of **H**emolysis, **E**levated **L**iver enzymes, and **L**ow **P**latelet count

A distinct subset of preeclampsia that occurs in 2%–12% of preeclampsia patients

Can occur without associated hypertension or proteinuria

Can occur antepartum or postpartum, usually within 48 hours; 30% of cases occur after delivery

What are its signs and symptoms?

Nausea
Vomiting
Malaise

Headache

Epigastric or RUQ pain

What are its differential diagnoses?

Gastritis

Hepatitis

Reflux

Cholecystitis

Pyelonephritis

Appendicitis

Thrombotic thrombocytopenic purpura

Immune thrombocytopenic purpura

Acute fatty liver of pregnancy

What are the etiologic factors of HELLP syndrome?

Unclear; clinical and pathologic manifestations result from an insult that leads to intravascular platelet activation and microvascular endothelial injury.

What laboratory findings are associated with HELLP syndrome?

Hemolysis:

Abnormal peripheral smear

Increased bilirubin > 1.2 mg/dl

Increased lactate dehydrogenase (LDH) > 600 IU/ml

Elevated liver enzymes:

Increased LDH

Low platelet count: < 150 ($10^3/\mu$l)

What are the complications of HELLP syndrome?

Perinatal and maternal mortality rates are significant.

Maternal morbidity includes complications from coagulopathy and liver disease

What is the treatment of HELLP syndrome?

Delivery

If immediate delivery is not feasible because of fetal immaturity and the aberrations are mild, steroids can be given to promote better neonatal performance. Steroids may temporarily reverse some of the laboratory findings.

Patients must be followed closely while being managed before delivery.

Rapid delivery is mandated by fetal instability; vaginal delivery is preferred, but C/S is not contraindicated.

Maternal condition should be assessed and stabilized, particularly coagulation abnormalities. Although seldom necessary, frozen plasma may be required to correct coagulation abnormalities.

Seizure prophylaxis with magnesium sulfate should be given.

ECLAMPSIA

What is eclampsia?

The occurrence of convulsions or coma, unrelated to other cerebral conditions, with signs and symptoms of preeclampsia

What is its incidence?

About 1 in every 1000 deliveries

What are the signs and symptoms of eclampsia?

Wide spectrum of signs and symptoms

Gradual onset with weight gain of approximately 2 pounds or greater per week in the last trimester

Hypertension: Hallmark; usually associated with significant proteinuria (> +2).

Seizures: Headache with visual disturbances may herald seizures.

What form of seizure occurs in eclampsia?

Tonic–clonic type (grand mal)

What is the onset of eclamptic seizures?

Can occur antepartum, intrapartum, or postpartum

Nearly all postpartum cases develop within 24 to 48 hours of delivery. Other diagnoses should be considered with onset of seizures after 48 hours postpartum.

Almost without exception, preeclampsia precedes onset of eclamptic seizures.

What is the epidemiology of eclampsia?

Primarily affects young primigravidas, but incidence is also increased in women older than 35 years of age.

Highest incidence occurs in low-income, nonwhite primigravidas.

What are the morbid sequelae of eclampsia?

Maternal:
　　Continued seizure activity despite appropriate magnesium sulfate therapy
　　Aspiration pneumonitis
　　Azotemia requiring dialysis
　　Sublethal intracranial hemorrhage resulting in hemiplegias
　　Massive intercerebral hemorrhage causing sudden death
　　Lactic acidosis
　　Blindness secondary to retinal detachment
Perinatal:
　　Abruptio placentae
　　Prematurity
　　IUGR
　　Hypoxic episodes during convulsions
　　Fetal death

What factors increase the risk for maternal death?

Early onset of preeclampsia in gestation (< 28 weeks)
Increased maternal age
Multiple gestations

What is the treatment of eclampsia?

Continuous intensive monitoring of mother and fetus
Large-bore IV access
Magnesium sulfate administration to control convulsions as previously outlined
Labetalol or hydralazine to control severe hypertension as previously outlined

Prevention of maternal injury during seizures

Maintenance of adequate airway and oxygenation; measures to minimize risk of aspiration

Correction of maternal acidemia

Delivery by induction of labor or C/S

Delivery should be attempted after seizures are controlled.

Some authorities recommend reevaluation of the patient after adequate anticonvulsant therapy is established to decide the necessity of delivery.

CHRONIC HYPERTENSION

What is chronic hypertension?

Hypertension present before pregnancy or diagnosed before 20 weeks' gestation

Hypertension that persists beyond 42 days after delivery

What is the etiology of chronic hypertension?

Primary hypertension:
  Also called essential or idiopathic hypertension
  Cause unknown
  Accounts for 90% of all cases of hypertension
Secondary hypertension:
  Renal hypertension (5%)
  Renal parenchymal disease (3%)
    Chronic pyelonephritis
    Acute/chronic glomerulonephritis
    Polycystic kidney disease
    Diabetic nephropathy
    Renin-producing tumors
    Renovascular disease
    Renal vascular stenosis
    Renal vascular infarction
  Endocrine hypertension (4%–5%)
    Oral contraceptive usage (4%)
    Primary aldosteronism (0.5%)

Aldosterone-secreting tumor
Pheochromocytoma (0.2%)
Cushing syndrome (0.2%)
Acromegaly
Hypercalcemia
Thyrotoxicosis
Miscellaneous
  Acute spinal cord accident
  Coarctation of the aorta
  Acute intermittent porphyria
  Drugs (alcohol)
Heredity: African-American race, male sex, and strong family history increase risk for development of hypertension.
Environmental factors such as obesity, high-stress occupations, smoking, and so forth play a role in etiology.

What are the target organs of chronic hypertension?

The major feature in hypertension is increased total vascular resistance, which in turn affects many organ systems:
Cardiac:
  Increased vascular resistance causes need for increased stroke volume, which in turn may cause left ventricular hypertrophy leading to CHF.
  Hypertension may lead to increased risk of myocardial infarction or CHF.
Retinal: Arterial hemorrhage, appearance of exudates, or papilledema may lead to blurred vision, scotomata, retinal detachment, and blindness.
CNS:
  The most serious neurologic complication is vascular occlusion leading to infarct and stroke.
  Other CNS complications include increased risk for arterial intracerebral hemorrhage and encephalopathy.

Renal: Arteriosclerotic lesions resulting from the damaging effects of hypertensive disease affect the afferent and efferent arterioles within the kidney, leading to decreased GFR and tubular dysfunction; renal failure is the ultimate result.

(Note: Because hypertension is a heterogenous disease, multiple factors affect its course. Eventually all hypertension results in end organ damage. Cardiomegaly, CHF, retinopathy, pulmonary edema, renal insufficiency are all possible. If left untreated, this disease is lethal.)

What are the complications of chronic hypertension in pregnancy?

Abruptio placentae
IUGR
IUFD
Increased risk of superimposed preeclampsia

What is the management of chronic hypertension in pregnancy?

Early prenatal care
Evaluation of the degree of hypertension
Adequate estimation of the severity of the individual's disease at initial visit
Education and appropriate counseling about potential risks that pregnancy imposes on the mother's medical condition, risks her disease imposes on her pregnancy, and the risks versus benefits of hypertensive medications during pregnancy
Close monitoring of prenatal course:
  Frequent follow-up should occur throughout prenatal course.
  In third trimester, fetus should be monitored with NST.
  At term, induction of delivery should be considered, if feasible; complications may dictate earlier intervention.

What are the important principles of pharmacologic management for chronic hypertension in pregnancy?

Patients with chronic hypertension who conceive while taking antihypertensive therapy may continue their medication if maintaining adequate control.

In general, studies have shown that mild to moderate hypertension does not require pharmacologic treatment in pregnancy. In patients with severe disease, however, pharmacologic therapy may reduce disease progression during pregnancy.

What is the pharmacologic management of chronic hypertension in pregnancy?

α-Methyldopa:

Remains a first-line agent in the United States, primarily because of its extensive use and well-documented fetal safety.

Initial dose is 1 g followed by a maintenance dose of 1–2 g/day.

Most common regimen is 250 mg three times a day or 500 mg four times a day.

Maximum dosage is 4 g/day.

Labetalol and atenolol (and other β-blockers):

β-Adrenergic blockers; labetalol hydrochloride has additional α_1 blocking capability.

Initial dose of labetalol is 100 mg by mouth twice daily, increased to a maximum dose of 300 mg twice daily or four times a day.

Initial dose of atenolol is 50 mg daily, increased to a maximum dose of 50 mg twice daily or 100 mg daily.

β-Blockers are contraindicated in asthmatic patients and should be used with caution in insulin-dependent diabetics because of their ability to mask symptoms of hypoglycemia.

Angiotensin-converting enzyme (ACE) inhibitors: CONTRAINDICATED IN PREGNANCY

ACE inhibitors have been associated with fetal hypocalvaria, fetal renal failure, oligohydramnios, IUGR, and fetal and neonatal death. These drugs induce vasodilatation by inhibiting the enzyme that converts angiotensin I to angiotensin II, and have been found to decrease uteroplacental blood flow in experiments with animals, leading to fetal death.

Thiazide diuretics:

Although often first-line medications in nonpregnant chronic hypertensives, they should probably not be initiated during pregnancy.

Commonly cause hypokalemia, hyponatremia, hyperglycemia, hypercalcemia, and elevated uric acid in the mother; a few cases of thrombocytopenia in fetuses have been reported.

Diuretics work by reducing both plasma and extracellular fluid volume, with a concomitant decrease in cardiac output, which theoretically could have adverse fetal effects.

PREGNANCY-AGGRAVATED HYPERTENSION

What is pregnancy-aggravated hypertension?

Superimposition of preeclampsia on chronic hypertensive disease during pregnancy; has a high perinatal morbidity and mortality rate

What are its signs and symptoms?

Typically manifests as a sudden rise in blood pressure that is almost always complicated by proteinuria

What is its progression?

Rapid progression of maternal hypertensive disease may occur.

What is its treatment?

It should be treated as preeclampsia.

16

Third Trimester Bleeding

INTRODUCTION

What is the definition of third trimester bleeding?

Any vaginal bleeding after 26 weeks' gestation

What are the most common causes of third trimester bleeding?

Vaginal—lacerations
Cervix—polyp, cervicitis, carcinoma
Intrauterine—Placenta previa (20%), placental abruption (30%), vasa previa
Preterm labor

How should third trimester bleeding be evaluated?

Take a history of:
-Abnormal PAP
-Coitus
-Pain
-Contractions
Monitor vital signs—maternal and fetal (fetal monitoring for decelerations)
Perform an **ultrasound** to determine placental location
Perform a sterile speculum exam to determine location and extent of bleeding, unless there is a placenta previa
Consider CBC and cross matching blood
Place an IV if indicated for fluid, drug, or drug administration or to deal with complications

PLACENTAL ABRUPTION

What is placental abruption?

Premature separation of a normally implanted placenta

What is the incidence of abruption?

1/200 deliveries

What is the perinatal

25%

mortality in placental abruption?

What risk factors are associated with abruption?	Prior abruption (risk of recurrence is 5%-15%; 25% with 2 prior abruptions) Hypertension Multiparity Smoking Cocaine use Trauma (direct and indirect) Rapid decompression of an overdistended uterus (multiple gestation, polyhydramniosis) Coagulation disorders
What is the etiology?	Hemorrhage into the decidua basalis leading to premature separation and further bleeding
How is the diagnosis of placental abruption made?	Clinical presentation Normal findings on **ultrasound** do not exclude this diagnosis
What is the usual clinical presentation of abruption?	Painful vaginal bleeding in the third trimester
What are 6 common symptoms associated with abruption?	Vaginal bleeding—extent of bleeding may vary Uterine contractions Abdominal pain Non-reassuring fetal status Hypertonic uterus Uterine tenderness
What maternal systemic complication is associated with abruption?	Consumptive coagulopathy
What is Couvelaire uterus?	Purplish or bluish appearance of uterus at time of cesarean delivery. It is caused by extravasation of blood into the uterine musculature and beneath the serosa.

What is always included in the management of abruption?	Resuscitation with crystalloid and transfusion of red cells sufficient to replace losses
What is the management of preterm abruption?	Expectant management, if mother and fetus are stable, can be considered in some circumstances
Management at term?	Prompt delivery [oxytocin (Pitocin) augmentation preferred to cesarean delivery unless there is evidence of fetal distress or hemodynamic instability]

PLACENTA PREVIA

What is the definition of placenta previa?	Abnormal location of the placenta over, or in close proximity to, the internal cervical os
What are the 4 types of placenta previa?	Total—covering entire cervical os Partial—margin of placenta extends across part of the os Marginal—edge of placenta lies adjacent to the os Low-lying placenta—located near but not directly adjacent to the internal os
What is the incidence of placenta previa?	1/250 deliveries
What is the etiology?	Abnormal vascularization leading to abnormal placement of the placenta
What are the risk factors associated with placenta previa?	Previous placenta previa Advancing maternal age Multiparity Prior cesarean delivery Uterine surgery (i.e., myomectomy) Smoking
How does placenta previa usually present?	Painless, bright red vaginal bleeding in the third trimester

What is the etiology of the bleeding?	Separation of part of the placenta from the lower uterine segment and cervix
What is the first episode of bleeding called?	*The Sentinel bleed*—usually ceases spontaneously but always recurs
What is the average gestational age at time of sentinel bleed?	29-30 weeks' gestation
How is the diagnosis of placenta previa made?	Ultrasound evaluation. **Do not perform digital exam** with vaginal bleeding until placental location is known!
What placental abnormality can be associated with placenta previa?	Placenta accreta—abnormal attachment of the placenta directly to the uterine muscle without intervening decidua. This condition, associated with 5%-10% of previas (but also occurring without previa), may lead to severe post partum hemorrhage. The incidence of placenta accreta is increased with a history of prior cesarean delivery.
What is always included in the management of placenta previa?	Initial hospitalization with hemodynamic stabilization
How is placenta previa managed preterm?	If bleeding ceases, expectant management until 37 weeks
How is it managed at term?	Cesarean delivery

VASA PREVIA

What is the definition of vasa previa?	Fetal vessels coursing through membranes and presenting at the cervical os
What is the common presentation of vasa previa?	A small amount of vaginal bleeding associated with significant fetal distress

**What test might confirm
this diagnosis?**

Apt test

Distinguishes between fetal and
maternal RBCs based on the marked
resistance to pH changes in fetal
RBCs

**What is the management
of vasa previa?**

Emergent cesarean delivery

17

Rh Isoimmunization and Blood Group Incompatibilities

How do maternal-fetal blood group incompatibilities produce disease?

Fetal erythrocyte antigens stimulate production of maternal antibodies which bind to fetal red blood cells, causing hemolysis and anemia.

What is hemolytic disease of the newborn?

The result of severe blood group incompatibility. Also known as erythroblastosis fetalis.

What are the characteristic symptoms?

Grave hemolytic anemia
Numerous erythroblasts in the fetal circulation
Generalized edema (hydrops fetalis)
Enlargement of the fetal liver and spleen in its most severe form

What is the most common antigen involved in serious blood group incompatibility?

The Rh-antigen. The Rhesus (Rh) blood group consists of three antigen pairs (Dd, Cd, and Ee), with Rh factor (RhO, the D antigen) being the most commonly involved in serious cases of fetal immune hemolytic anemia.

What are some other blood groups associated with blood group incompatibility?

D-antigen incompatibility and ABO group incompatibility, combined, account for 98% of all cases of hemolytic disease; but other blood groups (over 400 now identified) involved in incompatibility include:
Kell
Duffy
Kidd
MNSs
Diego
Lutheran

What is the incidence of blood group incompatibility-induced fetal hemolytic anemia?

Varies based on the prevalence of specific red cell antigens in different populations.

How does the prevalence of the D, or Rho, determinant of the CDE (Rhesus) blood group vary with race?

Asians express a 99% D-positive phenotype (either DD or Dd genotype)

African Americans are 92-93% D-positive

White Americans are 87% D-positive. The incidence of RH (D) incompatibilities is highest in white Americans due to the relatively higher percentage of the population who do not carry the D antigen on their red blood cells (hence, more Rh-negative mothers)

What role does the ABO group play in Rh isoimmunization?

Among D-positive fetuses, the risk of developing Rh isoimmunization is related to both the genetic makeup of the father (D-positive heterozygous or homozygous) and whether or not there is a simultaneous ABO-group incompatibility. For a known D-positive fetus with a known homozygous D-positive father, the risk of Rh isoimmunization in a D-negative mother is increased in fetuses with ABO-compatible blood groups (16% risk) versus ABO-incompatible blood groups (2% risk). ABO incompatibility decreases the number of fetal cells in maternal circulation available to stimulate maternal anti-D antibody production. The incidence of any single-antigen incompatibility which leads to production of anti-fetal-antigen antibodies is unknown, as many of these cases are probably mild and not clinically significant.

What role does the ABO group play in isoimmunization separate from Rh concerns?

While about 1 in 5 fetuses have an ABO group incompatibility, only 5% of these show evidence of hemolytic disease at birth, and this is usually manifest only as higher bilirubin and lower hemoglobin levels than unaffected infants.

What 5 factors determine the severity of hemolysis in blood group incompatibilities?

1. Antigenicity of the blood group
2. Maternal response to the antigen
3. Protection from isoimmunization by ABO incompatibilities
4. Quantity of fetal antigen passed from fetus to mother
5. Quantity of maternal antibody passed from mother to fetus

How do fetal cells gain access to the maternal circulation?

Disruption of the usually intact feto-maternal blood barrier (the placental villus) and leakage of fetal cells into the maternal bloodstream (leading to maternal antibody formation against non-self antigens on fetal red blood cells).

What mechanisms may cause this to occur?

Placenta previa
Placental abruption
Spontaneous or induced abortion
Amniocentesis
Trauma
Fetal death
Manual placental extraction
Cesarean section
Multiple pregnancy
Normal delivery

Which maternal immunoglobulin class causes fetal problems?

IgG antibodies

How do the problems occur?

Maternal IgG antibodies cross the placenta and hemolyze red blood cells (fetal red blood cell hemolysis from maternal antibody binding is the common pathway to all fetal and neonatal derangements in erythroblastosis fetalis and hydrops fetalis)

What are the effects of red cell hemolysis in the fetus?

Hyperbilirubinemia
Hemosiderin deposition in the liver
Bone marrow hyperplasia
Extramedullary hematopoiesis in the spleen and liver
Cardiac enlargement
Hepatomegaly
Splenomegaly
Pulmonary hemorrhages
Hydrops fetalis
Death

What is hydrops fetalis?

Hydrops fetalis is subcutaneous edema and effusions into serous cavities in the fetus.

How is it caused?

Not precisely known. Hypotheses include:
Cardiac origin from failure secondary to anemia
Vascular origin from leaky capillaries secondary to hypoxia
Hepatic origin from low oncotic pressure secondary to decreased protein synthesis

What is the incidence of stillbirths and hydrops fetalis with ABO group incompatibility?

In ABO blood group incompatibility the incidence of stillbirths is not increased and hydrops fetalis does not occur. Hemolytic disease does occur in fetuses with A, B, or AB blood types in mothers with blood group O, but is much milder than isoimmunization caused by Rho antigen and some others.

How are blood group incompatibilities diagnosed?

In the antepartum or postpartum period, the presence of clinically significant incompatibilities can be subtle or obvious depending on the severity of hemolytic disease (determined generally by the blood group involved).

On what evidence is the diagnosis based?

A clinically significant antibody in the maternal serum to an antigen not found on the maternal red blood cell (i.e., the presence of anti-Rh antibody in an Rh-negative woman's blood, given as an antibody titer correlating to the amount of antibody in the maternal blood)

Ultrasonographic evidence during the pregnancy may suggest fetal compromise from blood group incompatibility

Neonatal findings consistent with hemolytic disease may also confirm the diagnosis

What ultrasonographic findings suggest serious blood group incompatibility?

Subcutaneous edema with serous cavity effusions such as ascites and hydrothorax (*hydrops fetalis*, the hallmark of a severely affected fetus)

Cardiomegaly

Hepatomegaly

Splenomegaly

Abnormalities of Doppler flow velocity waveforms

Hydramnios

What neonatal or placental findings suggest hemolytic disease?

An edematous, pale infant at birth

Neonatal hepatomegaly

Neonatal splenomegaly

Neonatal hyperbilirubinemia

Neonatal anemia

Placental edema and enlargement

What has been the most significant advancement in the prevention of Rh disease?

The administration of anti-D immune IgG (RhoGam™,Rho (D) immunoglobulin, RhIg) to Rh-negative women. Given to Rh-negative women prophylactically at 28 weeks gestation, postpartum, and following events which may lead to fetomaternal hemorrhage in order to prevent maternal sensitization

What is the recommended dosage?

Women who are D-negative and nonimmunized should be given 300 μg of D-immunoglobulin at 28 weeks and following delivery (within 72 hours) of a D-positive infant. Implicit in the utilization of RhoGAM™ prophylactically is the testing of all women who present for prenatal care for blood group, Rh type (presence or absence of D antigen) and serum antibodies (via an indirect Coombs antibody screen test)

In addition to prophylactic administration and postpartum administration, in what other situations might RhoGAM™ be used?

After induced or spontaneous abortion (50 μg less than 13 weeks' gestation, 300 μg after 13 weeks)
Ectopic pregnancy (same dosing as for abortion)
Amniocentesis (standard, 300 μg dose)
Chorionic villus sampling (CVS)
Percutaneous umbilical blood sampling (PUBS)
External cephalic version
Any other case where feto-maternal hemorrhage is suspected

How can the extent of feto-maternal hemorrhage be determined if suspected?

If a large feto-maternal hemorrhage is suspected (e.g., massive trauma, fetal exsanguination), the quantity of fetal cells in the maternal circulation should be determined using the Kleihauer-Betke test and an appropriate (sufficient) dose of anti-D IgG given

What is the Kleihauer-Betke test?

The Kleihauer-Betke acid elution test detects and quantitates fetal red blood cells in the maternal circulation.

What is the severity of hemolytic disease

Treatment of hemolytic disease of the fetus or newborn is determined by the

associated with the common blood groups and how should each be managed?

severity of the disease. Management is guided by the maternal antibody type detected, which predicts the severity of disease and hence the aggressiveness of the intervention necessary

Generalizations can be made regarding the severity of disease and management for some specific blood group antigens as indicated in Table 17-1:

Table 17–1.

Blood Group	Antigen	Severity of Hemolytic Disease	Proposed Management
CDE (Rh)	D	Mild to severe/hydrops	Amnionic fluid studies
	C	Mild to moderate	Amnionic fluid studies
	C	Mild to severe	Amnionic fluid studies
	E	Mild to severe	Amnionic fluid studies
	E	Mild to moderate	Amnionic fluid studies
Lewis		Not a proven cause (IgM)	
Kell	K	Mild to severe/hydrops	Amnionic fluid studies
	K	Mild to severe	Amnionic fluid studies
Duffy	Fy^a	Mild to sever/hydrops	Amnionic fluid studies
	Fy^b	Not a cause	
Kidd	JK^a	Mild to severe	Amnionic fluid studies
	JK^b	Mild to severe	Amnionic fluid studies
MNSs	M	Mild to severe	Amnionic fluid studies
	N	Mild	Expectant
	S	Mild to severe	Amnionic fluid studies
	S	Mild to severe	Amnionic fluid studies
	U	Mild to severe	Amnionic fluid studies
Lutheran	LU^a	Mild	Expectant
	LU^b	Mild	Expectant

How can the severity of Lewis, Duffy, and Kell antibody detection be memorized?

"Lewis lives, Duffy dies, Kell kills"

Lewis antibody is the next most frequent antibody found on indirect Coombs testing other than D and is not a proven cause of hemolytic disease

Duffy antibody causes hydrops fetalis
Kell antibody is also associated with hydrops fetalis

What are the next steps in fetal evaluation after antibody titers are confirmed?

Ultrasound at 14–16 weeks to identify fetal ascites or edema and confirm gestational age
Titers should be followed every 2–4 weeks to evaluate for disease progression (titers less than 1:8 in an initial immunized pregnancy are generally associated with minimal fetal risk irrespective of the antigen)
Amniocentesis at 18–22 weeks to measure bilirubin, which correlates to the degree of hemolysis
Umbilical cord blood sampling can be used as a substitute for amniotic fluid assay. The fetal hemoglobin concentration can be directly measured.

What is the untreated mortality rate in Rh-sensitized pregnancies?

Sensitized D-negative women have a 30% perinatal mortality rate in an untreated pregnancy. Antibody titers are useful in determining prognosis:
With titers less than 1:8, it is unlikely that fetal death in utero will occur
Titers greater than 1:16, however, are considered clinically significant

How has treatment affected prognosis in isoimmunization?

Studies suggest that transfusion may sharply increase perinatal survival. For fetuses with disease severe enough to mandate transfusion in utero, studies at a major Canadian center indicate that fetal mortality rates after intraperitoneal transfusion have decreased from 55% in 1964 to 8% in 1988. Perinatal survival in a large North American study of intravascular transfusion was 86% (82% for hydropic fetuses and 90% for non-hydropic fetuses)

What problems may be associated with umbilical blood sampling?

Increased fetal loss compared to amniocentesis

Anamnestic immune response in mother secondary to fetal-maternal hemorrhage

What is the Liley curve and how is it useful?

The Liley curve is a graph which plots the ΔOD_{450} (a measurement of the change in optical density above baseline at 450 nm wavelength, reflective of the concentration of amnionic fluid bilirubin and red blood cell breakdown products, and hence the intensity of hemolytic disease), the y-axis, against the estimated gestational age in weeks, the x-axis. By determining the ΔOD_{450} at a known gestational age, the Liley graph allows one to categorize the severity of disease into one of three zones (Table 17-2). (From: Beckman CRB, Ling FW, Laube DW, Smith RP, Barzansky BM, Herbert WNP. Obstetrics and Gynecology, 4th Ed. Philadelphia: Lippincott Williams & Wilkins, 2002:168.)

Table 17–2.

Zone	Fetal Risk	Prognosis	Intervention
1	Low	Mild disease, if any	-Repeated amniocentesis every 2–3 weeks -Term delivery
2	Moderate-high	-Moderate to severe disease -Lower zone 2 fetal Hgb=11–13.9 -upper zone 2 fetal Hgb=8–10.9	-Repeated amniocentesis every 1–2 weeks -fetal blood sampling -early delivery -steroids (lung maturity)
3	High-critical	-severe to life-threatening -death within 1 week–10 days	-transfusion or delivery -steroids (lung maturity—see Preterm Labor section for more on lung maturity augmentation)

When should the fetus with hemolytic disease be delivered?

As always, assess the risks to the fetus in utero versus in the newborn intensive care unit. The decision whether or not to deliver is dependent upon gestational age and fetal condition. Consider the following variables:
- ΔOD_{450} value trends and/or measurements of fetal hemoglobin concentration
- Previous obstetric history
- Biophysical profile and fetal heart rate testing (in any infant with known hemolytic disease, a sinusoidal fetal heart rate portends a grim prognosis without immediate transfusion or delivery)
- Ultrasound and Doppler evaluation of the fetus
- Fetal lung maturity assessment
- Maternal cervical status

What if the fetus is very young and severely affected?

It can be transfused in utero

What are the two methods of fetal blood transfusion?

Intraperitoneal transfusion: first performed in 1964 and accomplished by transfusing blood into the fetal peritoneal cavity

Intravascular transfusion: first done in 1981 under fetoscopy and now performed under ultrasound-guided needle placement into the umbilical vein

18

Pulmonary Diseases in Pregnancy

ASTHMA

What is the incidence of asthma in pregnancy?

Asthma occurs in 3% to 5% of adults. It complicates 1% of pregnancies.

What is the pathophysiology of asthma?

Airway hyperreactivity and bronchoconstriction

What are the symptoms of asthma?

Wheezing
Chest tightness
Shortness of breath
May be episodic with various degrees of severity or chronic with persistent dyspnea

What are the criteria for a diagnosis of asthma?

Physical examination: Tachypnea, use of accessory muscles of respiration
Pulmonary examination: Hyperinflation of the chest, diffuse pulmonary wheezing, and rhonchi
Response to β-agonist or corticosteroid therapy

What are the etiologic factors of exacerbations?

The onset of asthma during pregnancy is rare; most cases of asthma during pregnancy are due to exacerbations of disease.
The etiologic factors of exacerbations in pregnancy are the same as those in the nonpregnant state (i.e., noncompliance with medications, respiratory tract infections, allergens, gastrointestinal reflux, and exercise).

What is the effect of pregnancy on asthma?

Improvement in asthma occurs in the first trimester of pregnancy.

Asthma improves in 69% of patients during pregnancy, worsens in 9%, and undergoes no change in 22%.

Worsening of asthma occurs in the sixth or seventh month of pregnancy;

The course of a patient's asthma in one pregnancy is not a predictor of the course of asthma in subsequent pregnancies.

The severity of a patient's asthma before pregnancy correlates with the severity of asthma in pregnancy; asthma usually worsens during pregnancy in women with severe asthma.

Certain obstetric medications (i.e., some prostaglandins and ergot derivatives) may exacerbate asthma and should be avoided.

Certain physiologic conditions associated with pregnancy (e.g., gastroesophageal reflux) may increase the frequency of asthma attacks.

What is the effect of asthma on the mother and developing fetus?

Mild or moderate asthma: No increase in the rate of fetal malformations or adverse effects

Severe asthma: Increased incidence of low birth weight, neurologic abnormalities, and pregnancy-induced hypertension

What is the management of asthma during pregnancy?

Differ little from therapy for nonpregnant patients

Avoidance of asthma triggers (e.g., allergens, exercise)

Yearly influenza vaccinations

Compliance with antiasthmatic medications

Metaproterenol, terbutaline, and albuterol are commonly given in two deep inhalations every 4–6 hours.

Teratogenicity or adverse effects on fetus?

Theorized risk of prolonged gestation and inhibition of labor

Dosage of oral corticosteroids in pregnancy?	Prednisone 60–100 mg; clinical improvement is usually seen within 6 hours of treatment.
Teratogenicity or adverse effects on fetus?	None
Why is prednisone the oral corticosteroid of choice in pregnancy?	Most of the drug is inactivated by placental 11-B-OL-dehydrogenase; only a small percentage of the ingested dose reaches the fetus.
When are intravenous (IV) steroids used in pregnancy?	Increased doses of IV steroids are used peripartum for the increased stress of labor in patients who are chronic users of oral agents.
What effects does steroid therapy have on neonatal adrenal function?	No evidence of neonatal adrenal suppression due to chronic maternal steroid use

PULMONARY EMBOLUS

What is the incidence of pulmonary embolus (PE)?	Occurs in 0.09–0.7/1000 pregnancies
Why is PE more common in pregnancy?	Increased incidence is related to the sixfold increase in development of a deep venous thrombosis (DVT) in pregnancy.
Incidence of thrombophlebitis (deep and superficial)?	Occurs in 1/70 pregnancies
When does thrombophlebitis most commonly occur during pregnancy?	In the immediate postpartum period; may occur antepartum
What are the risk factors for development of a PE?	Coagulation disorders Maternal age > 35 years

Obesity
Immobility
Cardiopulmonary disease
Diabetes
Prior history of DVT and/or PE
(5%–12% risk of recurrence)
Cesarean section (threefold increase)

What is a patient's course after the development of a PE?

Immediate result: Complete or partial obstruction of the pulmonary arterial blood flow to the distal lung
Partial obstruction: Decreased ventilation, pulmonary infarction
Complete obstruction: Circulatory collapse

What are the symptoms of PE?

Dyspnea (most common symptom)
Cough
Hemoptysis
Chest pain
Palpitations
Lightheadedness
Anxiety

What are the findings on physical examination?

Tachycardia, tachypnea, low-grade fever, pleural friction rub, rales, or decreased breath sounds
Findings may be deceptively normal because a pleural friction rub or evidence of pleural effusion is not present unless an infarction has occurred.
Patients may exhibit acute right ventricular strain with a right ventricular heave.

What are the laboratory findings?

Hypoxia
Arterial blood gas: Decrease in po_2 (usually < 80)
VTE D-Dimer has high negative predictive value
Chest x-ray: May show an infiltrate or pleural effusion

EKG:

> May show right axis shift or right bundle branch block
>
> Often, only a sinus tachycardia with nonspecific ST-T changes is seen.
>
> Confirming tests:
>
> > Ventilation–perfusion scan; if equivocal, pulmonary angiogram with abdominal shielding

What finding in the ventilation–perfusion scan is diagnostic of PE?

A V-Q mismatch showing normal ventilation but decreased perfusion

What conditions decrease the specificity of this test?

Congestive heart failure or chronic obstructive pulmonary disease

What is the maximum dose of radiation to the fetus in a ventilation–perfusion scan?

Fifty milliroentgen equivalents man (mrem), which is well below the level that raises concerns

What is the source of most of the radiation exposure, and how can this exposure be prevented?

The source of 85% of the radiation exposure is the maternal bladder.

A Foley catheter should be placed to empty the bladder.

What is the maximum dose of radiation to the fetus in a pulmonary angiogram?

With abdominal shielding, the radiation exposure may be kept under 0.05 cGy

Level that increases risk to fetus is > 5 cGy

What is the effect of pregnancy on PE?

Pregnancy increases the risk for DVT/ PE.

Because of stasis, hypercoagulability, and vascular injury.

> Pregnancy increases stasis secondary to compression by the uterus on the inferior vena cava.
>
> Pregnancy produces a hypercoagulable state; risk for DVT/PE is further increased in patients who are obese,

who have had pelvic surgery, or
who are on bed rest.
Pregnancy also causes an increase in
coagulation factors and a
suppression of the fibrinolytic
system.

**What are the most
common sites for a DVT?**

Venous sinuses within the soleus
Left iliofemoral venous segment

**What is the effect of PE on
mother and fetus?**

If mother is hemodynamically stable: No
adverse effect
If untreated: Maternal mortality rate
may approach 50% and is related to
the size of the lesion.

**What is the treatment for
PE?**

Heparin is the main therapeutic agent
used during pregnancy.
Risks to fetus: It does not cross the
placenta, does not increase the risk of
fetal malformations, and does not lead
to fetal anticoagulation.
Side effects: Hemorrhage (most common
side effect), bone demineralization
when used for more than 20 weeks,
anaphylaxis, alopecia, and
thrombocytopenia (usually mild and
dose/duration dependent)
Dosage: 80 U/kg IV, then 18 U/kg/hour
to maintain PTT at 60–90 sec.

**How long should
treatment continue?**

2–6 months following the embolus/DVT
Heparin is usually changed to coumadin
for the long run

**What is the most common
side effect of heparin
therapy?**

Hemorrhage

**What is the incidence of
thrombocytopenia that
results from heparin
therapy?**

Twenty percent

Why is Coumadin (warfarin) contraindicated in pregnancy?	It is teratogenic. It has been associated with hemorrhage in the fetus and placenta. It has been shown to produce nasal hypoplasia, stippling of bones, ophthalmologic abnormalities, intrauterine growth retardation, variable central nervous system (CNS) defects, anatomic defects, and mental delays.
What is the risk of perinatal hemorrhage as a result of Coumadin therapy?	Five percent to ten percent
What is the risk of congenital disease as a result of Coumadin therapy?	Fetuses exposed to the drug before 14 weeks' gestation have an estimated 10%–25% risk of congenital disease.
When do CNS defects occur as a result of Coumadin therapy?	At any time in the second or third trimester; may be related to bleeding
What coagulation workup should be considered in women with DVT during pregnancy?	Factor V deficiency Prothrombin gene mutation Protein C def Protein S def Antithrombin 3 def Antiphospholipid antibodies

PNEUMONIA

What are the symptoms of pneumonia?	Fever Chills Cough Purulent sputum Tachypnea
What are the etiologic factors of pneumonia?	Most common cause of pneumonia is *Streptococcus pneumoniae* infection.

Another common organism is *Mycoplasma pneumoniae*, which causes a "community-acquired pneumonia."

Other bacteria, such as *Haemophilus influenzae*, *Staphylococcus aureus*, and *Escherichia coli*, and viruses may produce pneumonia.

What are the criteria for diagnosis of pneumonia?

History:
   S. pneumoniae has a sudden onset, productive cough, and purulent sputum.
   M. pneumoniae has a gradual onset of symptoms with a nonproductive cough, headache, myalgias, and leukocytosis.
Physical examination: Rales and other signs suggestive of consolidation, such as decreased breath sounds, rhonchi, "e" to "a" changes, and percussive dullness
Chest x-ray:
   Lobar consolidation and air bronchograms are seen in *S. pneumoniae* infection.
   Unilateral or bilateral diffuse patchy infiltrates are seen in *M. pneumoniae*.
Gram stain of sputum and bacterial culture: In a healthy young woman, the trachea should be free of leukocytes and bacteria. Leukocytes and bacteria are consistent with infection.
Cold agglutin titers: Can help determine *M. pneumoniae* infection

What is the effect of pregnancy on pneumonia?

No effect

What is the effect of pneumonia on the mother and fetus?

Increased incidence of preterm labor in patients who have pneumonia near term

Perinatal mortality rate is < 10% in infants delivered during the acute phase of the disease and depends on the gestational age at birth.

What is the treatment for pneumonia?

IV or oral antibiotics, depending on the severity of the disease.

S. pneumoniae: ceftriaxone for 10 days

M. pneumoniae:
    Does not respond to either PCN or cephalosporins
    Azithromycin

What are the complications of pneumonia?

Poor outcome is related to involvement of more than two lobes, respiratory rate > 30, severe hypoxemia, hypoalbuminemia, and septicemia.

Pneumonia that progresses to adult respiratory distress syndrome has a 70% mortality rate.

Bacteremia may develop in up to 25% of patients.

Empyema and respiratory failure are other complications.

TUBERCULOSIS

What is the epidemiology of tuberculosis (TB)?

Incidence is increasing; it is the most common communicable disease among human immunodeficiency virus-infected individuals.

The risk of acquiring the infection is highest in large urban settings.

Overall, advanced disease develops in 5%–15%; of infected individuals.

What are the stages of TB?

Primary TB:
    Defined as first infection with tuberculosis agent
    May cavitate and heal spontaneously or progress (called progressive primary TB)

Secondary TB:
    Most common presentation in adults
    Represents a delayed reactivation of infection or exogenous reinfection

What are the symptoms of primary nonprogressive TB?

Most patients are asymptomatic, have no cough, and produce little sputum; only sign is a positive tuberculin skin test. Patients in cavitary stage have a chronic cough and produce mucopurulent sputum.

What are the manifestations of progressive primary TB?

Miliary tuberculosis, sometimes with meningitis; pulmonary disease of the apical and posterior segments of the upper lobes; or lower lobe disease

What are the symptoms of reactivation?

Night sweats
Chills
Fatigue
Fever from 39°C to 40°C occurring in the late afternoon and evening
Malaise
Weight loss
Hemoptysis

What is the etiologic factor of TB?

Infection with *Mycobacterium tuberculosis*

How is TB transmitted?

Inhalation of aerosolized droplets of liquid containing the bacteria from an infected patient with cavitary pulmonary tuberculosis

What is the pathophysiology of TB?

The bacteria travel to the lung alveoli. Once local invasion has occurred, the infection can be disseminated hematogenously, thereby seeding multiple organs and establishing latent foci. These latent foci are the sites of delayed reactivation.

What are the criteria for a diagnosis of TB?

Positive PPD test:
Defined as a wheal of induration of:
15mm in low risk population
>5mm in HIV positive patients

>10mm: abnormal CXR, steroid use, chronic illness, IV drug users, other high risk population

Suggests a history of exposure to TB but not necessarily active TB

False-negative reactions may occur in pregnant patients.

Chest x-ray:

In primary TB, shows patchy or lobular infiltrates in the anterior segment of the upper lobes or in the middle lobes, often with associated hilar adenopathy

In secondary TB, may show cavitary lesions with infiltrates

Acid-fast stain of the sputum: Definitive test

Culture: May also be performed but results take 6 weeks

Physical examination: Unremarkable or reveals dullness and rales in the upper lung fields

What is the effect of TB on mother and fetus?

TB has no adverse effect on pregnancy if adequate treatment is implemented.

Transplacental passage of TB is extremely rare.

Congenital infection of liver or regional lymph nodes may occur in the presence of maternal bacillemia.

What is the effect of pregnancy on TB?

No effect

What is the treatment for TB?

Two or three sputum samples for culture before starting antituberculous drug treatment

Baseline evaluation of liver function before the administration of potentially hepatotoxic drugs (isoniazid, rifampin, pyrazinamide)

Administration of multiple antimicrobials to prevent the growth of resistant organisms

What antibiotics are used to treat TB?

Isoniazid and rifampin for initial treatment in patients with susceptible organisms

How should a patient with positive PPd & negative CXR be treated?

Isoniazid post partum for 6 months

How long should antibiotic therapy last?

The current minimal acceptable duration of treatment for adults with culture-positive tuberculosis is 6 months.

What are the risks of TB medications to the fetus?

The risk of untreated tuberculosis is far greater to a mother and fetus than toxicities of medications.

Isoniazid: No increase in risk of congenital abnormalities

Ethambutol: No increase in risk of congenital abnormalities; the mother risks retrobulbar neuritis.

Rifampin: No associated fetal malformations are known; it readily crosses the placenta and may theoretically inhibit DNA-dependent RNA polymerase and injure the fetus.

Streptomycin: This drug should be avoided if possible in pregnancy because it may interfere with development of the ear, causing congenital deafness; it may be both ototoxic and nephrotoxic to the mother.

Is breast-feeding contraindicated during TB antibiotic therapy?

No, as long as the disease is not "active"

When is prophylactic therapy indicated in pregnancy?

If patient has a positive PPD and recent conversion

What agent is used for prophylaxis?

Isoniazid

19 Renal Diseases in Pregnancy

GENERAL

What normal renal changes occur in pregnancy?

Dilatation of the collecting system and ureters:Occurs as early as 10 weeks' gestation

Is due to both mechanical compression of the ureters by the enlarging uterus and the relaxing effect of progesterone on smooth muscle.

Increased renal plasma flow:
Exceeds prepregnant levels by 50%–75% at the end of the first trimester

Fifty percent increase in glomerular filtration rate (GFR)

Decreased renal threshold for glucose:
Sometimes causes glycosuria in patients with a normal blood glucose

Decreased serum levels of creatinine and blood urea nitrogen (BUN):
Nonpregnant levels are 0.8 mg/100 ml and 13 mg/100 ml.

Pregnant levels are 0.6 mg/100 ml and 9 mg/100 ml (mean values).

ASYMPTOMATIC BACTERIURIA

What is the incidence of asymptomatic bacteriuria in pregnancy?

Occurs in 2%–7% of all pregnancies

What are the criteria for diagnosis of asymptomatic bacteriuria?

Greater than 100,000 colonies/ml of a single organism in a clean-catch sample of urine

What is different about UTI in pregnancy?

Considered "complicated UTI"—requires 5–7 days therapy
Dysuria is often absent

Frequency, urgency & nocturia are common in pregnancy and do not necessarily suggest infection

What are the common organisms that cause asymptomatic bacteriuria?

Escherichia coli:
  Responsible for 75%–90% of bacteriuria cases during pregnancy
Other bacteria: *Klebsiella, Proteus,* and *Enterobacter* sp

What are the complications of asymptomatic bacteriuria?

If untreated, asymptomatic bacteriuria may lead to pyelonephritis or acute symptomatic cystitis in 25%–40% of patients.
Approximately 15% of patients treated for asymptomatic bacteriuria have a recurrence.

What is the treatment of asymptomatic bacteriuria?

Antibiotic therapy specific to the organisms involved

What antibiotics are commonly used in pregnancy?

Sulfa drugs (Sulfa-trimethoprim): Avoid using near term because they can cause kernicterus by competitively inhibiting the binding of bilirubin to albumin.
Nitrofurantoin:
  Contraindicated in patients with glucose-6-phosphate dehydrogenase deficiency

Who should be on prophylactic antibiotics?

History of pyelo in pregnancy
Multiple UTIs

PYELONEPHRITIS

What is the incidence of pyelonephritis?

Occurs in 1%–2% of all pregnancies
Most common serious medical complication of pregnancy
Right-sided in more than one-half of cases and bilateral in one-fourth

What are the symptoms of pyelonephritis?

Fever
Chills

Nausea
Vomiting
Anorexia
Dysuria
Flank pain
Frequency, urgency, and dysuria may
not be present.

What are the criteria for the diagnosis of pyelonephritis?

Physical examination: Costovertebral
angle tenderness and fever
Urinalysis: An increased number of
white blood cells and numerous
bacteria
Urine culture: Grows the infecting
organism.
Urine leukocyte esterase and nitrite:
Positive
(GFR: Temporarily decreased in ~25%
of patients
Blood creatinine: Temporarily increased
in ~25% of patients)

What are the etiologic factors of pyelonephritis?

The same organisms that cause
asymptomatic bacteriuria cause
pyelonephritis; pyelonephritis is an
ascending infection.

What is the effect of pregnancy on pyelonephritis?

Increased incidence of pyelonephritis in
pregnant women is related to the
increased incidence of asymptomatic
bacteriuria during pregnancy.
Increased urinary stasis caused by
dilatation and compression of the
urinary system during pregnancy
contributes to increased risk of
infection.

What is the effect of pyelonephritis on the mother and fetus?

Possible increased risk of preterm labor
Possible increased risk of fetal death and
intrauterine growth retardation
(IUGR) as a result of recurrent
pyelonephritis

What are complications of pyelonephritis?

Approximately 15% of patients with pyelonephritis have bacteremia.

Up to 2% of bacteremic patients develop endotoxin-mediated alveolar injury with resulting pulmonary edema or adult respiratory distress syndrome.

Some patients with pyelonephritis develop acute anemia as a result of endotoxin-induced hemolysis.

Some women have a considerable reduction in GFR that is reversed by effective treatment.

What is the treatment for pyelonephritis?

Intravenous (IV) hydration and IV antibiotic therapy for at least 24–48 hours; oral therapy may follow.

Empiric Rx with broad spec. antibiotic pending cultures (ceftraixone)

Lack of improvement by 72 hours suggests inadequate use or an underlying anatomic problem, renal US should be done.

UROLITHIASIS

What is the incidence of urolithiasis?

Occurs in 0.03% of pregnancies (same as that for the general population).

What are the symptoms of urolithiasis?

Colicky abdominal pain, hematuria; these symptoms are far less common in the pregnant patient.

What is the pathophysiology of urolithiasis?

Calcium salts make up about 75% of renal stones; in half these cases, idiopathic hypercalciuria is the most common predisposing cause.

Struvite stones are associated with infection, and *Proteus* is often cultured from the urine.

Uric acid stones are less common.

How is a diagnosis of urolithiasis made?

History and physical examination

Ultrasound can also be used to detect stones and hydronephrosis or urinary tract dilatation proximal to the stone.

The patient's urine can be strained for stones.

Patients with persistent pyelonephritis despite antibiotic therapy should be evaluated for a possible obstructing renal stone.

What is the effect of pregnancy on urolithiasis?

No effect

What is the effect of urolithiasis on mother and fetus?

No known adverse effects

Increased frequency of urinary infections

What is the management/ treatment of urolithiasis?

Expectant management

Acute event:

Hydration and narcotic analgesia

Because of the hydroureter that occurs in pregnancy, over one-half of patients spontaneously pass the stone.

Approximately one-third of patients with symptomatic stones need cystoscopy, ureteral catheterization, percutaneous nephrostomy, basket extraction, or surgical exploration for ureteral obstruction.

Lithotripsy: Contraindicated in pregnancy

Aggressive treatment for coexisting infection

GLOMERULONEPHRITIS

What is the incidence of glomerulonephritis in pregnancy?

Occurs in 1/40,000 pregnant women

What are the signs and symptoms of glomerulonephritis?

Hypertension
Edema (including periorbital edema)
Proteinuria
Hematuria (usually microscopic)
These signs and symptoms may be difficult to distinguish from those of preeclampsia.

How is glomerulonephritis diagnosed?

History, physical examination, and laboratory evaluation
Definitive test: Renal biopsy

How is glomerulonephritis distinguished from preeclampsia?

Patients with glomerulonephritis have red blood cell (RBC) casts in urine sediment and depressed serum complement levels.

What are the etiologic factors?

Acute glomerulonephritis:
    Usually but not always streptococcal in origin
    Other causes include other bacterial, viral, and parasitic infections; multisystem disease such as systemic lupus erythematosus; Henoch-Schönlein purpura; or primary glomerular disease.
Chronic glomerulonephritis: Secondary to a known episode of acute glomerulonephritis, IgA nephropathy, membranoproliferative glomerulonephritis, focal glomerulosclerosis, or systemic lupus erythematosus.

What is the effect of pregnancy on glomerulonephritis?

No effect; urinary protein excretion may transiently increase because of the increased renal plasma flow in pregnancy.

What is the effect of glomerulonephritis on the mother and fetus?

Increased incidence of fetal demise, IUGR, and preterm delivery
Fifty-two percent of patients have hypertension.
Fifteen percent have impaired renal function.

Patients with hypertension or impaired renal function (creatinine > 1.5) have a higher incidence of complications.

What are the complications of acute glomerulonephritis?

Chronic glomerulonephritis with resulting end-stage renal failure
Chronic proteinuria
Hypertension

What is the management/ treatment of glomerulonephritis?

Blood pressure control
Restriction of salt intake
Appropriate seizure prophylaxis if preeclampsia is suspected

CHRONIC RENAL DISEASE

What is chronic renal disease?

A syndrome that results from progressive and irreversible destruction of nephrons, regardless of cause

What is the criterion for a diagnosis of chronic renal failure?

Reduced GFR for at least 3 to 6 months

What are the criteria for a diagnosis of chronic renal disease?

Renal function may be normal.
Signs and symptoms include hypertension, proteinuria, or abnormal renal sediment.
Diagnosis is supported by the finding of bilateral reduction of kidney size.
Casts in the urinary sediment are consistent with chronic renal failure.
Proteinuria and hematuria are frequent but nonspecific findings. Other symptoms and laboratory values differ depending on the cause of the renal dysfunction:
Moderate proteinuria (< 2 g/day) is seen in glomerular disease (most commonly lipoid nephrosis), systemic lupus erythematosus, and in glomerulonephritis.

RBC casts and microscopic hematuria (RBCs > 1–2/hpf) are seen in glomerular disease or collagen vascular disease.

Cellular casts are seen in renal tubular disease.

What is the effect of chronic renal disease on mother and fetus?

In women with preexisting renal disease, the prognosis for a favorable pregnancy outcome is closely related to renal function at the time of conception.

Effects include increased incidence of hypertension, superimposed preeclampsia, IUGR, and preterm birth.

Obstetric outcome is usually successful provided renal function is only moderately compromised and hypertension is absent or minimal.

What is the effect of pregnancy on renal function?

Patients with baseline creatinine < 1.5: Pregnancy has little effect on long-term prognosis.

Patients with creatinine > 1.5: Deterioration of renal function is more frequent, especially in patients with diffuse glomerulonephritis.

If renal function deteriorates significantly during pregnancy, pregnancy termination may not reverse the initial process.

Hypertension:

Fifty percent of patients with chronic renal disease have worsening hypertension.

Patients with diffuse proliferative glomerulonephritis and nephrosclerosis are at greatest risk for development of severe hypertension.

Increased incidence of pyelonephritis

What are the causes of sudden deterioration of renal function?

Infection
Dehydration
Obstruction

What is the management/ treatment of chronic renal disease?

Frequent urine monitoring for creatine clearance and protein excretion

Frequent visits

Serial ultrasonography to evaluate possible IUGR

Antepartum fetal heart rate testing

Anemia secondary to chronic renal disease: Erythropoietin

Hypertension: Methyldopa, β-blockers

When is dialysis indicated?

Severe abnormalities in fluid and electrolyte balance such as fluid overload, acidosis, and hyperkalemia

Symptoms of uremia

Renal function 5% or less of normal, regardless of symptoms

What precautions should be taken during dialysis of the pregnant patient?

Avoidance of sudden volume shifts

Continuous fetal heart rate monitoring in late pregnancy

Avoidance of prolonged periods in the supine position due to compression of the vena cava

What are the complications of dialysis during pregnancy?

Polyhydramnios

Preterm birth

Other common problems: Clotting and infection of the vascular access

PREGNANCY IN THE INDIVIDUAL WITH A RENAL TRANSPLANT

Which individuals with a renal transplant should attempt pregnancy?

Individuals in whom surgery was performed 2 or more years previously (risk of graft rejection is greatest during first 2 years)

Individuals with no evidence of rejection, hypertension, or proteinuria

Creatinine < 2

What is the effect of a renal transplant on pregnancy?

Ninety percent of pregnancies that continue beyond the first trimester have a successful outcome.

Increased incidence of:
Preeclampsia (1/3 of patients)
Preterm labor (1/2 of patients)
IUGR
Premature rupture of membranes
Urinary and viral infections
Cephalopelvic disproportion due to pelvic osteodystrophy
Fifteen percent of patients experience a significant decrease in renal function in late pregnancy that usually reverses after pregnancy.

What is the effect of pregnancy on a renal transplant?

The incidence of rejection is 9%, which is the same as that in the nonpregnant population.

What two conditions can the symptoms of rejection mimic?

Acute pyelonephritis or severe preeclampsia

What test can distinguish rejection from acute pyelonephritis or severe preeclampsia?

Renal biopsy

What is the management/ treatment of the renal transplant patient?

Continuation of immunosuppressive therapy (glucocorticoids, azathioprine, and cyclosporin)
Frequent assessment of renal function
Monitoring for worsening of underlying hypertension and superimposed preeclampsia
Urinalysis at each prenatal visit
Urine culture each trimester
Bacteriuria: Requires aggressive treatment; the transplanted kidney is denervated and therefore the patient may have pyelonephritis or urosepsis without pain

What is the cesarean section rate in this population?

Fifty percent

Why does obstruction of labor occasionally occur in this population?

The transplanted kidney is located in the pelvis and can obstruct labor.

What are the risks to the fetus associated with immunosuppressive therapy?

Glucocorticoids are metabolized in the placenta and are not known to cause any adverse fetal effects.

Azathioprine has reported fetal complications of IUGR and a decrease in IgG and IgM in the fetus.

Cyclosporin may cause hypertension and is associated with IUGR.

Concerns persist about the possibility of late effects in offspring subjected to immunosuppressive therapy in utero, including malignancy, germ cell dysfunction, and malformations in the offspring's children.

ACUTE RENAL FAILURE IN PREGNANCY

What is acute renal failure?

The production of < 400 ml of urine in a 24-hour period

What is the incidence of acute renal failure?

Occurs in 1/10,000 pregnancies

When do most acute renal failure cases occur during pregnancy?

Postpartum

What are the etiologic factors of acute renal failure in pregnancy?

Sudden, severe volume depletion due to blood loss occurring in placenta previa, placental abruption, and postpartum uterine atony

Marked volume contraction due to preeclampsia and acute fatty liver of pregnancy

Sepsis

Complicated preexisting renal problems

What are the most common obstetric causes of acute renal failure?	Placental abruption and preeclampsia
What are the signs and symptoms of acute renal failure?	Oliguria followed by a period of polyuria Increased BUN and creatinine Acidosis Uremia
What are the complications of acute renal failure?	The immediate maternal mortality rate with acute renal failure is 20%. Acute renal failure with mild ischemia: Quickly reversible prerenal failure With prolonged ischemia: Reversible acute tubular necrosis With severe ischemia: Irreversible acute cortical necrosis
Incidence of acute cortical necrosis?	Occurs in 15%–30% of all cases of acute renal failure in pregnancy
Mortality rate of acute cortical necrosis?	One hundred percent if untreated
Treatment of acute cortical necrosis?	Dialysis
How is acute cortical necrosis differentiated from early acute tubular necrosis?	Differentiation is not possible.
What is the management/ treatment of acute renal failure?	Correction of underlying cause of acute volume loss Balance of volume and electrolytes Prompt treatment of acidosis, if present Dialysis if the patient has hypernatremia, hyperkalemia, severe acidosis, volume overload, or worsening uremia
Why should diuretics be avoided?	They increase urine flow without correcting the cause, and may contribute to volume depletion.

20

Teratogenicity

What is teratogenicity?

Strict definition: Production of physical defects in the developing embryo. The definition over time has expanded to include functional and behavioral deficits.

What is the incidence of major congenital malformations in a newborn?

Three percent

What are the causes of developmental defects in humans?

Genetic transmission: 20%
Chromosomal aberrations: 5%
Environmental
  Ionizing radiation: 1%–2%
  Infections: 1%–2%
  Maternal metabolic imbalances:
    1%–2%
  Drugs and environmental chemicals:
    4%–6%
Unknown: 65%–70%

What is the incidence of drug use during pregnancy?

Eighty-six percent of women take medications during pregnancy.
They take an average of five medications.

What are the most commonly used drugs in pregnancy?

Analgesics
Antibiotics
Antacids
Diuretics
Laxatives

What two stages described fetal exposure to medications?

Preimplantation and implantation

What is the usual effect of a drug on the embryo preimplantation?

Any chemical present in the tubal or uterine fluids potent enough to cause irreparable injury usually kills the affected embryo.

What determines the effect of drugs on the fetus after implantation?

Placental transfer: Because most drugs have a molecular weight of 250–500 daltons, placental transfer is readily accomplished.

Fetal dosage

Duration of exposure of fetus to drug

Gestational age at time of exposure

During embryogenesis (2–8 weeks' gestational age), teratogens can cause structural defects; an example is neural tube defect.

After embryogenesis, drugs mainly cause adverse effects in the fetus.

How can teratogenic effects be identified antenatally?

Amniocentesis is normally **not** helpful because most drugs do not damage the fetal chromosomes.

α-Fetoprotein testing of maternal serum can detect 85% of all open neural tube defects.

Ultrasound may be able to detect malformations or intrauterine growth retardation (IUGR).

What steps can be taken to decrease congenital anomalies from medications?

Minimize drug exposures

Avoid polydrug regimens

Use lowest drug dose for shortest duration possible

For what purpose are the Food and Drug Administration (FDA) Use-in-Pregnancy Ratings intended?

To provide guidelines on the use of drugs during pregnancy and discourage medication use

What are the different FDA Use-in-Pregnancy ratings?

A: Controlled studies show no risk

B: No evidence of risk in humans

C: Risk cannot be ruled out

D: Positive evidence of risk

X: Contraindicated in pregnancy

For each medication below, list its teratogenicity and/or adverse effect.

Phenytoin

Teratogenicity: Ten percent of newborns may have cleft lip and palate, heart disease, and microcephaly.

Children born to mothers with seizures receiving no medications also have an increased incidence of congenital anomalies.

Considerable controversy exists about the true incidence of teratogenicity from phenytoin, if any.

Carbamazepine

Teratogenicity: Growth and developmental delay, minor craniofacial anomalies, neural tube defects in the first trimester ($< 1\%$ incidence)

Valproic acid

Teratogenicity: Neural tube defects (1%–3% incidence), developmental delays, and craniofacial anomalies

Metronidazole

Teratogenicity: Mutagenic in bacteria, but no problems have been reported in humans

Because of this **theoretical** risk, it should be given only for clear-cut indications.

Ciprofloxacin

Teratogenicity: Not recommended in pregnant women and children

Human studies have **not** shown an association between quinolone use in the first trimester and an increased risk of malformations or musculoskeletal problems.

However, immature dogs and guinea pigs treated with quinolones have developed arthropathy.

Sulfamethoxazole/ trimethoprim

Adverse effect: When given in the third trimester, may compete with bilirubin for albumin-binding sites and contribute to increased risk of hyperbilirubinemia

Tetracycline (doxycycline, minocycline, tetracycline)

Teratogenicity: Staining of fetal teeth when used after 20th week; enamel hypoplasia and inhibition of fibula growth in premature infants

Aminoglycosides

Adverse effect: Hearing loss appears to be dose related; if used, maternal serum levels should be monitored and the course of therapy kept short.
No toxicity noted with gentamycin, only kanamycin and streptomycin

Other antibiotics (penicillins, cephalosporins, erythromycin, nitrofurantoin and clindamycin)

Teratogenicity: none is known

Warfarin

Teratogenicity: When used in the first trimester can cause fetal warfarin syndrome (nasal hypoplasia, bone stippling, and ophthalmologic abnormalities); when used beyond first trimester, blindness and mental retardation can occur.

Heparin

Because it is a large molecule and does not cross the placenta, it is the drug of choice for anticoagulation in pregnancy.
Teratogenicity: none is known
Adverse effects: Bleeding (2% incidence), bone demineralization with doses > 20,000 U/day

Enoxaparin

Because it is a large molecule, it does not cross the placenta.
Teratogenicity: Appears safe, but not as much information exists about this drug as exists for heparin.

Alcohol

Teratogenicity: Fetal alcohol syndrome (IUGR, mental retardation, as well as ocular, facial, and skeletal anomalies) occurs when large amounts of alcohol are ingested.

A threshold for safety has not been established, and it is best to avoid any exposure.

Antihistamines

Teratogenicity: none is known

Decongestants

Teratogenicity: none is known

Ventral wall defects have been reported with pseudoephedrine use in the first trimester.

If a decongestant is necessary, a topical nasal spray subjects the fetus to lower doses than a systemic medication.

Because antihistamines and decongestants provide only symptomatic therapy for the common cold, other remedies such as a humidifier, rest, and fluids should be recommended.

If drugs are necessary, only one should be used.

Meclizine

Teratogenicity: none is known

Dimenhydrinate

Teratogenicity: none is known

Metoclopramide

Teratogenicity: none is known

Trimethobenzamide

Teratogenicity: none is known

Promethazine

Teratogenicity: none is known

Acetaminophen

Teratogenicity: none is known when used as an antipyretic and analgesic

Aspirin

Teratogenicity: none is known

Adverse effects: Inhibits prostaglandin synthesis and can decrease uterine

contractility and cause delayed onset
and longer duration of labor
May also decrease platelet aggregation in
newborn

**Nonsteroidal anti-
inflammatory drugs**

Teratogenicity: none is known, but when
used in third trimester may prolong
labor and cause premature closure of the
fetal ductus arteriosus

Codeine

Teratogenicity: none is known
Adverse effect: Fetal/newborn addiction
   with prolonged use

**Narcotic analgesics
(morphine,
hydrocodone,
oxycodone, meperidine,
hydromorphone)**

Teratogenicity: none is known
Adverse effect: Fetal/newborn addiction
   with prolonged use; at term may cause
   neonatal respiratory depression

Methyldopa

Teratogenicity: none is known

Hydralazine

Teratogenicity: none is known

Digoxin

Teratogenicity: none is known

Nifedipine

Teratogenicity: none is known
Experience in human pregnancy is
   limited.

β-Blockers

Teratogenicity: none is known

**Angiotensin-converting
enzyme inhibitors**

Teratogenicity: **Contraindicated** in
   pregnancy
Use of these drugs in the second and
   third trimesters has been associated
   with fetal injury and death.
Risks to the fetus include potential fatal
   hypotension, anuria, and renal failure.
Decreased renal function can lead to
   oligohydramnios, which can result in
   fetal limb contractures, craniofacial
   deformities, and hypoplastic lung
   development.

Caffeine

Teratogenicity: none is known
Conservative consumption is
recommended.

Hydrochlorothiazide

Teratogenicity: none is known

Furosemide

Teratogenicity: none is known

Diuretics

Adverse effects: Fetal electrolyte
disturbances have been observed in
some cases when used in the third
trimester.
Diuretics are normally not
recommended during pregnancy
because of interference with maternal
blood volume.

Progesterone (natural)

Teratogenicity: none is known

Medroxyprogesterone

Teratogenicity: none is known

Estrogens

Teratogenicity: none is known
Controversy exists.

Diethylstilbestrol (DES)

Teratogenicity: **Contraindicated** in
pregnancy
Female fetuses exposed to DES have an
increased risk of adenocarcinoma of
the vagina and cervix.
May also cause uterine anomalies
affecting reproductive capacity.
DES may also affect the reproductive
tract of exposed male fetuses.

Oral contraceptives

Teratogenicity: none is known
Controversy exists.
Patient should be informed that a
possible risk to the fetus exists if the
drug is continued during pregnancy.

Vaccines (general)

Most vaccines contain toxoids or killed
organisms and present a low risk to
the fetus.

Vaccines containing live attenuated viruses present a slightly higher **theoretical** risk.

If a vaccine or a toxoid is indicated during pregnancy, it should be given during the second or third trimester.

In general, the advantages of immunization usually outweigh the potential risks.

The best time to receive immunizations is before pregnancy.

Measles, mumps, and rubella (MMR) vaccine

Teratogenicity: Although the recommendation is not to give during pregnancy, evidence does not support vaccine-associated malformations.

Give immediately postpartum.

Influenza vaccine

Teratogenicity: none is known

Women who will be beyond the first trismester during influenza season should be vaccinated because of increased risk for influenza related complications.

Hepatitis B vaccine

Teratogenicity: Pregnancy should **not** be considered a contraindication.

Tetanus and diphtheria vaccine

Teratogenicity: none is known

Docusate

Teratogenicity: none is known

Docusate/casanthranol

Teratogenicity: none is known

Serotonin reuptake inhibitors (general)

Experience is limited.

Unanswered questions include effects on infant behavior and intellect or problems with newborn adaptation.

Fluoxetine

Teratogenicity: none is known

Sertraline — Teratogenicity: none is known

Paroxetine — Teratogenicity: none is known

Smoking — Teratogenicity: Associated with IUGR and preterm labor, but not malformations.
Children may also be at increased risk for sudden infant death syndrome, although the data do not make it clear if smoking before pregnancy, after pregnancy, or both, is the cause.

Corticosteroids (general) — Teratogenicity: none is known
All steroids cross the placenta to some degree.

Prednisone / Prednisolone — Teratogenicity: none is known
Both drugs are inactivated by the placenta, and less than 10% of the drug reaches the fetus.
Drug of choice for diseases such as asthma

Betamethasone/ dexamethasone — Teratogenicity: none is known
These drugs cross the placenta and are preferred for stimulating fetal lung maturity.

List the therapeutic or adverse effect associated with the following agents: — CMV: Hydrocephaly, microcephaly, chorioretinitis, mental retardation
Rubella: Microcephaly, mental retardation, cataracts, deafness, heart defects
Varicella: Scarring, chorioretinitis, cataracts, microcephaly, muscle atrophy, hypoplasia of hands & feet
Toxoplasmosis: Central nervous system maldevelopment

21   Diabetes in Pregnancy

GENERAL

What is the most common medical complication of pregnancy?	Diabetes mellitus
What is the incidence?	Three percent
What is the perinatal mortality rate in diabetic pregnancy?	Approximately the same as that of nondiabetic pregnancy
How is nongestational (preexisting) diabetes classified?	As Type I (insulin-dependent diabetes mellitus) or Type II (non–insulin-dependent diabetes mellitus)
What is gestational diabetes mellitus?	Carbohydrate intolerance first recognized during pregnancy and not persisting after delivery
How is diabetes that predates pregnancy classified?	According to the degree of maternal metabolic control and the presence or absence of vasculopathy

PREEXISTING DIABETES IN PREGNANCY

What are the benefits of normalization of maternal blood glucose levels during diabetes in pregnancy?	Decreased congenital anomaly rate (otherwise increased fourfold) if the diabetes is established before conception Decreased risk of neonatal macrosomia Decreased mortality and morbidity rates
Why do infants of diabetic women have high anomaly rates?	Glucose is a teratogen

What specific anomalies are associated with diabetes in pregnancy?

Cardiac anomalies
Transposition of great vessels
Ventricular septal defect
Atrial septal defect
Neural tube defect
Renal anomalies
Anal/rectal atresia

What are the risks associated with preexisting Type 1 diabetes mellitus during pregnancy?

Higher risk of preeclampsia
Higher risk of pyelonephritis
Hypoglycemia (with tight glucose control)
Progression of proliferative retinopathy (but not progression of renal disease)

What are the goals of maternal metabolic control?

Glucose levels that do not exceed 90 milligrams per deciliter (mg/dL) at fasting or 105 mg/dL prior to meals
One hour postprandial values not to exceed 120 mg/dL
Hemoglobin A or A_{Ic} within the normal range

How can these goals be achieved?

Patient glucose monitoring
Carefully regulated dietary intake
Carefully regulated insulin administration usually requiring multiple injections of variously acting insulins; insulin pumps can be used

Why are oral hypoglycemic agents avoided during pregnancy?

They may produce fetal hyperinsulinemia and they may cause increased rates of congenital malformations if used during early pregnancy.

What is a carefully regulated dietary intake for a woman with diabetes in pregnancy?

Total caloric intake of 30–35 kcal/kg of ideal body weight
55% carbohydrates
20% protein
25% fat with less than 10% saturated fat

Consumption: 25% of calories at breakfast, 30% at lunch, 30% at dinner, and 15% as a bedtime snack
Day-to-day consistency in dietary behavior and activity

What should the prenatal workup of a woman with preexisting diabetes consist of?

History and physical examination
Standard prenatal laboratory tests
Twenty-four-hour urinalysis for creatinine clearance and protein excretion (usually requires a repeat test)
Ophthalmologic examination
Thyroid function tests

What does the fetal work-up consist of?

Early ultrasound to clearly establish gestational age
Ultrasound at approximately 20 weeks' gestation to screen for anomaly
α-fetoprotein (maternal serum) to screen for neural tube defect
Fetal echocardiography (controversial)
Surveillance for fetal well-being (in the third trimester)
  Nonstress test (NST)
  BPP
  Ultrasound
  Kick count
  Determination of lung maturity when delivery is considered
See Table 21-1.

Table 21–1. Pre-Existing Diabetes

Diabetes Classification	Mode/Timing of Test
<10 years duration and no other risk factors	NST twice weekly; begin at 34 weeks
>10 years or other risk factors	NST twice weekly; begin at 32 weeks
H/O prior IUFD	NST twice weekly; begin at 2 weeks before ???

Why is fetal surveillance necessary?	Intrauterine death from placental insufficiency is common in women with poor glucose control. Surveillance prevents unnecessary early delivery of a healthy fetus.
When should the fetus be delivered?	When fetal maturity is determined Prematurely, when risk in utero exceeds neonatal risk, i.e., when the fetus appears ill by surveillance techniques (Table 21-2)

Table 21–2. Timing of Delivery

Diabetes Classification	Timing
Pre-existing DM of <10 years	After amnio at 38 weeks
Pre-existing DM >10 years or other risk factors	After amnio at 36-37 weeks

How is maturity determined?	By amniotic fluid assay
How is amniotic fluid assessed?	Lecithin/sphingomyelin ratio is the standard assessment. (≥2.0 is mature). The presence of phosphatidylglycerol is helpful. Both are assayed by thin-layer chromatography.
What is the preferred method of delivery?	Vaginal, although rates of cesarean section are high
How is labor managed?	Cervical ripening techniques (prostaglandin) are probably acceptable but are used infrequently. Oxytocin induction is often used. Maternal euglycemia can be maintained with insulin/glucose infusion (usually 1–2 units per hour with 125 milliliters of 5% dextrose in Ringer's lactate solution or normal saline). Frequent blood glucose assays should be performed, with a goal of approximately 100 mg/dL.

What complications of delivery are associated with diabetes in pregnancy?	Cephalopelvic disproportion Shoulder dystocia (while not predictable, anticipation allows preparation) Trauma
How should the woman be managed postpartum?	The patient should return to her preconception insulin dose and hypoglycemia should be avoided.
What newborn complications can occur?	Hyperbilirubinemia Hypoglycemia Hypocalcemia
What contraception methods are appropriate for women with diabetes?	Oral contraceptive pills can be used but with caution in women with vasculopathy. The IUD is usually not recommended in diabetes because of the increased risk of infection. The Paragard IUD insert lists diabetes as a contraindication. Barrier methods are probably optimal. Bilateral tubal ligation is acceptable for permanent contraception.

GESTATIONAL DIABETES MELLITUS

Because it is asymptomatic, how is gestational diabetes mellitus detected?	With a modified glucose tolerance test
How is the modified glucose tolerance test performed?	A 50-gram (g) oral glucose load is given. Blood is then sampled for glucose measurement 1 hour after the glucose load.
When is this test usually performed?	At approximately 28 weeks' gestation
What is an abnormal blood glucose level result of the modified glucose tolerance test?	> 140 mg/dL

Is this result diagnostic of gestational diabetes?	No
What test is used to diagnose gestational diabetes?	Standard glucose tolerance test
How is this test performed?	A 100-g glucose load is given after morning fasting. To ensure accurate test results, the patient must be healthy and eating an appropriate diet. Blood samples are taken immediately following the glucose load (fasting value) and at 1, 2, and 3 hours after the glucose load.
What are the normal values of a glucose tolerance test?	Fasting: < 105 mg/dL 1 hour: < 190 mg/dL 2 hour < 165 mg/dL 3 hour < 145 mg/dL
What results are diagnostic of gestational diabetes?	Abnormal fasting value or two abnormal values in either the 1-, 2-, or 3-hour samples
What are the risk factors for gestational diabetes?	Obesity Age > 30 History of large infant(s) History of unexplained stillbirth Ethnicity (American Indians)
Who should be screened for gestational diabetes?	Women with risk factors Some experts advocate universal screening.
How is gestational diabetes managed?	Dietary and/or insulin management to achieve euglycemia See Table 21-3

Table 21–3. Gestational Diabetes

Diabetes Classification	Mode/Timing of Test
Diet therapy with adequate control	NST weekly; begin at 40 weeks
Diet therapy with poor control	NST twice weekly; begin at 37 weeks
Insulin with adequate control	NST twice weekly; begin at 37 weeks
Insulin with poor control or other risk factors	NST twice weekly; begin at 34 weeks
H/O prior IUFD	NST twice weekly; begin at 2 weeks before

What percentage of women with gestational diabetes "become" Type II diabetics?	Fifty percent if obese and stay that way
How is diabetes after pregnancy diagnosed?	With a modified or standard glucose tolerance test at 6-8 weeks' postpartum (Table 21-4)

Table 21–4. Timing of Delivery

Diabetes Classification	Timing
GDM; good control on ???	By 42 weeks
GDM; all others	By 40 weeks

22

Obstetrics Infections

INTRODUCTION

What are the "TORCH" infections?

"TORCH" is an acronym for the common nonbacterial congenital infections that can lead to a variety of fetal and neonatal problems.

T = Toxoplasmosis
O = Other [e.g., varicella-zoster virus (VZV), parvovirus, and other organisms]
R = Rubella
C = Cytomegalovirus (CMV)
H = Herpes simplex virus (HSV)

What is the incidence of TORCH infections?

Cause disease in about 1% of all births and lead to serious disease in about 10% of infected infants

What are the characteristic neonatal signs and symptoms of TORCH syndrome?

Prematurity
Intrauterine growth retardation (IUGR)
Microcephaly
Hepatosplenomegaly with jaundice
Thrombocytopenia
Hemolytic anemia
Chorioretinitis
Adenopathy
Rash

How are perinatal infections diagnosed?

By isolating or detecting the organism in question from tissue obtained from amniocentesis or chorion villus sampling (By culture, PCR, ELISA)
By documenting seroconversion (the presence of antibodies to the organism in question) in maternal or fetal blood
By ultrasound in combination with the clinical picture

What are possible consequences of infection to the fetus?

Interference with organogenesis with consequent structural anomalies with infection in the first trimester

Neurologic impairment secondary to interference with nervous system development (generally occurs throughout the pregnancy and thus impairment can occur late in pregnancy)

Depression and acidosis at birth

Poor sucking reflex, vomiting, or abdominal distension at birth

Respiratory insufficiency at birth

Lethargy or jitteriness at birth

Hypothermia at birth

Depressed total leukocyte or neutrophil counts at birth

Via which immunoglobulin does the fetus respond to infection?

The fetus synthesizes IgM as the primary response to infection.

Development of fetal cell-mediated and humoral immunity begins at 9 to 15 weeks' gestation.

How does the mother contribute to fetal immunocompetence?

Maternal IgG passes transplacentally and provides passive immunity.

Transfer of IgG begins at 16 weeks' gestation.

By 26 weeks, $[IgG]_{fetal} = [IgG]_{maternal}$.

By what routes can the fetus/neonate become infected?

Some agents (e.g., VZV, rubella, and CMV) move transplacentally to cause intrauterine infection.

Other routes of access include ascending chorioamnionitis (intrauterine), maternal exposure (intrapartum), external contamination (intrapartum), and neonatal human or nosocomial exposure.

TOXOPLASMOSIS

What is toxoplasmosis?

A protozoal infection that can be transmitted from mother to fetus (*Toxoplasma gondii*).

Where is *Toxoplasma gondii* found?

In undercooked meat as infective tissue cysts and in cat feces as oocysts, which can become aerosolized

How is *Toxoplasma gondii* transmitted?

By ingestion of infected meat or exposure to infected cat feces

How common is infection in adults and in pregnancy?

Approximately 15% to 40% of adult women in the United States have toxoplasmosis antibodies (IgG) and, hence, immunity.

About 1 in 1000 pregnancies are affected by acute toxoplasmosis infection.

How does congenital infection and outcome differ in the first and third trimesters?

In general, congenital infection in the third trimester is more common, whereas infection in the first trimester is more severe.

Third-trimester infection is associated with a 60% congenital infection rate, with most infections subclinical or mild.

First-trimester infection is associated with a 10% congenital infection rate, but two-thirds of these fetuses have severe symptoms. Five percent of first-trimester infections result in perinatal death or stillbirth.

Second-trimester infection is associated with a 25% risk of transmission.

What are the maternal signs and symptoms of toxoplasmosis?

Usually asymptomatic, but careful documentation can reveal a mononucleosis-like syndrome with symptoms such as fever, chills, headache, fatigue, muscle pains, and lymphadenopathy in 60% to 90% of patients.

What are the fetal and neonatal signs and symptoms of toxoplasmosis?

The classic triad of hydrocephalus, intracranial calcifications, and chorioretinitis is rarely seen.

Seventy-five percent of infected newborns are asymptomatic at birth.

Twenty-five percent of infected newborns have low birth weight, hepatosplenomegaly, icterus, anemia, convulsions, intracranial calcifications, hydrocephaly or microcephaly, microphthalmia, and chorioretinitis.

How is toxoplasmosis diagnosed in the mother?

Toxoplasma antibodies indicate acute disease or prior infection.

Antibodies can be detected using hemagglutination, immunofluorescence, or ELISA techniques.

Anti-toxoplasma IgG antibody titers can be obtained, but cannot differentiate between a prior toxoplasmosis infection (which confers immunity) and an infection acquired during pregnancy (which can pose a threat to the fetus).

High IgG titers suggest recent or current infection, whereas lower titers should be followed to determine if a rise in titer occurs, which suggests active infection (a fourfold increase in IgG titer over 2–3 weeks).

Toxoplasma-specific IgM testing can differentiate acute illness from prior exposure.

How is toxoplasmosis diagnosed in the fetus?

Culture and serologic testing of fetal blood and amnionic fluid (cord blood IgM is indicative of fetal infection)

Serial fetal brain ultrasound

PCR assays, which may soon be commonly employed to study amnionic fluid when infection is suspected

Placental culture (positive in 90% of infections)

How is toxoplasmosis prevented?

Avoidance of undercooked meat, unpasteurized goat's milk, and cat litter or feces

| How is toxoplasmosis treated? | Proper antimicrobial therapy: either spiramycin alone or pyrimethamine plus sulfadiazine |

| What are the recommendations for prenatal screening of toxoplasmosis? | Routine prenatal screening of toxoplasmosis is not recommended except for pregnant women with HIV. |

RUBELLA

| What is rubella and what is another name for the virus? | Also known as German measles, rubella is caused by a single-stranded RNA togavirus capable of causing severe fetal and neonatal problems.
Infection is not threatening in the nonpregnant state. |

| Why is rubella infection so rare today? | The incidence of rubella in the United States has decreased as a result of vaccination. |

| Is the incidence of congenital rubella syndrome (CRS) increasing or decreasing? | Data suggest a recent resurgence of cases of CRS from an all-time low of 225 cases in 1988 to annual totals of 1093 cases from 1988 to 1990. |

| What may account for this change in incidence? | Six percent to eleven percent of postpubertal women remain seronegative despite attempts at uniform vaccination, according to premarital screening programs.
Greater than 50% of CRS cases may be caused by missed testing or vaccination opportunities. |

| What are the signs and symptoms of maternal rubella infection? | Rash can be the sole presenting symptom.
The remainder of cases are asymptomatic (25%–50% of infections are subclinical despite viremia and embryo or fetal infection). |

Outcomes of maternal infection include normal infant, spontaneous abortion, or CRS.

What are the signs and symptoms of fetal rubella infection (CRS)?

Cataracts and other eye problems (chorioretinitis, microphthalmia)

Cardiac malformations (patent ductus arteriosus, septal defects, and pulmonary artery hypoplasia)

Sensorineural deafness (detected after 1 year of age)

Central nervous system (meningoencephalitis, microcephaly, psychomotor retardation, brain calcifications)

Symmetric IUGR

Hematologic problems (thrombocytopenia, hemolytic anemia)

Hepatic problems (hepatitis, hepatosplenomegaly, jaundice)

Chronic interstitial pneumonitis

Bony changes

Chromosome abnormalities

What are the signs and symptoms of childhood rubella infection?

Panencephalitis and type I diabetes (extended rubella syndrome) in up to one-third of infants asymptomatic at birth

May not develop until second or third decade of life

When is maternal rubella infection most likely to result in congenital infection?

The congenital infection rate with maternal rash/infection in the first trimester is 80% to 90%.

The risk of congenital infection at 13 to 14 weeks' gestation is 54%.

The risk of congenital infection by the end of the second trimester is 25%.

When is maternal rubella infection most likely to result in congenital defects?

Infected fetuses are most prone to develop serious defects from infection prior to 11 weeks' estimated gestational age.

Fetuses infected between 13 and 16 weeks' gestation have a 35% risk of utero defect formation.

No studies have demonstrated congenital defects when maternal infection occurred after 20 weeks' gestation.

How is rubella diagnosed?

Diagnosis in the pregnant state is usually made after the appearance of a rash with conversion from absent rubella antibodies to positive titers.

Viremia precedes clinically evident disease by 1 week.

What is the temporal relationship between infection and antibody detection?

Peak antibody titers occur 1 to 2 weeks after rash or 2 to 3 weeks after viremia.

IgM and IgG antibody titers increase with rash onset; IgM disappears by 1 to 2 months, whereas IgG is present for life.

What specific serologic findings are diagnostic of maternal rubella infection?

Either a fourfold increase in acute and convalescent sera of total of IgG rubella antibody titers over 2 weeks, or the presence of rubella IgM antibody

What specific serologic findings are diagnostic of maternal rubella infections?

High IgG antibody titers are present in 15% of the normal population.

Acute IgG titers should be saved and tested later in parallel with convalescent specimen of IgG titers to determine a rise in IgG titer.

Why is rubella-specific IgM useful in diagnosis of rubella?

Rubella-specific IgM may distinguish acute rubella from prior immunization or infection (peaks at 7 to 10 days after onset of illness and persists for 4 weeks).

How are IgG and IgM antibodies quantitated?

Hemagglutination inhibition
ELISA
Indirect immunofluorescent assays

How is rubella diagnosed in the fetus?

Fetal IgM can be detected in cord blood (sensitivity, 98%; specificity, 100% after 22 weeks' gestation)

Amniotic fluid isolation of the virus has been used.

RNA identification via in situ hybridization or PCR is a promising technique to detect rubella.

When should prenatal diagnosis be undertaken?

Between weeks 8 and 18 gestation, if infection is suspected

Establishment of a diagnosis is not necessary if infection occurs after midgestation, as fetal complications are rare.

Does the absence of rubella-specific IgM antibody rule out active infection?

Absence of IgM does not definitively rule out acute rubella infection.

In the presence of acute infection, it is possible to have a false-negative IgM titer because the antibody may decrease initially.

In women with previously documented rubella-specific antibody presence, a rise in rubella IgG antibody titer in the absence of detectable IgM should be interpreted as potential reinfection and consultation with a clinical virologist or other expert in diagnosis of rubella is warranted.

Does the presence of rubella-specific IgM antibody rule in active infection?

False-positive IgM assays, although rare, are possible with indirect assays such as ELISA or indirect fluorescent immunoassay.

Diagnosis of acute rubella infection should be based on the appropriate clinical scenario in conjunction with IgG and IgM testing.

How is rubella infection screened for and prevented?

All pregnant women should be screened for rubella immunization at their first prenatal visit and non-immune women should be given the vaccine postpartum.

Non-immune women should be given the live attenuated rubella vaccine at routine medical, gynecologic, and family planning clinic visits and after childbirth and abortion.

Children 12 to 15 months of age should be vaccinated and all school children without record of previous rubella vaccination should be vaccinated.

Infants born with congenital rubella syndrome should be isolated from other infants to prevent spread of rubella.

Because the vaccine contains live, attenuated virus, it cannot be administered shortly before (pregnancy should be delayed for three months after receiving vaccine) or during pregnancy.

What are the risks of administering rubella vaccine to pregnant women?

All women with positive rubella-specific antibody documentation prior to pregnancy can be presumed to be immune.

Although there is no proven risk of vaccine administration to pregnant women, this recommendation that pregnant women should not be vaccinated remains on theoretic grounds.

Can women vaccinated postpartum breast-feed?

Postpartum vaccination should not prevent breast-feeding, although vaccine virus may be excreted in milk and cause infant seroconversion.

How is rubella infection treated?

There is no known treatment for active rubella infection.

Abortion can be offered with early infection.

CYTOMEGALOVIRUS

What is cytomegalovirus (CMV)?

CMV is a member of the DNA herpesvirus family.
It is a commonly acquired infection in daycare centers.

How is CMV transmitted?

Horizontally by droplets, saliva, and urine
Vertically from mother to fetus (via transplacental infection, delivery, and breast-feeding)
Via sexual contact and through blood transfusions

How common is CMV?

It is the most common cause of perinatal infection (0.5% to 2% of all neonates).
The risk of seroconversion in susceptible women during pregnancy is 1% to 4%.
One percent to two percent of all infants excrete CMV in their urine.
Thirty percent to sixty percent of school-age children and sixty percent of all pregnant women are seropositive.

What important factor predisposes adults to CMV infection?

Risk is increased in immunocompromised individuals.

What are the maternal signs and symptoms of CMV infection?

A mononucleosis-like syndrome (fever, pharyngitis, lymphadenopathy, and polyarthritis) is present in 15% of cases.
The remainder of cases are asymptomatic.
Presentation is not affected by pregnancy.

What are the fetal and neonatal signs and symptoms of CMV infection?

Fetal (cytomegalic inclusion disease): symmetric IUGR, nonimmune hydrops, low birth weight, microcephaly, hydrocephaly, microphthalmia, intracranial calcifications, chorioretinitis, psychomotor retardation, deafness, hepatosplenomegaly, jaundice, hemolytic anemia, and thrombocytopenic purpura

Neonatal: 90% of infected newborns are asymptomatic at birth, but may have later onset of hearing loss, mental retardation, visual impairment, or delayed psychomotor development.

How often do infected infants manifest evidence of congenital CMV syndrome?

Congenital cytomegalovirus infection (cytomegalic inclusion disease) leads to syndrome in 10% of 40,000 infected neonates born annually and later onset of hearing loss and intellectual impairment in 10% to 15%.

How does CMV infection vary with socioeconomic status?

Approximately 55% of high-income pregnant women are immune to CMV.

Approximately 85% of low-income pregnant women are immune to CMV.

Why is it important to determine if the infection is primary or recurrent?

Most congenital infections are acquired from maternal reactivation.

Recurrent infection is associated with a low (.15%–2%) risk of transmission and a small number (.1%) of infants with clinically apparent disease or sequelae.

Primary infection is associated with an approximately 40% to 50% transplacental transmission rate; 10% to 20% of these infants are symptomatic at birth.

High-income women have a high risk of developing primary infection and thus are more susceptible to having infants with clinically apparent disease.

How is CMV screened for and diagnosed in the mother?

Primary infection is suggested by fourfold increased IgG titers in paired acute and convalescent sera measured simultaneously.

IgM detection in maternal serum is also generally predictive of primary infection, as IgM is usually not produced in recurrent infection (peaks 3–6 months after infection and disappears in 1 to 2 years).

How is CMV screened for and diagnosed in the fetus?

Ultrasound: intracranial calcifications, symmetric IUGR, nonimmune hydrops or ascites and CNS anomalies (nonspecific findings)

Amniotic fluid culture

Total IgM (CMV-specific) and elevated γ-glutamyl transferase by cordocentesis

CMV-specific DNA in chorionic villi (PCR)

CMV-specific IgM may not be a reliable test; amniotic fluid cultures are probably the best test (80%–100% sensitivity) while DNA results show good correlation with cultures and clinical outcome.

How is CMV infection treated?

There is no effective treatment for maternal infection, although intrauterine treatment with ganciclovir or other antiviral agents may prove safe and effective.

Abortion is an option.

How can CMV infection be prevented?

Serologic screening for CMV during pregnancy is not recommended.

Good hygiene and hand-washing practices, avoidance of kissing and nuzzling infants, and use of latex gloves may prevent transmission among health care workers.

Can personnel in dialysis and neonatal units work while pregnant?

There is no evidence that transfer to another unit or to a different patient population decreases the risk of CMV infection.

Compliance with universal precautions should be emphasized.

Routine screening of hospital employees for serologic testing of CMV is not recommended.

HERPES SIMPLEX VIRUS

What is herpes simplex virus (HSV)?

HSV is a herpesvirus and can be either type 1 (HSV-1) or type 2 (HSV-2).

Approximately what percentage of HSV infections are caused by type 1 and type 2?

Approximately 85% of primary genital herpes infections in adults are caused by HSV-2 and the remainder by HSV-1. HSV-1 causes most nongenital herpetic infections.

Neonatal infection is more commonly caused by HSV-2 (75%); approximately 25% of isolates from infected neonates are HSV-1.

What is the incidence of HSV in the general population?

A national study of serology revealed that 25% of all women have HSV-2 antibodies.

What are the risk factors for presence of HSV antibodies?

African-American race
Previous marriage

How is HSV transmitted?

Via intimate mucocutaneous contact

How common is HSV infection in pregnancy?

HSV infection is thought to have the same frequency in pregnancy as in the nonpregnant state.

Estimates vary from shedding in 0.1% to 0.4% of all deliveries to positive cultures in 0.2% to 7.4% of asymptomatic women.

Does pregnancy alter the course of HSV infection?

No

What is the typical duration of primary versus recurrent HSV outbreaks?

Primary HSV infections last approximately 2 to 3 weeks.
Recurrent HSV infections have a shorter 5 to 10 day course.
Asymptomatic infections also occur and their course is unknown.

How does the neonate acquire HSV?

Proposed mechanisms include the following:
During delivery (passage through infected birth canal)
Prior to delivery [ascending infection (90% of cases), especially with rupture of membranes or via transplacental passage of virus]
After delivery (close contact with an infected mother, relative, or health care worker)

Does neonatal risk of HSV infection vary in primary versus recurrent HSV?

Primary infection is associated with 50% transmission to the neonate in vaginal delivery.
Recurrent infection is associated with only a 4% transmission rate.
This difference may be related to virus shedding for 1 to 2 weeks during primary infection compared with 3 to 6 days during recurrent infection, or to the protective effect of maternal antibodies in recurrent infection.
Overall, neonatal herpes occurs in 0.01% to 0.04% of deliveries (two-thirds of which are preterm infants).

What is the mortality rate of neonatal HSV?

Approximately 60% in infants infected with HSV delivered vaginally by a mother with a primary outbreak

What is the incubation period for HSV?

Prodromal symptoms after primary infection with HSV occur within 3 to 6 days of infection.

What are the varied maternal signs and symptoms of HSV infection?

Asymptomatic

Prodrome: tingling, burning, or pruritus in vulvar area

Inguinal adenopathy and flu-like symptoms

Painful vesicular lesions on an erythematous base that eventually ulcerate primarily on the labia minora, but can be found anywhere on the vulva, vagina, or cervix

Urinary retention if pain is significant

Disseminated disease: rare and has a high mortality rate; may result in hepatitis, thrombocytopenia, coagulopathy, meningitis, and encephalitis

What complications of pregnancy are associated with HSV infection?

Spontaneous abortion and preterm labor

What are the fetal signs and symptoms of HSV infection?

Death (60% of those infected at vaginal delivery from a mother with primary HSV infection)

Disseminated infection involving major viscera

Sequelae include microcephaly, mental retardation, seizures, microphthalmia, retinal dysplasia, chorioretinitis, meningitis, encephalitis, hypertonicity, apnea, and coma

How is HSV diagnosed?

Clinical diagnosis is made by identification of the typical lesion.

Viral isolation by tissue culture is highly accurate, with a sensitivity of 95% and few false-positive results.

Occasionally, the Pap smear report will cite cytopathic effects consistent with HSV, but these effects are not as accurate as direct isolation of the virus.

Likewise, the Tzanck preparation (scrapings from the lesion base) can be used for rapid diagnosis (findings include large multinucleated cells and eosinophilic viral inclusion bodies), but it is not as accurate as viral culture.

Antibodies appear within 7 days of the primary outbreak, peak in 2 to 3 weeks, and remain for life.

ELISA assays are available, but have low sensitivity, and PCR techniques are on the horizon.

What special tests should be done during prenatal care for women with a history of HSV?

Weekly surveillance cultures from 36 weeks' gestational age to term and amniocentesis to detect intrauterine infection are currently not recommended because they do not decrease the incidence of neonatal HSV and are not cost-effective.

Current recommendations are to obtain viral cultures of an active lesion on any pregnant woman with a reported history of HSV infection not proven by cultures or with new onset of a characteristic herpetic genital lesion for the first time in pregnancy.

How are women with a history of HSV managed in labor and delivery?

Careful internal and external genital examination to rule out the presence of any vulvo-vaginal lesions is extremely important.

Any woman with a lesion in labor or with ruptured membranes should undergo cesarean delivery to decrease the risk of neonatal HSV.

If no lesions are present, culture is not necessary and vaginal delivery is acceptable.

Should women with ruptured membranes undergo cesarean section?

This topic is controversial.

The "four hour rule" suggests that if the membranes have been ruptured for more than 4 hours in a woman in whom herpes infection is strongly suspected, cesarean section should not be performed because the fetus has already been exposed to the virus through an ascending route from the vagina into the uterus.

However, practitioners now perform cesarean sections in cases of suspected infection regardless of the duration of membrane rupture because a clear cause–effect relationship between the duration of membrane rupture and neonatal infection has not been established.

How is HSV infection treated?

Because herpes virus resides in nerve ganglia, it is currently impossible to be completely "cured" of the virus.

Acyclovir has been used to treat primary HSV infections, recurrent HSV infections, and as prophylaxis against developing recurrent infections.

Because of uncertainty regarding teratogenicity in pregnancy, acyclovir is currently recommended in pregnancy only for life-threatening infections.

Disseminated HSV should be treated with parenteral acyclovir.

Symptoms such as urinary retention or pain may be treated with a Foley catheter or lidocaine gel if needed and may require hospitalization.

OTHER VIRAL INFECTIONS

VARICELLA-ZOSTER VIRUS

What is varicella-zoster virus (VZV)?

Varicella-zoster virus (VZV) is 1 of 6 human herpesviruses.

It is comprised of double-stranded DNA surrounded by a lipid and protein envelope.

How is VZV infection transmitted?

It is highly contagious and is transmitted via household contacts and other routes of exposure (respiratory secretions and droplets, direct contact, indirect contact with secretions).

The attack rate of VZV is 90%.

Enters the host via the conjunctivae and mucosa. Moves into the bloodstream and replaces the skin via capillaries, and finally enters the dorsal root ganglia of sensory nerves where it remains latent.

What diseases does VZV cause?

Varicella (chickenpox) and herpes zoster (shingles, a reactivation of the virus)

How common is chickenpox in general and in pregnancy?

Chickenpox is the second most commonly reported communicable disease in the United States.

It is uncommon in pregnancy (it occurs approximately 1 in 7500 pregnant women).

Prenatal serology shows that 95% of women in the United States are immune.

What is the mortality rate of infection in nonpregnant adults?

Approximately 50/100,000

What is the incubation period of VZV?

Ten to twenty-one days

What are the maternal signs and symptoms of VZV infection in pregnancy?

Prodrome (2–3 days): fever, malaise, myalgia, arthralgia, and headache

Lesions: initially vesicular and intensely pruritic maculopapular lesions that break open and crust over, causing pustules and scabs on the face, scalp, and trunk

Pneumonia: may develop 1 to 6 days after rash with cough, dyspnea, fever, pleuritic chest pain, hemoptysis; chest x-ray reveals diffuse bilateral infiltrates

Encephalitis: potential complication in infected adults

VZV has been implicated in preterm labor.

What are the fetal signs and symptoms of VZV infection?

Can result in asymptomatic seroconversion, congenital varicella syndrome, or neonatal varicella

Congenital varicella syndrome (varicella embryopathy) affects the following systems:

Extremities: hypoplasia or contractures

Skin: cutaneous scars

Eye: chorioretinitis, microphthalmia, cataracts

Central nervous system: cervical or lumbosacral cord involvement, cerebral cortical atrophy, microcephaly

Gastrointestinal system

Genitourinary system: hydronephrosis

Can also cause mental retardation and death

What are the neonatal signs and symptoms of VZV infection?

Disseminated visceral and central nervous system disease, which can be fatal if untreated

What is the infection rate of neonates if delivered to a VZV-infected mother?

Twenty-five percent to fifty percent of neonates are infected.

Neonatal infection is possible if the mother develops a rash in the 5 days preceding or 2 days following parturition.

What are typical incubation periods in maternal and neonatal infection?

Maternal incubation period: 11 to 21 days (mean 15 days)

Average incubation period in the neonate: 11 days

When is the fetus most susceptible to maternal VZV infection?

Twenty-five percent to fifty percent of fetuses are infected during maternal infection with a 2% to 5% risk of congenital varicella syndrome (the risk is 10% if VZV is acquired in the first trimester).

Most cases of congenital varicella syndrome result from maternal infection occurring at less than 20 weeks' gestation.

When is the infectious period of VZV infection?

From 2 days prior to the appearance of the rash until all lesions are crusted

How common is varicella pneumonia in pregnancy and why is it so important?

It occurs in 10% to 30% of all cases of VZV infection in pregnancy.

Mortality rates for varicella pneumonia in pregnancy have been quoted as high as 20% to 40%.

How is VZV diagnosed in the mother?

Clinical assessment

Tzanck prep (multinucleated giant cells with intranuclear inclusions for varicella, zoster, and HSV)

Culture: vesicular fluid within 3 to 4 days of appearance of rash (virus grows easily in culture)

Fluorescent antibody to membrane antigen of ELISA techniques to determine varicella serology and confirm a prior infection

What are the typical changes in antibody titers in VZV infection?

IgM rises within 2 weeks of infection.

IgG rise in paired sera taken 2 weeks apart indicates infection.

How is VZV diagnosed in the fetus?

Ultrasound (microcephaly, limb deformities, polyhydramnios, liver hyperechogenicities, fetal hydrops)

VZV-specific IgM in fetal cord blood (cordocentesis)

Amniotic fluid culture

CVS with PCR

How is VZV diagnosed in the neonate?

Characteristic findings include limb hypoplasia, cutaneous scars, chorioretinitis, cataracts, cortical atrophy, microcephaly, and symmetric IUGR.

How is VZV infection treated?

All pregnant women with acute VZV infection require chest x-ray to rule out pneumonia.

Treatment is recommended for maternal infection with visceral involvement (pneumonia or encephalitis) or high fever using acyclovir (12.4 mg/kg or 500 mg/m^2 every 8 hours) within 72 hours of rash onset or onset of respiratory symptoms.

Some advocate abortion if desired by the mother in the presence of limb abnormalities on a 20-week ultrasound.

All women without a history of chickenpox should be passively immunized with varicella-zoster immune globulin (VZIG) within 96 hours of an exposure to chickenpox.

Neonates exposed peripartum should receive VZIG and/or acyclovir within 72 hours of birth if born to mothers with infection onset from 5 days before until 2 days after delivery.

Exposed infants should be isolated.

How can VZV infection be prevented?

Avoidance of persons known to have chickenpox

Isolation of the affected patient from other pregnant women if hospitalized

Isolation of the neonate from an infected mother

Passive immunization (VZIG) in susceptible patients within 96 hours of a significant exposure

How effective is VZIG in preventing VZV infection?

Eighty percent of susceptible patients given VZIG remain symptom-free.

Eighty-nine percent of susceptible patients not given VZIG have symptoms.

Varicella vaccine is a live attenuated virus and should not be given in pregnancy.

HUMAN IMMUNODEFICIENCY VIRUS

What is human immunodeficiency virus (HIV)?

HIV is an RNA retrovirus that uses reverse transcriptase to transcribe DNA from its native RNA.

HIV DNA is incorporated into the infected cell's genome.

It enters cells via the CD4 antigen.

The primary target cells of HIV are the T-helper lymphocytes, but macrophages, CNS neurons, and even placental cells can be infected.

What are risk factors for HIV infection in women?

Illicit drug abuse (especially IV drug use)

Current or previous multiple sexual partners or prostitution

Transfusion of blood products prior to 1985

Sexual intercourse with bisexual men or IV drug users

Origin in endemic countries (e.g., West Africa)

History of or current sexually transmitted diseases (STDs)

What is the significance of the CD4 count?

The CD4 count is inversely related to the immunocompetence of the HIV-infected individual.

The lower the CD4 count, the less cell-mediated immunity and the more likely the risk of acquiring opportunistic infections that attack the immunosuppressed susceptible individual.

The Centers for Disease Control (CDC) has designated a CD4 count lower than 200 as one definition of "AIDS."

What constitutes the diagnosis of AIDS?

Serologic evidence of HIV infection and a history of characteristic, ARDS-related opportunistic infections, or

Pathognomonic-associated illnesses without serologic evidence of HIV, or

A CD4 count of less than 200

What are some opportunistic infections associated with AIDS?

Extrapulmonary cryptococcus (i.e., cryptococcal meningitis)

Cryptosporidiosis-associated diarrhea

Disseminated *Mycobacterium avium* complex (**MAI**)

Tuberculosis

Pneumocystis carinii pneumonia (PCP)

Cerebral toxoplasmosis

Disseminated coccidioidomycosis

CMV retinitis

Disseminated histoplasmosis

Esophageal or pulmonary candidiasis

Persistent herpes simplex or zoster

Condyloma accuminata

What are some neoplasms commonly associated with AIDS?

Kaposi's sarcoma

Brain lymphoma

Small noncleaved cell lymphoma

Some non-Hodgkin's lymphomas

What noninfectious, nonmalignant conditions are associated with HIV?

Progressive multifocal leukoencephalopathy

HIV encephalopathy ("HIV dementia"; "AIDS dementia")

HIV wasting syndrome ("slim disease")

What serologic tests are used to diagnose HIV infection?

ELISA testing for HIV antibody (sensitivity > 99%)

Western blot assay for HIV antibody (sensitivity = 99% and specificity = 99.8%); used to confirm a positive ELISA test

"HIV-positive" status requires either two positive ELISA tests followed by a positive Western blot or a positive HIV antigen test or a positive HIV culture.

What is the "window phase"?

The time between initial HIV infection and demonstration of antibodies in the blood of the infected individual

The appearance of HIV antibodies typically occurs 6 to 12 weeks after infection, but may take up to 6 months or longer.

What are the initial signs and symptoms of HIV infection?

Can be asymptomatic or associated with an acute mononucleosis-like syndrome that may be associated with an aseptic meningitis

How is HIV virus acquired?

Through parenteral exposure to blood, sexual activity, and vertical transmission from mother to fetus

What is the prevalence of HIV in pregnant women?

A 1991 study suggested 1.5/1000 pregnant women were HIV positive, but this number may be much greater today.

Is prenatal HIV testing compulsory?

Prenatal compulsory screening for HIV has not yet been accepted by society.

Some states have laws that require offering HIV testing to all pregnant women and explaining the possible benefits to the patient and her fetus with treatment.

Screening should be offered to all pregnant women.

How does pregnancy affect HIV-infected patients?

Pregnancy does not affect disease progression, immune status, or morbidity or mortality rates.

Rates of preterm birth, low-birth–weight neonates, and complications in pregnancy likewise have not been proven to be markedly different in asymptomatic HIV-infected individuals compared with individuals not infected with HIV.

Adverse pregnancy outcomes are common in HIV-infected women with

CD4 of less than 14%. Rate of preterm birth = 20%. IUGR = 24%. Still births with maternal HIV infection may be increased.

How is HIV passed from mother to fetus?

Unknown, but may be transmitted by both transplacental and intrapartum pathways

What is the perinatal transmission rate of HIV from mother to fetus?

Maternal–fetal transmission of HIV infection occurs in 25% to 35% of pregnancies.

The transmission rate may be increased in women with low CD4 counts and advanced disease.

How does zidovudine (ZDV) affect the perinatal transmission rate of HIV?

A monumental study in 1994 found a 67.5% decrease in risk of HIV transmission from mother to infant with antepartum and intrapartum use of zidovudine.

The 25.5% transmission rate in the placebo group was reduced to 8.3% in the treated group.

Women included in the study had CD4 counts greater than 200 and had not received previous antiretroviral therapy.

ZDV was administered orally from the end of the first trimester until delivery and intravenously during labor and delivery.

Neonates were given ZDV for 6 weeks from 12 hours of life.

Should cesarean section be performed in HIV-positive women?

Scheduled C-section should be discussed & recommended for HIV-infected women with an HIV-RNA load of greater than 1000 copies.

This is whether or not antiretroviral therapy is ongoing.

Scheduled delivery may be done as early as 38 weeks to lessen the chance of membrane rupture.

Are scalp monitors, episiotomies, and forcep deliveries appropriate for HIV-positive women?

Currently, no consensus exits about whether or not scalp monitor placement, episiotomy, or delivery via forceps affects maternal–fetal transmission.

On theoretic grounds, use of these invasive procedures should be limited as much as possible in HIV-infected parturients.

HEPATITIS VIRUSES

What are the hepatitis viruses?

A group of viruses, both DNA and RNA, that cause perturbation of liver function by preferentially invading hepatocytes and causing acute and chronic problems and sometimes death

All but hepatitis B are RNA viruses.

Responsible for the most common serious liver disease in pregnancy

How is hepatitis infection diagnosed clinically?

Symptoms of acute hepatitis include malaise, fatigue, anorexia, nausea and vomiting, headache, and right upper quadrant or epigastric pain.

Physical examination may reveal jaundice, upper abdominal tenderness, and liver enlargement.

Encephalopathy and coagulopathy may be present in severe cases.

What are common laboratory findings in viral hepatitis?

Elevated liver aminotransferase (AST and ALT) levels (400–4000 U/L) and elevated serum bilirubin levels (5–20 mg/dl) in acute hepatitis

Coagulation abnormalities and hyperammonemia in severe cases

The peaks of AST or ALT do not correspond to disease severity.

What illness associated with pregnancy must be

Acute fatty liver of pregnancy, a rare condition characterized by nausea,

**ruled out with liver-
associated symptoms?**

vomiting, malaise, anorexia, epigastric pain, and jaundice and commonly associated with hypertension, proteinuria, edema, and coagulopathy in late pregnancy should always be differentiated from viral hepatitis.

The maternal mortality rate of 25% and fetal mortality rate of 50% in acute fatty liver of pregnancy emphasize the need for proper diagnosis.

Differentiation can be made by serologic studies and liver biopsy (viral hepatitis is characterized by a pattern of extensive hepatocellular injury and inflammatory infiltrate, whereas acute fatty liver of pregnancy causes microvesicular fat deposition) if needed.

Marked hypoglycemia is common.

Hepatitis A virus (infectious hepatitis)

**What is hepatitis A virus,
how is it transmitted, what
is the incubation period,
and what is the incidence
in pregnancy?**

Hepatitis A virus is an RNA picornavirus and causes approximately one-third of all cases of acute hepatitis in the United States

Transmission: usually via fecal–oral contamination and is increased with poor hygiene, poor sanitation, and intimate contact

Incubation period-2–7 weeks.

Incidence in pregnancy: affects about 1/1000 pregnancies.

**How is hepatitis A
diagnosed serologically?**

Hepatitis A virus IgM antibodies

Demonstration of IgG hepatitis A antibodies suggest prior infection.

**How is hepatitis A
infection prevented and
treated?**

An inactivated hepatitis A vaccine is effective in >90% of cases.

The vaccine appears to be safe for use in pregnancy and should be administered to women with risk factors for infection.

Immunotherapy with hepatitis A virus immune globulin is also used in both nonpregnant and pregnant women, especially those traveling to endemic areas and for postexposure prophylaxis.

What is the perinatal transmission rate of hepatitis A infection?

Associated with perinatal transmission

Hepatitis B virus (serum hepatitis)

What is hepatitis B virus, how is it transmitted, and what is the incidence in pregnancy?

Hepatitis B virus is a DNA hepadnavirus that causes approximately 40% of hepatitis cases in the United States.

Transmission: The virus is carried in vaginal secretions, semen, blood, saliva, and breast milk and is transmitted via contact with body secretions; risk factors include IV drug use, sexual promiscuity, and exposure to blood (health care workers, hemodialysis technicians, transfusion recipients), especially in endemic areas (Asia and Africa).

Incidence in pregnancy: occurs in 1 to 2/ 1000 pregnancies acutely, and 5 to 15/ 1000 pregnant women are hepatitis B virus carriers in the United States.

What is the composition of the hepatitis B virus and the associated antigens?

The hepatitis B virus, also known as the Dane particle, is composed of an outer shell, a middle portion, and the viral genome.

Hepatitis B surface antigen (HBsAg) is found on the outer viral shell, but can also circulate free in the serum and is the first marker of infection.

Hepatitis B core antigen (HBcAg) lies in the middle portion of the Dane particle and is found only in hepatocytes (it does not circulate freely like HBsAg).

Hepatitis B e antigen (HBeAg) has its messenger RNA transcribed on the same part of the genome as the core antigen, and it is found when a significant amount of Dane particle is present in the serum; thus, HBeAg correlates with infectivity.

How is hepatitis B infection diagnosed serologically?

Acute infection is diagnosed by an immunoglobin M response to the core antigen (anti-HBc) and the presence of the surface antigen.

Detection of HBeAg in acute infection implies severe infection.

Chronic infection is suggested by detecting HBsAg without an IgM antibody response to the core antigen.

What is the perinatal transmission rate of hepatitis B virus?

Women who test positive for the hepatitis B surface antigen have a 10% to 20% risk of transmitting the virus to the fetus in pregnancy.

Ninety percent of women with HBeAg transmit the virus to the fetus.

What is the mechanism for fetal and neonatal infection?

The majority of cases of perinatal transmission are the result of exposure of the fetus during labor to blood and vaginal secretions.

Other mechanisms for infection that occur less frequently include transplacental infection, breastfeeding, and close contact between the neonate and mother.

What are the maternal effects of hepatitis B infection?

Death in approximately 1% of cases

Resolution of symptoms and complete recovery in 85% of cases

Chronic infection in 14% of cases

Hepatitis and cirrhosis in about 10% to 30% of persons with chronic infection with persistently high HBeAg levels

Chronic infection is a significant risk factor for hepatocellular carcinoma.

What are the fetal/ neonatal effects of hepatitis B infection?

Fulminant hepatitis (rare)

Prematurity, low birth weight, and death

Eighty-five percent to ninety percent become chronic carriers.

Twenty-five percent ultimately develop hepatocellular carcinoma and cirrhosis.

How is hepatitis B infection prevented and treated?

Hepatitis B virus vaccine is the most effective method to prevent infection and is recommended for high-risk women, especially health care workers.

Vaccine administration is believed to be safe during pregnancy.

Hepatitis B immune globulin (HBIG) should be administered after high-risk contact in the pregnant or nonpregnant state.

All infants should receive hepatitis B vaccine after birth, with the second and third vaccine doses given to the infant at 1 and 6 months of age.

Administration of active (hepatitis B vaccine) and passive (HBIG) immunization within 12 hours of birth to neonates of carrier mothers decreases the perinatal transmission rate by 80% to 90%.

Interferon may also be used to treat acute hepatitis.

What are current prenatal screening recommendations?

Both the American College of Obstetrics and Gynecology (ACOG) and the CDC recommend universal hepatitis B screening of pregnant women at an early prenatal visit or at the first opportunity in a woman who presents later in pregnancy or in labor with no prenatal care.

High-risk women should be rescreened in the third trimester if the initial screen is negative.

Liver enzyme (AST and ALT) levels and a hepatitis panel should be tested in women who test positive.

Hepatitis B vaccine should be encouraged in women who test negative and have risk factors for infection.

Hepatitis C virus

What is hepatitis C virus, how is it transmitted, and what is the incubation period?

Hepatitis C virus is a single-stranded RNA virus of the flaviviridae family; it causes a parenterally transmitted non-A, non-B hepatitis.

It is responsible for 10% to 20% of cases of hepatitis in the United States.

Transmission: transmitted parenterally; risk factors for infection include a history of blood transfusions, use of IV drugs, and sex with an infected partner (transmission is the same as that of hepatitis B)

Incubation period: approximately 15 weeks

How is hepatitis C diagnosed serologically?

Demonstration of hepatitis C virus antibody

It is possible for the antibody production to be delayed for 2 to 4 months after the initial hepatitis flare.

What is the risk of perinatal transmission of hepatitis C?

Can be transmitted vertically, but the vertical transmission rate varies between 3–6%.

How is hepatitis C infection treated?

With interferon-α

Improvement occurs in 30% to 40% of patients, but relapse occurs in half of these patients.

Newborns can be given immune serum globulin in cases of seropositive mothers, although good data are not available regarding its effectiveness.

Hepatitis D virus

What is hepatitis D virus, how is it transmitted, and what is the incidence in pregnancy?

Hepatitis D (delta) virus is an RNA virus that requires hepatitis B virus infection to exert its effects on the host.

It is composed of a hepatitis B surface antigen and a delta core.

It coinfects about 1 in 4 patients infected with hepatitis B simultaneously.

It can cause superinfection (acute hepatitis D infection in a chronic hepatitis B carrier) with sequelae of chronic hepatitis, cirrhosis, and portal hypertension with a 25% mortality rate.

Transmission: same as that of hepatitis B virus

Incidence: rarely affects pregnancy

How is hepatitis D infection diagnosed serologically?

Presence of D antigen in liver tissue or blood and anti-hepatitis D IgM antibody

Chronic infection with hepatitis D is diagnosed with continued D antigen presence in the presence of IgM anti-D antibody.

How is hepatitis D infection prevented and treated?

Prevented with vaccination and immune prophylaxis against hepatitis B infection

Is hepatitis D infection transmitted vertically?

Can be transmitted vertically in pregnancy

Prevention tactics are the same as those used for hepatitis B (hepatitis B vaccination and immune globulin administration).

PARVOVIRUS B19

What is parvovirus B19?

A single-stranded DNA virus
The only known host of this virus is human beings.

What disease does parvovirus B19 cause, what are its symptoms, and what is its incubation period?

Causes erythema infectiosum, or "fifth disease"
Symptoms include a red macular facial rash, trunk rash, flu-like symptoms, and symmetric polyarthralgias (especially the hands)
Twenty percent of infections are asymptomatic.
The incubation period for parvovirus infection is about 1 week.

How is parvovirus transmitted?

Can be found in respiratory secretions and is thought to be transmitted via these secretions and hand-to-mouth contact, as well as possibly by infected blood products or transplacentally.

How is parvovirus infection diagnosed?

The presence of parvovirus IgM antibodies suggests current infection (IgM antibodies persist for several months) and they appear 2 weeks after infection.
The presence of IgG antibodies suggests a history of parvovirus exposure and immunity in the absence of IgM; they appear 3 weeks after infection.

How common is parvovirus infection and how often is it transmitted to the fetus?

Approximately 50% of pregnant women show parvovirus immunity.
About 1% of pregnant women seroconvert to show parvovirus IgG antibodies during pregnancy.
The transmission rate of parvovirus infection during pregnancy is estimated to be 20%.
Parvovirus is most commonly transmitted between 10 to 20 weeks' gestation.

What are fetal effects of parvovirus infection in pregnancy?	Associated with spontaneous abortion in the second trimester following maternal first-trimester infection Also linked to the rare development of nonimmune hydrops fetalis, which can resolve spontaneously or lead to fetal death Typically, the fetus is not affected by maternal parvovirus infection.
How is parvovirus-associated hydrops treated?	Intravascular transfusion may have a beneficial effect on parvovirus-associated nonimmune hydrops fetalis.

BACTERIAL INFECTIONS

GROUP B STREPTOCOCCUS

What is group B streptococcus (GBS) and what is its importance in perinatology?	Group B streptococcus (*Streptococcus agalactiae*) is a bacterium commonly found in the vagina and rectum of pregnant women. It is responsible for more life-threatening neonatal infections than any other organism. It is also a common pathogen in chorioamnionitis and postpartum endomyometritis.
What is the incidence of GBS colonization in pregnancy?	Estimates for vaginal GBS colonization range from 3% to 30%, depending on the population studied. Approximately 1 in 4 women has vaginal GBS colonization in pregnancy.
Where does colonization occur?	Primarily occurs in the rectum, with secondary genitourinary (bladder, vagina, and cervix) colonization; colonization of the throat and skin also occurs in healthy women
What are the signs and symptoms of maternal GBS colonization?	Usually asymptomatic
What are the fetal effects?	None are known

What are the maternal–neonatal transmission rates of GBS?

Range from 35% to 70%

Heavily colonized women are at greater risk of transmission.

It is important to differentiate fetal colonization (the presence of GBS without ill effects) from fetal infection

Preterm infants colonized with GBS have a 10% risk of developing sepsis; sepsis causes 90% of deaths reported from this disease.

Term infants colonized with GBS have only a 1% to 2% risk of sepsis.

Although preterm or low-birth weight infants are at highest risk, more than half of cases of neonatal sepsis are in term neonates.

What are the neonatal effects of GBS infection?

GBS infection in the neonate can lead to respiratory distress, neonatal sepsis, pneumonia, meningitis, shock, and death.

The mortality rate of early-onset (within 7 days of birth) infections is approximately 25%.

Thirty percent of infants with early-onset GBS sepsis and eighty percent of infants with late-onset GBS sepsis develop meningitis.

One-third of survivors of neonatal meningitis have long-term neurodevelopmental sequelae.

The majority of early-onset neonatal infections are diagnosed within 6–12 hours of birth.

What are the attack rates and modes of transmission of early-onset versus late-onset neonatal GBS infection?

Early-onset neonatal sepsis:

Attack rate: 1–2/1000 live births

Transmission: primarily via colonization at birth

Late-onset neonatal sepsis:

Attack rate: 0.5–1/1000 live births

Transmission: via intrapartum exposure (50%) and nosocomial or community exposure

What are the maternal effects of GBS colonization?

Can lead to GBS infection with chorioamnionitis, endomyometritis (20% of all cases, with onset within 48 hours of delivery and typical fulminant course), wound infection, and early postpartum febrile morbidity

Heavy colonization of the genitourinary tract increases the risk of infection for both the mother and fetus.

Presence of GBS in the urine implies heavy vaginal colonization, which increases the rate of neonatal infection to 10/1000 live births.

How is GBS colonization diagnosed?

Culture and latex agglutination or ELISA identification of the characteristic polysaccharide antigen

Cultures are accurate, but time-consuming and thus are not suitable for immediate decision making in labor and delivery

Rapid immunoassays appear inadequate for intrapartum detection of GBS as they are limited by low sensitivities.

How are cultures performed for GBS?

It is not necessary to culture samples from the cervix.

The lower vagina and rectum should both be swabbed and the swab placed in a selective culture medium.

What are the risk factors for neonatal GBS infection?

GBS colonization with each of the following:

Multiple gestation

Preterm labor (< 37 weeks)

Preterm premature rupture of the membranes (< 37 weeks)

Prolonged rupture of the membranes (> 18 hours)

Sibling affected by symptomatic GBS infection

Maternal fever during labor

What is the rationale for intrapartum antibiotic prophylaxis against GBS?

Neonatal GBS infection can have grave consequences (15% mortality rate; 33% risk to long-term neurodevelopmental problems after meningitis).

The attack rate is increased tenfold in neonates born to mothers with perinatal vaginal colonization.

Group B streptococcus is the most prevalent cause of serious neonatal infection.

Intrapartum antibiotic use decreases the risk of early-onset GBS disease by thirtyfold.

Antibiotics are inexpensive and have few side effects.

What are current recommendations regarding GBS prevention in neonates from ACOG, the CDC, and by the American Academy of Pediatrics (AAP)?

Culture-based strategy: intrapartum antibiotic use based on late prenatal culture (35–37 weeks' gestation) as the primary risk determinant; antibiotics given with positive cultures or if the mother has had a previous infant with invasive GBS disease, GBS bacteriuria in the current pregnancy.

What is the drug of choice for chemoprophylaxis of GBS?

Intravenous penicillin G, 5 million units initially followed by 2.5 million units every 4 hours

Ampicillin is an acceptable alternative and is given as an initial 2-g dose followed by 1 g every 4 hours.

LISTERIA MONOCYTOGENES

What is *Listeria monocytogenes?*

A gram-positive aerobic rod found in soil, water, sewage, unpasteurized milk or milk products, and carrier animal (pig and chicken) feces

How is *Listeria* transmitted and what is the incidence of infection?

Listeria can be transmitted via food products including cabbage, pasteurized milk, and fresh Mexican-style cheese.

Vertical transmission from mother to fetus occurs via transplacental passage, intrapartum, and via ascending infection.

Listeriosis affects 2 to 3 million people annually.

What are the maternal signs and symptoms of *Listeria* infection?

Asymptomatic

A general febrile illness that can be confused with the flu or pyelonephritis, usually mild and selflimited

Can be associated wtih preterm labor, chorioamnionitis (murky brown amniotic fluid), and spontaneous abortion

What are the signs and symptoms of *Listeria* infection?

Stillbirth

Respiratory infection and pneumonitis

Sepsis and disseminated infection

Granulomatous lesions with microabscesses

Meningitis, conjunctivitis, and skin rash

What is the mortality rate of neonatal listeriosis and how is late-onset disease manifest?

The neonatal mortality rate for listeriosis has been estimated at 50%.

Late-onset disease is characterized by meningitis about 1 month after delivery.

How is *Listeria* screened for and diagnosed?

Listeria is relatively rare in pregnancy and does not have a characteristic clinical presentation; thus, it is often difficult to diagnose.

It is often diagnosed via blood or other cultures (with selective media) sent with a high index of suspicion in a pregnant patient.

It should be suspected in the presence of an unusual illness in a pregnant woman.

Women who ingest contaminated food should have vaginal, rectal, stool, cerebrospinal fluid (CSF), urine, and blood cultures.

How is *Listeria* infection treated?

Either ampicillin and gentamicin or Bactrim in penicillin-allergic patients

SEXUALLY TRANSMITTED DISEASES

SYPHILIS

What is *Treponema pallidum*?

Treponema pallidum is the spirochete responsible for causing the chronic infection known as syphilis.

Venereal Disease Research Laboratory (VDRL) and rapid plasma reagin (RPR) test nonspecific antibodies and have good sensitivity 4 to 6 weeks after infection but lack specificity.

The fluorescent treponemal antibody absorption test (FTA-ABS) and the microhemagglutination assay for antibodies to *Treponema pallidum* (MHA-TP) are specific tests that confirm a positive VDRL or RPR test.

What are recommendations for screening in pregnancy?

Screening for syphilis in pregnancy is required by law.

CDC recommend an additional screening in the third trimester in women at high risk for syphilis infection.

What are risk factors for syphilis in pregnancy?

Drug abuse (especially crack use) and lack of prenatal care

The incidence of syphilis in the U.S. declined 85% from 1990–1998; It is currently increasing.

What is the transmission rate for syphilis in pregnancy?

Fifty percent to eighty percent; occurs transplacentally

What are the effects of *Treponema pallidum* on pregnancy and on the fetus/neonate?

Infection in pregnancy has been linked to preterm labor, fetal death, and neonatal infection via transplacental or intrapartum transmission.

Early congenital syphilis is characterized by infection of fetal organs, which leads to marked hepatomegaly, ascites, nonimmune hydrops, anemia and thrombocytopenia, skin lesions, rash, osteitis and periostitis, pneumonia and hepatitis and is associated with a 50% perinatal mortality rate.

Late congenital syphilis (after 2 years of age) causes dental abnormalities, saber shins, nasal septum destruction, interstitial keratitis, cranial nerve VIII deafness, and failure to thrive.

The placenta becomes large and pale with a decrease in the number of blood vessels.

How is *Treponema pallidum* treated in pregnancy?

Penicillin is used to treat syphilis; treatment is aimed at maternal cure and prevention of congenital syphilis.

Benzathine penicillin G is the CDC drug of choice and use of alternative nonpenicillin therapy is discouraged with recommendations for penicillin desensitization and subsequent penicillin treatment.

Follow-up VDRL or RPR titers should be obtained.

Infants symptomatic for syphilis, seropositive for syphilis, or with CSF studies suggestive of infection should also be treated with penicillin.

GONORRHEA

What is *Neisseria gonorrhoeae* and how is it detected?	The causative organism of gonorrhea infection It is detected via an endocervical swab, which can be used for DNA probe analysis or culture on selective media (e.g., Thayer-Martin medium)
To what drug is the organism resistant?	Penicillin and tetracycline
What are the effects of *Neisseria gonorrhoeae* on pregnancy?	Has been linked to septic spontaneous abortion, stillbirth, preterm delivery, premature rupture of the membranes, chorioamnionitis, postpartum infection, first-trimester pelvic inflammatory disease [(PID); rare], and maternal disseminated gonorrhea Maternal disseminated disease can lead to gonococcal arthritis, dermatitis, endocarditis, and meningitis. Fetal infection occurs in 25% to 50% of cases in pregnancy if not treated. Neonatal gonococcal ophthalmia, sepsis, and arthritis may result.
How is *Neisseria gonorrhoeae* treated in pregnancy?	High penicillin resistance in Neisseria strains mandates treatment with ceftriaxone or spectinomycin. Erythromycin or azithromycin should also be prescribed if chlamydia cultures are not performed due to high coincidence of infection with chlamydia. Infants should all be given prophylactic ophthalmic erythromycin or silver nitrate to prevent possible blindness from gonococcal ophthalmia neonatorum.

CHLAMYDIA

What is *Chlamydia trachomatis* and how is its presence diagnosed?

An obligatory intracellular bacterium that attaches to columnar or transitional cell epithelium

It is the most common sexually transmitted bacteria in the United States.

Diagnosis is made with culture on selective media (cycloheximide-treated McCoy cells), rapid antigen detection, or DNA probe analysis.

What are risk factors for chlamydia infection?

Age less than 25 years
Unmarried status
Inner-city population
Multiple sexual partners
History or presence of other sexually transmitted diseases

What are the effects of *Chlamydia trachomatis* on pregnancy?

Most cases are asymptomatic.

Mothers can have chlamydial cervicitis, urethritis, proctitis, salpingitis (rare), or conjunctivitis.

Neonates manifest infection primarily as conjunctivitis, pneumonitis, and otitis media.

Links have been suggested to antepartum chlamydia infection and preterm labor, premature rupture of membranes, increased perinatal mortality, and late postpartum metritis.

How is *Chlamydia trachomatis* treated in pregnancy?

Pregnant women should be treated with erythromycin or azithromycin to prevent teratogenic consequences of tetracycline-based therapy (fetal teeth and long bone anomalies).

Should receive erythromycin ophthalmic ointment or silver nitrate drops to treat chlamydial conjunctivitis/ ophthalmia neonatorum.

23

Neurologic Disorders in Pregnancy

GENERAL

In general, how does pregnancy affect preexisting neurological disease?

Most neurologic disorders are compatible with normal pregnancy. Pregnancy seldom exacerbates neurologic disease.

USE OF NEUROLOGIC IMAGING TECHNIQUES DURING PREGNANCY

Is computed tomography (CT) safe to use during pregnancy?

Yes, with appropriate abdominal shielding

When is CT is most useful?

To evaluate acute intracerebral hemorrhage

Is magnetic resonance imaging (MRI) safe to use during pregnancy?

Because MRI does not employ radiation, it has no known fetal risk.

When is MRI most useful?

To diagnose atrioventricular malformations, posterior fossa lesions, and spinal cord disease

Is angiography safe to use during pregnancy?

Can be used if necessary, with shielding of the abdomen

Is positron emission tomography (PET) safe to use during pregnancy?

No, because PET uses radioisotopes

SEIZURE DISORDERS

What is the prevalence of seizure disorders in pregnancy?

Four in every 1000 pregnancies

For each type of seizure disorder, give its distribution (in percentages) in pregnancy.

Complex partial: 60%
Generalized tonic–clonic: 30%
Petit mal (absence): 5%

What causes seizure disorders?

Injury
Structural lesion
Drugs
Biochemical
Idiopathic

Does pregnancy worsen seizures?

No

Is pregnancy outcome adversely affected by seizure disorders?

Some data indicate increases in:
  Pregnancy-induced hypertension
  Preterm delivery
  Low-birth–weight infants
  Cerebral palsy
  Seizure disorders in children
  Mental retardation
  Congenital anomalies

How should management of seizures be changed when the patient is pregnant?

Drug use should be minimized but must be effective.

For each of the following seizure medications, list the possible adverse effects in pregnancy:
  Phenytoin

Interferes with vitamin K-dependent clotting factors and contributes to impaired clotting mechanism in the newborn
May cause craniofacial anomalies, although it is not clear whether these abnormalities result from the drug or the seizure disorder

  Carbamazepine

Associated with a 1% risk of neural tube defect

Phenobarbital   Has not been associated with anomaly

Valproic acid   Associated with a 2% risk of neural tube defect

CEREBROVASCULAR DISEASE

What percentage of maternal deaths are caused by cerebrovascular accident?

Ten percent

Are ischemic or hemorrhagic strokes more commonly associated with pregnancy?

Hemorrhagic

What condition is associated with thrombotic stroke during pregnancy?

The presence of lupus anticoagulant

What two conditions are associated with hemorrhagic strokes during pregnancy?

Hypertension or atrioventricular malformation

MIGRAINE HEADACHES

What is the definition of migraine headache?

Periodic, hemicranial, throbbing headaches usually accompanied by nausea, paresthesia, and scotomata

Does pregnancy influence incidence or severity?

Yes; both commonly improve

Can ergot derivatives be used during pregnancy?

No

Can beta-blockers and calcium channel–blockers be used during pregnancy?

Yes

Can sumatriptan be used in pregnancy?	The safety of sumatriptan during pregnancy has not been evaluated.

MULTIPLE SCLEROSIS

Does multiple sclerosis worsen during pregnancy?	Yes, in 10% of affected women
Does multiple sclerosis impair pregnancy outcome?	No
Can epidural anesthesia be used in women with multiple sclerosis?	Yes

MYASTHENIA GRAVIS

Does pregnancy affect the course of myasthenia gravis?	Yes. Myasthenia gravis worsens in one-third of affected women and improves in two-thirds of women.
Is magnesium sulfate contraindicated?	Yes, except under extreme circumstances
What neonatal problems may occur as a result of myasthenia gravis during pregnancy?	Fifteen percent have neonatal muscle function impairment.

NEUROPATHIES

Does the incidence of Bell's palsy increase during pregnancy?	Yes
What is the incidence of carpal tunnel syndrome during pregnancy?	Twenty-five percent of women have some symptoms of median nerve compression.
What serious complication of cord injury is especially important in pregnancy?	Autonomic dysreflexia

What circumstances trigger this complication?

Labor and bladder or bowel distention

What consequence of this complication is extremely dangerous to the mother and fetus?

Hypertension

24

Autoimmune Disease in Pregnancy

RHEUMATOID ARTHRITIS

What is the prevalence in pregnant women?

2%

What are the symptoms?

Rheumatoid arthritis is a chronic disease. Symptoms may include:
morning stiffness
pain on motion of a joint
malaise
fatigue
anorexia
other constitutional symptoms

What is the pathophysiology?

Rheumatoid arthritis is an autoimmune disease and has a genetic predisposition. There is a propensity for cartilage destruction, bony erosions, and joint deformities. It primarily affects the synovial fluid-lined joints. The peripheral joints are most affected.

What are the clinical manifestations?

Rheumatoid nodules occur in 20% of patients and may occur in the heart, lungs, and along any extremity.
Pericarditis, myocarditis, and vasculitis are also occasionally seen.
Rarely affects the kidneys.
There are usually intermittent periods of acute exacerbations and remissions of joint inflammation.

How is the diagnosis made?

History and physical examination
Physical examination will show soft tissue swelling and tenderness.
Subcutaneous nodules may be found.
Laboratory evaluation will confirm the presence of rheumatoid factor and

IgM and IgG antibodies directed against the Fc fragments of IgG.

The severity of disease is related to the rheumatoid factor titers.

Anti-nuclear antibody (ANA) is also found in 20% of cases.

Patients may have a normochromic normocytic anemia and an elevated sedimentation rate.

Radiographs will show juxta-articular osteopenia and soft tissue swelling with subsequent marginal joint erosions, joint-space narrowing and subluxation.

What is the effect of pregnancy in a patient with rheumatoid arthritis?

70% of patients experience a substantial improvement in disease during pregnancy with a decrease in pain, swelling, and stiffness.

Remission during one pregnancy usually predicts further remission during subsequent pregnancies; however, more than 90% relapse within 6–8 months postpartum.

The majority of relapses occur between 2 and 10 weeks postpartum.

What is the effect of the disease on pregnancy?

There is no obvious adverse effect on pregnancy outcome.

Caution should be taken in intubating patients with spinal involvement as subluxation is possible.

Contracted pelvises and severe hip deformities predispose such patients to having a C-section.

What is the treatment?

The goals are pain relief, reduction of inflammation, and preservation of function.

Why is it important to treat rheumatoid arthritis?

Cartilage loss is irreversible

While physical therapy and occupational therapy are important components of the treatment plan,	Pharmacological agents used include:
	  -aspirin
	  -NSAIDS
	  -gold
	  -immunosuppressive agents
	  -penicillamine

What is the is the cornerstone of pharmacologic treatment during pregnancy for patients with rheumatoid arthritis?	Aspirin and other NSAID therapy
What pharmacologic agents are not routinely used in pregnancy?	Azathioprine, cyclosporine, gold, penicillamine, and methotrexate are fetotoxic.
What complications may be associated with salicylate use throughout pregnancy?	Prolonged gestation Long labor Increased blood loss at delivery Postpartum hemorrhage
What complications may be caused by use of indomethacin in late pregnancy (>32 weeks)?	Premature closure of the fetal ductus Renal insufficiency
What pregnancy complication may be caused by use of NSAIDS over a long period of time?	Oligohydramnios

MYASTHENIA GRAVIS

What is myasthenia gravis?	An autoimmune disease caused by circulating antibodies that damage acetylcholine receptors lying within the postsynaptic muscle membrane
What is the prevalence?	Occurs in 1/25,000 pregnant women

What are the symptoms?	Symptoms include weakness and fatiguability. Weakness usually begins in the extraocular muscles with ptosis and diplopia. Other bulbar muscles may be affected leading to difficulty swallowing, chewing, or speaking. Limb muscles also may be involved.
What are the complications of the disease?	Respiratory weakness alone or in combination with swallowing paralysis may occur. All symptoms are exacerbated by fatigue or infection.
What is the effect of pregnancy on myasthenia gravis?	There is an exacerbation of disease in 41%, a remission in 28%, and no change in 31%. Postpartum relapses occur in 40% of patients.
What is the effect of disease on pregnancy?	Neonatal myasthenia occurs in 10–25% of infants. It is thought to be secondary to transplacental passage of IgG antibodies directed against acetylcholine receptors. Preterm labor occurs in 25–60% of patients. It is thought that anti-acetylcholinesterase agents may have an oxytocic action.
Describe the course and symptoms of neonatal myasthenia.	It does not exist at birth but is usually evident within the first two days of life. Affected infants have bulbar weakness which manifests as feeding problems, floppy limbs, and a feeble cry. Symptoms subside within a week to a month. Neonates of mothers with myasthenia gravis must be watched for at least four days.
What is the treatment for myasthenia gravis?	Anticholinesterase drugs (Neostigmine and Pyridostigmine) increase

acetylcholine concentration by preventing its breakdown. These drugs do not cross the placenta and are safe in pregnancy. Plasmapheresis improves disease by removing circulating antibodies.

Thymectomy suppresses antibody production. Steroids may also be used as an immunosuppressive agent.

How should myasthenia gravis be managed in a pregnant patient?

1. Patients should continue taking acetylcholinesterase inhibitors; they have been shown to be safe in pregnancy.
2. Magnesium sulfate therapy is absolutely contraindicated because of its neuromuscular blockade; it will precipitate a myasthenic crisis.
3. Because myasthenia gravis affects striated muscle only, the uterus usually is not affected. The first stage of labor progresses normally. The second stage is impaired as it involves the use of voluntary pushing and the use of skeletal muscles.
4. Some patients are sensitive to narcotics and thus their use should be limited if possible.
5. Aminoglycosides can block the motor end plate and cause a myasthenic crisis and should not be used.

SYSTEMIC LUPUS ERYTHEMATOSUS

What is systemic lupus erythematosus (SLE)?

An autoimmune disease of unknown etiology. The pathogenesis involves the production of autoantibodies and immune complexes.

What is the prognosis for patients with lupus?

The 10-year survival for patients without nephritis is 87% and 65% for patients with nephritis. The leading causes of death are infections and renal failure.

How is systemic lupus erythematous diagnosed?

A patient needs to have at least four of the following criteria to be diagnosed with SLE:
1. malar or discoid rash
2. photosensitivity
3. oral ulcers
4. arthritis
5. serositis
6. renal disorder (persistent proteinuria >0.5g/day or cellular casts)
7. neurological disorder (seizures or psychosis)
8. hematological disorders (hemolytic anemia with reticulocytosis, or leukopenia <4,000/mm^3 or lymphopenia <1500/mm^3 or thrombocytopenia <100,000)
9. Immunologic disorder (presence of antibody to native DNA, anti-smith antibody, false positive serologic test for syphilis or antinuclear antibodies (ANA) in a titer of at least 1:80)

How does pregnancy affect SLE?

Pregnancy does not affect the long-term prognosis of patients with SLE who do not have renal involvement. Patients with renal involvement (Cr >1.5, proteinuria >3g/day) have a 7% incidence of a permanent increase in renal dysfunction and a 30% incidence of transient renal dysfunction in the third trimester. The incidence of exacerbations in pregnancy is not increased and is 10–15%.

How does the disease affect pregnancy?

Ideally, the patient should be in remission for at least 6 months.

There is an increased incidence of fetal loss, stillbirth, preterm delivery preeclampsia, and IUGR.

What are some predictors of fetal loss in a pregnant patient with SLE?

Prior history, the activity level of the lupus, the presence of renal disease, and the presence of anti-phospholipid antibodies (lupus anti-coagulant and anti-cardiolipin antibodies).

With what other complications are anti-phospholipid antibodies associated?

Increased incidence of venous and arterial thrombosis, hemolytic anemia, and thrombocytopenia. Increased risk of recurrent abortions/fetal wastage, IUGR, preterm labor, preeclampsia, and fetal distress in the second trimester.

What is the prevalence of preeclampsia in a pregnant patient with SLE?

Preeclampsia occurs in 30% of patients with a history of renal disease.

How can you differentiate between lupus nephritis and preeclampsia?

It may be difficult to distinguish between preeclampsia and a lupus flare. Both preeclampsia and lupus nephritis will present with hypertension, edema, and proteinuria. CNS lupus may produce seizures. Lupus nephritis may be distinguished by the fact that it can occur anytime in pregnancy, whereas preeclampsia usually occurs after the 24th week. Lupus nephritis is suggested by extrarenal symptoms and significant hematuria and cellular casts. Lupus nephritis begins with proteinuria alone. Some believe that a lupus flare is associated with low C3 and C4 levels.

What implications are there for the fetus of a mother with SLE?

Increased incidence of congenital heart block
Neonatal lupus

What factors contribute to the increased incidence of congenital heart block?

It is related to the presence and transplacental passage of maternal anti-SSA(Ro) and anti-SSB(La) antibodies. There is a diffuse myocarditis and fibrosis in the region between the bundle of His and the AV node. These antibodies are not always present in patients with SLE. Infant mortality with congenital heart block is 5% and the risk of recurrence is 25%.

What factors contribute to the development of neonatal lupus?

This syndrome involves cutaneous lupus (erythematous lesions of the face, scalp, and upper thorax), thrombocytopenia, and hemolysis. The syndrome is due to transplacental passage of maternal antibodies, including anti-SSA and anti-SSB. The syndrome resolves in a few months. The risk is 1/60 but increases to 1/20 with the presence of anti-SSA antibodies.

What is the treatment of SLE?

Glucocorticoids are the cornerstone of treatment. They may be used in the same doses as before pregnancy. They have been found to produce no other fetal abnormality other than decreased birth weight. Azathioprine may be used if the patient has a steroid-resistant nephropathy. Cyclosporine is avoided unless life-threatening complications develop.

How should patients with SLE be managed in pregnancy?

The patient should have good renal function with a creatine <1.5, and continue taking her steroids throughout pregnancy.

Patients who are on chronic steroid therapy should be given additional stress doses of steroids peripartum.

Hematologic, liver function tests, and renal function should be assessed early in pregnancy and then renal function should be evaluated each month.

If the patient has antiphospholipid antibodies, she should be placed on low dose (80 mg) aspirin and low dose prednisone, or low dose aspirin and low dose heparin, daily. Some authors believe that the low dose aspirin–heparin therapy is more effective.

Check for the presence of anti-SSA or anti-SSB antibodies. If positive, the patient should have a fetal echo performed at 22 weeks. In addition, a fetal heart rate of approximately 60 bpm with no baseline variability suggests heart block. If a patient is on corticosteroid therapy, a 1-hour glucose tolerance test should be performed at 20, 28, and 32 weeks since hyperglycemia may be a side effect of therapy.

Ultrasonography should be performed to rule out intrauterine growth retardation. The IUGR is usually asymmetric and occurs after 20 weeks. Some authors believe that antenatal fetal surveillance with NSTs should begin at 28 weeks.

25

Thyroid Diseases in Pregnancy

NORMAL PREGNANCY

What is the thyroid state of a healthy pregnant woman?

Euthyroid, but changes in thyroid function test values occur.

What is the significance of an enlarged thyroid (goiter) in pregnancy?

Mild thyroid enlargement is normal and results from glandular hyperplasia and increased vascularity. Development of a true goiter during pregnancy signifies thyroid disease.

Should pregnant women in the United States take iodine supplements during pregnancy?

No. The renal clearance of iodine almost doubles during pregnancy secondary to a rise in cardiac output and the ensuing rise in glomerular filtration rate. Although this increased iodine loss can lead to deficiency in areas of the world with borderline iodine intake, in the United States the average iodine intake is substantially above the minimum requirement (150 g/day).

What are the changes in thyroxine-binding globulin (TBG), thyroid-stimulating hormone(TSH), and free thyroxine (T_4) and triiodothyronine (T_3) levels during pregnancy?

TBG levels rise in response to elevated estrogen levels.
Rise in TBG levels is associated with a parallel but smaller increase in total T_4 and T_3 levels; therefore, free (i.e., functional) T_4 and T_3 levels are slightly reduced but remain within the normal range.
TSH remains normal.

Should pregnant women be screened for thyroid disease?

Thyroid nodules should be investigated to rule out malignancy
There is insufficient data to warrant routine screening of asymptomatic pregnant patients for hypothyroidism

Thyroid function should be checked in women with a history of thyroid disease or symptoms of thyroid disease

What is a normal result of a thyroid uptake test administered during pregnancy?

Low, which reflects the increase in thyroid hormone binding capacity

What effect does human chorionic gonadotropin (hCG) have on thyroid function?

Because hCG and TSH have the same α-subunit, hCG can stimulate thyroid hormone production in a manner similar to TSH. As hCG levels increase early in pregnancy, the level of T_4 increases and the level of TSH decreases. However, because hCG is a less potent stimulator of thyroid hormone production than TSH, thyrotoxic T_4 levels are unusual in normal pregnancy. Thyrotoxic levels may occur in gestational trophoblastic disease, which is associated with very high hCG levels.

Do thyroid hormones cross the placenta?

The fetal hypothalamic-pituitary-thyroid axis develops autonomously. It does appear that TRH, T_4 and T_3 cross the placenta. Neonates without a thyroid still have low levels of thyroid hormone. TSH does not cross the placenta. Iodine does cross the placenta and pregnant women should not be treated with radioactive iodine or with inorganic iodine.

Which thyroid-active drugs cross the placenta?

Iodine
Thionamides
β-blockers
Somatostatin
Thyrotropin-releasing hormone
Dopamine agonists and antagonists

THYROID DYSFUNCTION AND INFERTILITY

How does hypothyroidism affect fertility?

In hypothyroidism, libido and fertility are decreased. The mechanism is unclear. It has been hypothesized that decreased activity of the central dopaminergic system may be responsible for the increased prolactin and luteinizing hormone levels associated with hypothyroidism. The increased levels of these hormones cause amenorrhea, anovulation, and, in rare cases, galactorrhea, which may be associated with hypothyroidism.

What is the relationship between spontaneous abortion and hypothyroidism?

Women with hypothyroidism have been shown to have a higher incidence of recurrent spontaneous abortions than euthyroid women. Early T_4 replacement therapy improves fetal outcome in this setting.

Does hyperthyroidism affect fertility?

Mild hyperthyroidism does not seem to affect fertility. Thyrotoxicosis is rare in early pregnancy, implying a negative effect on fertility. The exact mechanism is unknown but probably involves alterations in sex hormone levels. Most women with mild to moderate thyrotoxicosis do ovulate, and the evaluation of amenorrhea in such patients should include a pregnancy test.

HYPERTHYROIDISM AND PREGNANCY

What is the incidence of hyperthyroidism in pregnancy?

Occurs in 1 of every 1000 pregnant women

What signs and symptoms are common to both pregnancy and thyrotoxicosis?

Signs and symptoms of hyperthyroidism include:
Heat intolerance
Diaphoresis and warm skin

Fatigue
Anxiety and emotional lability
Tremulousness
Tachycardia

What signs and symptoms differentiate thyrotoxicosis from normal pregnancy?

Signs seen in thyrotoxicosis but usually not in pregnancy include:
Weight loss
Onycholysis
Diarrhea
Proximal myopathy
Tachycardia that is unresponsive to Valsalva maneuver
Thyromegaly and ophthalmopathy may also be present, but do not necessarily indicate active disease.

What thyroid function test results indicate hyperthyroidism?

Suppressed TSH levels in the absence of pituitary disease are diagnostic.
Increased free T_4 levels are frequently seen.
Occasionally, T_4 levels may be normal; in this case, an isolated elevation of T_3 levels should be sought.

What other laboratory abnormalities may be seen in hyperthyroidism?

All of the following abnormalities may be associated with thyrotoxicosis, especially Graves' disease:
Normochromic normocytic anemia
Mild neutropenia
Elevated liver function test results (alkaline phosphatase, transaminases, and bilirubin)
Mild hypercalcemia
Hypomagnesemia

What is the most common cause of hyperthyroidism during pregnancy?

Graves' disease (90% of cases)

What are other causes of hyperthyroidism during pregnancy?

Less frequent causes include:
Toxic multinodular goiter
Toxic adenoma

Gestational trophoblastic disease
Pituitary adenoma
Metastatic follicular cell carcinoma
de Quervain's thyroiditis
Struma ovarii

What physical findings are commonly associated with Graves' disease?

Some or all of the following may be seen in Graves' disease:
Nontender goiter that is diffusely enlarged and firm
Exophthalmos, which is associated with retraction of the upper eyelids, widened palpebral fissures, lid-lag on downward gaze, and infrequent blinking
Pretibial myxedema or clubbing, or both

What tests support the diagnosis of Graves' disease?

Increased level of free T_4
Decreased level of TSH
Increased level of thyroid-stimulating immunoglobulin (TSI)
Radioactive thyroid scan normally shows increased uptake by the thyroid gland; however, this study is contraindicated during pregnancy.

What is the cause of Graves' disease?

Production of autoimmune antibodies against the TSH receptor
These antibodies usually have a stimulatory effect; however, inhibitory action has also been reported.

Describe the course of Graves' disease during pregnancy.

The same poorly understood mechanisms responsible for immunotolerance of the mother to the fetoplacental unit are thought to play a role in the improvement of the course of Graves' disease during pregnancy. Initially, as the hCG levels rise, thyrotoxicosis may worsen, but as the pregnancy progresses, TSI levels fall and signs and symptoms improve.

When should Graves' disease be treated?

Best fetal outcome is achieved when thyrotoxicosis is treated before conception.

If treatment is not an option before conception, thyrotoxicosis should be treated during pregnancy.

Why should Graves' disease be treated?

Hyperthyroid women have a higher risk of complications during labor and delivery.

Hyperthyroidism is associated with an increased incidence of minor fetal anomalies.

The risks of preterm delivery, perinatal mortality, and maternal heart failure are significantly increased among inadequately treated or untreated thyrotoxic pregnant women.

What is the goal of treatment of hyperthyroidism in pregnancy?

Control the maternal hyperthyroidism while avoiding fetal or neonatal hypothyroidism (because drugs used in treatment of hyperthyroidism cross the placenta).

The maternal T_4 level should be maintained in the high normal to slightly elevated range normally seen in pregnancy.

What drugs are available for the treatment of hyperthyroidism?

Usual agents are the thionamides: Propylthiouracil (PTU) and carbimazole (metabolized to methimazole).

Mechanism of action of thionamides?

Inhibits iodination of thyroglobulin and thyroglobulin synthesis by competitively inhibiting the enzyme peroxidase

PTU also inhibits the conversion of T_4 to T_3; methimazole does not.

Risk to fetus with methimazole?

Methimazole has been reported to cause fetal aplasia cutis of the scalp.

How soon after initiating thionamide therapy does the patient's condition improve?

Because thionamides work by inhibiting new hormone synthesis, response is seen after thyroid follicle stores are depleted. Most patients begin to show improvement after about 1 week of therapy.

How should patients taking thionamides be monitored?

Free T_4, free T_3, and TSH levels should be monitored monthly to maintain a euthyroid state using the smallest dose of thionamide.

What are the main maternal side effects of thionamides?

Uncommon and include:
Pruritus
Rash
Drug fever
Metallic taste
Nausea
Oral ulcerations
Hepatitis
Agranulocytosis (rare)

In what percentage of patients taking thionamides does agranulocytosis occur?

0.1%

How should patients be monitored for agranulocytosis?

A baseline white blood cell count should be obtained in all patients at the onset of therapy and repeated periodically.

What are the fetal effects of thionamide therapy and how can they be prevented?

Most important fetal effect is hypothyroidism, because antithyroid drugs cross the placenta (methimazole crosses four times more efficiently than PTU). Hypothyroidism can lead to development of neurologic impairment.
The fetus should be closely monitored for signs of hypothyroidism (goiter, bradycardia, and intrauterine growth retardation).

When is additional therapy necessary for the treatment of hyperthyroidism?

Because thionamides do not have an immediate onset of action, additional agents may be necessary for treating severe thyrotoxicosis. In this setting, labor and delivery, cesarean section, infection, or eclampsia can precipitate thyroid storm.

What drugs are used to treat severe thyrotoxicosis?

β-blockers are useful for treating the sympathetic symptoms of thyrotoxicosis such as tachycardia, although they have no effect on hormone production.

Iodides (e.g., potassium iodide) can be used in conjunction with β-blockers in cases of severe hyperthyroidism, although not during pregnancy. They decrease serum T_4 and T_3 levels by inhibiting the release of stored thyroid hormone.

What is the goal of therapy with β-blockers and iodides?

Short-term control of severe hyperthyroidism while awaiting the effects of thionamide therapy

For what condition is it necessary to be cautious when prescribing β-blockers?

Heart failure

Can radioactive iodine be used to treat thyrotoxicosis during pregnancy?

No; contraindicated in pregnancy because it crosses the placenta and is concentrated in the fetal thyroid gland

What treatment option is reserved for patients who fail thiomide therapy?

Thyroidectomy

HYPOTHYROIDISM AND PREGNANCY

What is the incidence of hypothyroidism during

Occurs in about 1 in every 170 pregnancies

pregnancy in the United States?

Severe hypothyroidism is rare because of its association with infertility.

What risks are associated with hypothyroidism during pregnancy?

Increased risks of preeclampsia, placental abruption, and low-birth weight and stillborn infants. These outcomes improve with early thyroxine replacement therapy.

What signs and symptoms are associated with hypothyroidism?

Most are insidious in onset and may be masked by signs and symptoms associated with pregnancy:

Modest weight gain or inability to lose weight while dieting
Decreased exercise ability
General lethargy
Cold intolerance
Menorrhagia
Hoarseness
Constipation
Bradycardia
Goiter
Hair loss

What information in the history can alert the physician to the possibility of hypothyroidism?

Personal or family history of thyroid disease
History of head and neck irradiation
Past or present treatment with lithium- or iodine-containing drugs

How is hypothyroidism diagnosed?

History
Physical examination
Measurement of serum TSH and free T_4 levels

What is primary hypothyroidism and what abnormalities are seen in the thyroid function tests?

The thyroid gland is not producing enough thyroid hormone to maintain a euthyroid state.
TSH level is elevated and T_4 level is usually low.

What is subclinical hypothyroidism and in what patients is it prevalent?

Form of primary hypothyroidism
Elevated TSH level in the presence of T_4 levels within the normal range
Prevalent in pregnant women and is thought to be autoimmune in nature

What is secondary hypothyroidism and what thyroid function test abnormalities are associated with it?

Also called pituitary hypothyroidism
Inadequate TSH secretion by the pituitary gland
Low T_4 levels

What other laboratory abnormalities may be associated with hypothyroidism?

Elevated serum creatine phosphokinase, serum glutamic oxaloacetic transaminase, lactic dehydrogenase, cholesterol, and prolactin levels
Anemia secondary to menorrhagia and other, poorly understood causes

What group of patients is at particular risk for development of hypothyroidism during pregnancy?

Women with insulin-dependent diabetes mellitus (type I)

What is the most common cause of hypothyroidism during pregnancy in the United States?

Hashimoto's (chronic lymphocytic) thyroiditis

What is the second leading cause of hypothyroidism during pregnancy in the United States?

Prior treatment of Graves' disease with radioactive iodine or thyroidectomy

What are other, less frequent causes of hypothyroidism during pregnancy in the United States?

Acute (suppurative) thyroiditis
Subacute (viral) thyroiditis
Iatrogenic causes: Thionamide, iodide, and lithium therapy

Is iodine deficiency a cause of hypothyroidism in the United States?

No

What is the typical presentation of a patient with Hashimoto's thyroiditis?

Firm, diffusely enlarged, usually painless goiter

Histology reveals infiltration of the gland with lymphocytes, although a biopsy is seldom necessary.

What are the characteristic immunologic findings associated with Hashimoto's thyroiditis?

Antimicrosomal antibodies: Almost all patients

Antithyroglobulin antibodies: 70% of patients

How does pregnancy affect the course of Hashimoto's thyroiditis?

As in Graves' disease, the immunotolerance associated with pregnancy improves the course of Hashimoto's thyroiditis. During the course of pregnancy, antimicrosomal and antithyroglobulin antibody titers and the size of the goiter decrease. However, relapse frequently occurs after delivery.

What are the signs and symptoms of subacute thyroiditis?

May present in the setting of an ongoing viral illness as a firm, mildly tender goiter

This illness tends to have a variable clinical course, starting with a hyperthyroid state which gradually becomes euthyroid and progresses to a hypothyroid state in 20% of patients.

What is the cause of subacute thyroiditis?

Thought to be viral

What is the treatment of subacute thyroiditis?

The duration of illness is 6 weeks to 6 months, and it tends to be self-limited.

What is the treatment of hypothyroidism during pregnancy?

Replacement with levothyroxine should be initiated promptly. Initial dosage is 0.1–0.15 mg/day; dosage should be increased every 4 weeks until TSH level decreases to the low-normal range.

POSTPARTUM THYROIDITIS

What is the course of postpartum thyroiditis?

Starts with a brief hyperthyroid state about 3 months postpartum, which lasts a few weeks and evolves into a hypothyroid state

The hypothyroid phase persists for a few months.

Most patients return to euthyroid state by about 12 months after delivery.

In what percentage of patients with postpartum hypothyroidism does permanent hypothyroidism develop?

10% to 30%

What is a hallmark of this disease?

Transient nature of thyroid dysfunction associated with it

What are its signs and symptoms?

Thyrotoxic phase: Fatigue, palpitations, dizziness, and weight loss; patients may assume that these signs and symptoms are normal in the postpartum period.

Hypothyroid phase: Weight gain, constipation, cold intolerance, and dry skin. A goiter develops in 50% of the patients; an increased incidence of depressive symptoms is associated with this phase.

What is the cause of postpartum thyroiditis?

Postpartum thyroiditis is a lymphocytic thyroiditis involving antimicrosomal antibodies, similar to Hashimoto's disease. The cause is poorly understood, but it is thought to involve both genetic and environmental factors.

How is postpartum thyroiditis diagnosed?

Increased TSH and decreased free T_4 levels with positive antimicrosomal antibody titers in the postpartum period

Section II

Gynecology

26 Gynecologic Glossary

Abdominal Incisions

The abdominal incision may be either vertical or transverse.

Cherny: the rectus bellies are dissected off pubic symphysis

Mayllard-transverse: divides the rectus bellies horizontally to increase the diameter of the incision

Midline-vertical: used most commonly in gynecologic oncology to allow access to the upper abdomen

Pfannenstiel (low transverse): most common for cesarean section; performed approximately two fingerbreadths above the pubic symphysis

Adenomyosis

Endometrial tissue within the myometrium

Adnexa

The fallopian tubes, ovaries, and other structures attached to the uterus

Adrenarche

Normal development of axillary and pubic hair as a result of increases in 17-ketosteroids, dehydroepiandrosterone (DHEA), and dehydroepiandrosterone sulfate (DHEA-S)

Barr bodies

One less than the number of X chromosomes in a cell

Bartholin gland

Vulvar-vaginal glands located at both sides of the fourchette; analogous to the bulbourethral glands in the male

Blighted ovum

Gestational sac with diameter > 3 cm with absence of fetal pole

Culdocentesis

Diagnostic maneuver in which the

peritoneal cavity is entered through the posterior cul-de-sac; used in the diagnosis of pelvic inflammatory disease and ectopic pregnancy

Curettage Scraping of the uterine lining (endometrium); used diagnostically in the event of bleeding to evaluate pathology and therapeutically after abortions to remove products of conception

Danazol Derivative of 17-ethinyl testosterone used to create a "pseudomenopause" in endometriosis therapy

D&C Dilation and curettage

Dysmenorrhea Pain with menstrual periods

Dyspareunia Pain with intercourse
Multiple etiologic factors, including psychosocial, secondary to endometriosis, scar tissue from obstetric trauma, and sexual dysfunction

Decidua basalis Area of endometrium that separates the placenta from the myometrium and maintains the embryo during early pregnancy

Ectopic pregnancy Any pregnancy located outside of the uterine cavity

Endometriosis Condition in which endometrial glands are located outside the uterine cavity

ERT Estrogen replacement therapy; also known as hormone replacement therapy

Fibroid (leiomyoma) Common benign muscle cell tumors that occur in approximately 50% of African-

	American women and 25% of white women; associated symptoms include bleeding, pain, dyspareunia, dysuria, premature labor, and infertility
Fitz-Hugh–Curtis syndrome	Perihepatic adhesions most often secondary to chlamydia or gonorrhea infection
FSH	Follicle-stimulating hormone
GnRH	Gonadotropin-releasing hormone
HPV	Human papillomavirus
HSG	Hysterosalpingogram
Hysteroscopy	Fiberoptic evaluation of the endometrial cavity
Imperforate hymen	Occlusion of the outflow tract of the vagina; possible cause of primary infertility, and may be associated with hematocolpos (vaginal cavity filled with blood)
IUD	Intrauterine device used for contraception
Kallmann syndrome	Inappropriate GnRH secretion that may be associated with anosmia; a cause of primary amenorrhea
Kleinfelter syndrome	47XXY male; associated with tall stature, mental retardation, small testes, decreased testosterone, and increased FSH and LH
Koilocytosis	Cellular changes associated with HPV infection consisting of perinuclear cavitation

Krukenberg tumor

Metastatic signet-ring cell ovarian tumor; primary tumor located in gastrointestinal tract; other locations include breast, cervix, and bladder

Laparoscopy

Fiberoptic evaluation of the peritoneal cavity

Laparotomy

Surgical entry into the peritoneal cavity

LH

Luteinizing hormone

Meigs' syndrome

Benign ovarian tumor, most likely an ovarian fibroma; also associated with ascites and pleural effusions

Menarche

Onset of menses

Menopause

Cessation of menses secondary to ovarian failure or removal
The perimenopausal period is associated with other complaints, such as insomnia, mood swings, fatigue, forgetfulness, depression, and hot flushes

Mittelschmerz

"Middle pain"; abdominal pain associated with ovulation

Necrotizing fasciitis

Anaerobic infection that affects the underlying layers of fascia; occurs most commonly in diabetic patients with perineal infections

OCP

Oral contraceptive pill

Pap

Papanicolaou smear (cervical cytology) used as a screening test for cervical and uterine malignancy

PID

Pelvic inflammatory disease

PCO

Polycystic ovary

POF	Premature ovarian failure
Premarin	PREgnant MARe urINe; a form of estrogen most commonly used for hormone replacement therapy
Provera	Medroxyprogesterone acetate
Puberty	Physical changes and sexual maturation occurring as a result of the maturation of the hypothalamic–pituitary axis and its effects on the gonads
RKH	Rokitansky-Küster-Hauser syndrome; also called Mayer-Rokitansky-Küster-Hauser syndrome; uterovaginal agenesis leading to amenorrhea
Spinnbarkeit	Clinical test performed on cervical mucus to evaluate the degree of estrogenization
Stein-Leventhal syndrome	Polycystic ovary syndrome
Tanner staging	Tanner defined five stages of breast and pubic hair development Refer to Chapter 34
Testicular feminization	Androgen insensitivity (male pseudohermaphrodite) XY karyotype; characterized by blind vaginal canal, absent uterus, primary amenorrhea, and the presence of male gonads
Thelarche	Onset of development of breast tissue
TOA	Tubo-ovarian abscess
Vaginitis	Inflammation of vaginal mucosa due to infection, contact or chemical irritation, or atrophy
Vaginismus	Involuntary constriction of the outer muscles of the vagina, which can lead to sexual dysfunction and dyspareunia

27

Gynecologic Infections

INFECTIONS OF THE LOWER GENITAL TRACT

ACUTE URETHRAL SYNDROME AND BACTERIAL CYSTITIS

What are the three classic symptoms?	Dysuria, frequent urination, and urinary urgency
Diagnosis?	Pelvic exam to rule out dysuria secondary to vulvovaginitis Urinalysis Urine culture with antibiotic sensitivities
How is acute urethral syndrome differentiated from bacterial cystitis?	Acute urethral syndrome: Dysuria, urinary frequency, and $< 10^2$ organisms/ml Bacterial cystitis: Dysuria and $> 10^2$ organisms/ml
What is the most common cause of acute urethral syndrome?	*Chlamydia trachomatis*
What is the treatment for acute urethral syndrome?	Seven days of a tetracycline
What are the most common organisms that cause cystitis?	*Escherichia coli, Klebsiella* sp, *Pseudomonas* sp, and *Proteus* sp
What is the treatment for bacterial cystitis?	Single dose or 3-day course of: Trimethoprim–sulfamethoxazole Nitrofurantoin Amoxicillin or ampicillin First-generation cephalosporin Ciprofloxacin Phenazopyridine hydrochloride (Pyridium) may be used as a urinary analgesic

INFECTIONS OF THE BARTHOLIN GLANDS

Where are the Bartholin glands located?	At the vaginal introitus at 5 and 7 o'clock Normally not palpable
What are the three main causes of clinical enlargement?	1. Cystic dilatation: Usually due to continued secretion of glandular fluid after duct obstruction 2. Abscess: Also follows duct obstruction and is often polymicrobial 3. Adenocarcinoma (rare)
What are the differential diagnoses?	Mesonephric cyst, epithelial inclusion cysts, lipoma, fibroma, hydrocele
Diagnosis of Bartholin gland cyst?	Usually asymptomatic and found on exam
Treatment?	Excision in older women to rule out cancer
Diagnosis of Bartholin gland infection?	Presents with acute vulvar pain and dyspareunia
Treatment?	Simple incision and drainage are associated with a high rate of recurrence. If true abscess has not yet developed, treat with antibiotics and soaks. If abscess is present, marsupialization creates a permanent opening and prevents recurrence.

PARASITES

Describe two parasitic conditions associated with gynecologic symptoms.	1. Pediculosis pubis: Infestation by the crab louse, *Phthirus pubis* 2. Scabies: Infestation by the itch mite, *Sarcoptes scabiei*
What are the symptoms of pediculosis pubis and scabies?	Constant itching, particularly over the mons pubis Scabies symptoms are often worse at night.

How are pediculosis pubis and scabies diagnosed?	Visualization of the eggs (nits), excreta, or parasite itself
What are the treatments for pediculosis pubis and scabies?	Permethrin (Nix Cream) or lindane (Kwell)

MOLLUSCUM CONTAGIOSUM

What is molluscum contagiosum and its cause?	An asymptomatic, benign skin disease of the vulva caused by the poxvirus
What are the signs of molluscum contagiosum?	Characteristic lesions are small nodules or papules, 1–5 mm in diameter, with an umbilicated center.
What are the treatments for molluscum contagiosum?	Excision, cryosurgery, or electrocautery of lesions

CONDYLOMA ACUMINATUM

What is condyloma acuminatum?	Genital warts The most common sexually transmitted disease
What is the cause of condyloma acuminatum?	The highly contagious human papillomavirus (HPV subtypes 6, 11) Virus has been detected in 50% of sexually active females
What areas are affected?	Vulva, vagina, perineum, anus, and cervix
What lesions are associated with condyloma acuminatum?	Pedunculated, warty excrescences
What is the characteristic cell on Pap smear?	The koilocyte, a cell with a perinuclear clearing or halo
Why is colposcopy important after the finding of the characteristic cell on Pap smear?	Koilocytosis is often associated with atypia and dysplasia.

What are the treatment options for condyloma acuminatum?

Small, external lesions: Topical podophyllin, trichloroacetic acid, imiquimod, or 5-fluorouracil

Cryotherapy, electrocautery, or laser therapy

What is recurrence rate?

Recurrence are common.

Treatment does not eradicate the HPV infection from surrounding tissue.

Is is associated with cervical cancer?

HPV infection is the most important risk factor for cervical disease.

HPV subtypes 6, 11 are usually associated with mild dysplasia.

GENITAL HERPES

What is the cause of genital herpes?

The highly contagious herpes simplex virus (HSV)

HSV type II is more common than HSV type I as a cause of genital herpes.

What is the incubation period of HSV?

Two to seven days

What are the duration and symptoms of primary infection with HSV?

Duration: About 10 days

May be accompanied by systemic symptoms of malaise and fever

Lesions:

Multiple vesicles that may coalesce and become superficial ulcers

Associated with severe vulvar pain and exquisite tenderness

Often simultaneously involves the vagina and cervix

Possible urinary retention secondary to vulvar pain

Often associated with inguinal adenopathy

Fifty percent of infected people never experience the "typical primary outbreak" and are thus unaware that they harbor this virus.

How is the diagnosis of genital herpes made?	Physical examination: Typical appearance of vesicles and ulcers History: Typical clinical syndrome Cytologic smear (tzank-Prep) and culture of lesions. High rate of false-negative results, depending on the activity of the lesion
What are the characteristics of recurrences?	Less severe and shorter in duration than primary infection Vary widely in incidence; the virus lies dormant in S2, S3, and S4 nerve roots between recurrences. Viral shedding may occur for several weeks after lesions appear.
What is the treatment for genital herpes?	Oral acyclovir can reduce viral shedding and shorten the clinical course. Severe cases may require intravenous (IV) acyclovir, especially if patient is immunocompromised. Oral acyclovir for prophylaxis is used if frequent episodes occur. Therapeutic procedures include sitz baths, Lidocaine jelly, and vulvar rinses with Burow solution.

GRANULOMA INGUINALE

What is granuloma inguinale?	Chronic, ulcerative infection of the vulva The lesion is a painless nodule that progresses to a beefy-red ulcer. It is uncommon in the United States and more frequent in the Caribbean.
What is the cause of granuloma inguinale?	The bacterium *Calymmatobacterium granulomatis*
What is the classic diagnostic finding?	The lesion smear shows Donovan bodies, deep-staining bacteria with a bipolar appearance resembling a safety pin.
What is the treatment for granuloma inguinale?	Oral tetracycline

LYMPHOGRANULOMA VENEREUM (LGV)

What is LGV?	Chronic infection of lymphatic tissue in the genital region, including the vulva, urethra, rectum, or cervix Rarely seen in the United States except in the tropical areas
What is the cause of LGV?	*C. trachomatis* subtypes L-1, L-2, L-3
What are the three phases of infection?	Primary infection: Shallow, painless ulcer on labia Secondary: Painful adenopathy in inguinal and perirectal areas If untreated, buboes (matted nodes that adhere to overlying skin) form. Classic sign is the double genitocrural fold or "groove sign." Tertiary: Rupture of bubo, leading to formation of multiple sinuses/fistulas Edema leads to fit fibrosis and elephantiasis
How is the diagnosis of LGV made?	Polymerase chain reaction for C. *trachomatis* DNA obtained by swab from lesion
What is the treatment for LGV?	Oral tetracycline or erythromycin for 2–3 weeks

CHANCROID

What is chancroid?	Acute, ulcerative disease of the vulva Typically, a painful ulcer with ragged edges Solitary or multiple lesions
What causes chancroid?	*Haemophilus ducreyi*
How is a diagnosis of chancroid made?	Gram stain shows classic streptobacillary chains.

What is the treatment for chancroid?	Oral trimethoprim–sulfamethoxazole or erythromycin

SYPHILIS

What is the cause of syphilis?

Treponema pallidum

How is a diagnosis of syphilis made?

Definitive: Dark-field microscopy reveals spirochetes.

What serologic screening tests are available?

Nonspecific: Venereal Disease Research Laboratory (VDRL) test and rapid plasma reagin (RPR) test
Easy and cheap to perform
High rate of false-positive results
Must confirm with specific test
Specific:FTA-ABS (fluorescent-labeled *Treponema* antibody absorption)
MHA-TP (microhemagglutination assay for antibodies to *T. pallidum*)
HATTS (hemagglutination treponemal test for syphilis)

What are the three clinical phases of syphilis?

Primary: Hard chancre or painless ulcer
Secondary: Hematogenous dissemination causing systemic disease
Classic rash of red macules and papules on palms and soles of feet
Condyloma latum, or large, raised, gray areas on vulva or other mucous membranes
Latent phase ranges from 2 to 20 years.
Tertiary: Optic atrophy, tabes dorsalis, paresis, aortic aneurysm, gummas (necrotic abscesses) of skin and bone

What is the treatment for syphilis?

Lumbar puncture for women with syphilis of > 12 months' duration to rule out neurosyphilis
Penicillin:
Drug of choice

Different regimens for different stages
of syphilis:
Disease < 1 year Benzathine pen G
2.4 mu 1M x 1
Disease > 1 year 2.4 mu 1M q w 3
Neurosyphilis pen G x 14 d
Tetracycline: For patients allergic to
penicillin
Pregnant patients:
Penicillin regimen appropriate for
stage
Skin testing and desensitization if
patient has a history of penicillin
allergy

BACTERIAL VAGINOSIS (NONSPECIFIC VAGINITIS)

What is bacterial vaginosis?

A symbiotic infection of anaerobic bacteria and *Gardnerella vaginalis*

What are the symptoms of bacterial vaginosis?

Presenting symptom: Vaginal odor described as "fishy" or "musty"
Discharge: Thin and grayish white without associated vulvar irritation, pH > 5, amine-like odor when mixed with potassium hydroxide (KOH; positive whiff test)

How is bacterial vaginosis diagnosed?

A saline wet smear reveals clue cells, vaginal epithelial cells with bacteria clusters that adhere to the epithelial cell surface.

What is the treatment for bacterial vaginosis?

Oral metronidazole
If pregnant, clindamycin or ampicillin

TRICHOMONIASIS

What is trichomoniasis?

A protozoan vaginal infection
The most prevalent nonviral sexually transmitted disease

What is the cause of trichomoniasis?	The anaerobic, flagellated protozoan *Trichomonas vaginalis*
What are the symptoms of trichomoniasis?	Presenting symptoms and signs: Profuse discharge; erythema and irritation of vulva; vulvar pruritus; dysuria; "strawberry cervix" Discharge: Large amount; often frothy and bubbling; malodorous; pH > 5
How is the diagnosis of trichomoniasis made?	Light microscopy of vaginal fluid mixed with saline reveals mobile, flagellated organisms and many white blood cells.
What is the treatment for trichomoniasis?	Oral metronidazole 2 g orally in a single dose or 500 mg twice daily for 7 days If pregnant, the same treatment is used but deferred until the second trimester Treatment of sexual partners

CANDIDIASIS

What is candidiasis?	Yeast infection
What is the cause of vaginal candidiasis?	Primarily *Candida albicans* Other species: *Candida glabrata* and *Candida tropicalis*
What factors predispose a patient to candidiasis?	Antibiotic treatment that alters the normal vaginal flora Depressed immunity [corticosteroids, acquired immunodeficiency syndrome (AIDS)] Hormonal changes associated with pregnancy and menstruation Diabetes mellitus
What are the symptoms of vaginal candidiasis?	Presenting symptoms: Pruritus, burning, external dysuria, extreme vulvar erythema Discharge: White; highly viscous; often with clumps or plaques; pH < 5

How is vaginal candidiasis diagnosed?	Light microscopy of vaginal fluid mixed with KOH reveals filamentous forms or pseudohyphae.
What is the treatment for vaginal candidiasis?	Topical antifungals such as miconazole, clotrimazole, and terconazole as a 3- or 7-day course of intravaginal suppositories inserted at bedtime; can also be used externally for itching Oral fluconazole as a single 150-mg dose in nonpregnant women

INFECTIONS OF THE CERVIX

What are the two diagnostic criteria for mucopurulent cervicitis?	1. Direct visualization of yellow mucopurulent material on a swab of the cervix 2. Presence of 10 or more leukocytes on Gram-stained smears from cervix
What are the symptoms of cervicitis?	Presenting symptoms: Vaginal discharge, dyspareunia, and postcoital bleeding
Signs?	Erythema, edema, or friability
What are the major causes of cervicitis?	*C. trachomatis* (most common) *Neisseria gonorrhoeae* *Mycoplasma hominis* (rare) *C. trachomatis* and *N. gonorrhoeae* are often found simultaneously.
What kind of organism is *C. trachomatis*?	An obligate intracellular bacterium
How is a diagnosis of *C. trachomatis* infection made?	DNA probe for the organism in epithelial cells removed from the endocervical canal
What is the treatment for *C. trachomatis* infection?	Oral doxycycline 100 mg bid for 10 days (or azithromycin 1 gm PO as a single dose or erythromycin or ofloxacin) Treatment of sexual partners

What kind of organism is N. gonorrhoeae?

Gram-negative, intracellular diplococci

How is a diagnosis of N. gonorrhoeae infection made?

DNA probe for the organism in epithelial cells removed from the endocervical canal

Cultures of rectum, pharynx, or urethra may be indicated.

Test for sensitivity to penicillin because of high rate of resistance

What is the treatment for N. gonorrhoeae infection?

Recommended regimen treats both *C. trachomatis* and *N. gonorrhoeae* infections: (50% of N.g. patients have both N.g. and C.t.

Ceftriaxone 250 mg intramuscularly once, or

Ofloxacin 800 mg by mouth once, or

Cefixime 400 mg PO x1 or

Cipro 500 mg PO x1

Plus

Doxycycline 100 mg by mouth twice a day for 7 days (for possible coexisting *C. trachomatis* infection) should be given with any of the above

Azithromycin 1 ng PO x1

Repetition of cultures following therapy to ensure response after treatment of either or both

INFECTIONS OF THE UPPER GENITAL TRACT

PELVIC INFLAMMATORY DISEASE (PID)

What is PID?

An infection that ascends from the vagina and endocervix along the mucosal surface

May involve any or all of the following sites: Endometrium (endometritis), oviducts (salpingitis), ovary (oophoritis), uterine wall (myometritis), broad ligaments (parametritis), and the pelvic peritoneum

What pathogens cause PID?

Most common pathogens: *N. gonorrhoeae, C. trachomatis*

C. trachomatis often causes a longer standing infection with a more indolent course.

C. trachomatis infection may lead to more sequelae because treatment is often not initiated quickly.

Other pathogens:

Facultative aerobes such as *E. coli*, coagulase-negative staphylococcus, and group B streptococcus

Anaerobes such as *Bacteroides* and *Peptococcus*

Genital mycoplasmas such as *Mycoplasma hominis*

Key point: PID is almost always a polymicrobial infection.

What are the risk factors for PID?

Menstruation: Most episodes occur after menses because of mucosal susceptibility during this event.

Multiple sexual partners without barrier protection

Young age and early onset of sexual behavior

Previous PID

Invasive procedure that penetrates the mucosal barrier (i.e., iatrogenic)

History of other sexually transmitted diseases

What are the symptoms of PID?

Often nonspecific and can vary from mild to severe

High rate of false-positive and false-negative results occur when diagnosis is based on history, physical examination, and laboratory results.

How is a diagnosis of PID made?

Laparoscopy is the ultimate standard for making the diagnosis by visualization of the infection and subsequent cultures.

Often, the physician must rely on history, physical examination, and laboratory results because laparoscopy may be inappropriately invasive.

The main diagnostic criteria (required for diagnosis) are

Diffuse lower abdominal pain and tenderness with or without rebound

Cervical motion tenderness

Adnexal tenderness, can be bilateral or unilateral

Minor criteria:

Fever

Leukocytosis

Purulent material in cul-de-sac

Purulent cervical discharge (defined as > 6 white blood cells/hpf)

Pelvic abscess or mass detected by physical examination or ultrasound (although this obviously is not a minor problem, it is not an essential criterion for diagnosis)

Elevated erythrocyte sedimentation rate

Positive gonorrhea or chlamydia tests from endocervix

What is Fitz-Hugh–Curtis syndrome?

Perihepatic inflammation with associated right upper quadrant pain

Occurs in 5%–10% of PID cases

What other tests should be considered?

β-Human chorionic gonadotropin assay to rule out ectopic pregnancy

Complete blood count with differential

Cervical cultures

Ultrasonography to investigate any masses

Culdocentesis to evaluate fluid in the peritoneal cavity

What are the differential diagnoses of PID?

Ectopic pregnancy

Acute appendicitis

Urinary tract infection

Adnexal torsion

Endometriosis

Bleeding corpus luteum
Diverticulosis

**What are the criteria for
hospitalization?**

Suspected pelvic or tubo-ovarian abscess
Pregnancy
Temperature > 38°C
Uncertain diagnosis
Nausea and vomiting precluding oral
    medications
Upper peritoneal signs, suggesting
    spread of peritonitis
Failure to respond to outpatient
    antibiotics within 48 hours

**What is the inpatient
treatment of PID?**

Inpatient and outpatient treatment both
    require multiple antimicrobials
    because no single agent is active
    against entire spectrum of possible
    pathogens.
Anaerobic coverage is very important:
    Cefoxitin IV 2 g q6h plus doxycycline
    100 mg q12h by mouth or IV (or
    third-generation cephalosporin)
Clindamycin IV 900 mg q8h plus
    gentamicin IV 1.5 mg/kg q8h
Imipenem/cilastin IV
Treatment of sexual partners

**What is the outpatient
treatment of PID?**

Ceftriaxone [250 mg intramuscularly
    (IM)] or cefoxitin (2 g IM) plus
    doxycycline by mouth for 10–14 days
Ofloxacin 400 mg orally bid for 14 days
    plus either clindamycin 450 mg orally
    four times a day or metronidazole 500
    mg orally two times a day for 14 days
Reexamination of the patient within 48
    to 72 hours

**What are the complications
of PID?**

Infertility
Ectopic pregnancy
Chronic pelvic pain
Adhesions
Hydrosalpinx
Dyspareunia

What are preventive measures for PID?

Barrier methods of contraception: Mechanical and chemical

Oral contraception: Thickens the cervical mucus and decreases the duration of menstrual flow, limiting the interval for bacterial colonization

Treatment of sexual partners

TUBO-OVARIAN ABSCESS

With what disease are tubo-ovarian abscesses often associated?

PID; significantly increases the mortality rate from PID

What are some common findings on physical examination?

Patients are very ill with severe pelvic and abdominal pain, high fever, nausea and vomiting, and possible septic shock.

Tachycardia

Abdominal rigidity and guarding

Rebound tenderness

Manual examination of adnexa is usually difficult because of extreme adnexal tenderness, but it may be possible to appreciate an adnexal mass.

How is a tubo-ovarian abscess diagnosed?

Ultrasound

Computed tomography scan

Exploratory laparoscopy

What are the differential diagnoses of tubo-ovarian abscess?

Septic incomplete abortion

Acute appendicitis

Diverticular abscess

Adnexal torsion

What are the treatment options for tubo-ovarian abscess?

Conservative treatment with bed rest in the hospital, adequate hydration, analgesics, and IV antibiotics (clindamycin and an aminoglycoside; or imipenem/cilastin)

Surgery if no improvement or rupture occurs; often requires total abdominal hysterectomy and bilateral salpingo-oophorectomy

ACTINOMYCOSIS

What is actinomycosis?

Infection with *Actinomyces* sp

What species of *Actinomyces* causes infection in the urogenital tract?

Actinomyces israelii

What birth control method is associated with *Actinomyces* abscesses?

Intrauterine device

What are characteristic gross and histologic findings?

"Sulfur granules"
Fistula formation
Chronic draining sinuses

What is the treatment for actinomycosis?

Penicillin

TUBERCULOSIS (TB)

What is the cause of genital tract TB?

Mycobacterium tuberculosis or *Mycobacterium bovis* that has spread hematogenously from either the lung or gastrointestinal tract

What are the symptoms of TB?

Infertility, abnormal uterine bleeding, and abdominal pain

How is a diagnosis of TB made?

Should be suspected when patient does not respond to conventional PID therapy
Confirmed by endometrial biopsy and culture

What is the treatment of TB?

Isoniazid and rifampin. Secondary agents may be necessary when resistance occurs.

OTHER INFECTIONS

TOXIC SHOCK SYNDROME (TSS)

What is TSS?

An acute, febrile illness leading to multiorgan system failure
Fifty percent of cases are associated with menses and tampon use.

What is the cause of TSS?

A bacterial exotoxin from *Staphylococcus aureus* (streptococcal TSS-Group A-is associated with invasive disease such as necrotizing fasciitis)

What are the signs and symptoms of TSS?

Presenting signs and symptoms: Abrupt onset of high fever, headache, myalgia, vomiting, diarrhea, generalized skin rash, and often hypotension
Characteristic rash begins as an intense "sunburn" that evolves into flaky desquamation and sloughing of the skin.

What is the treatment for TSS?

Intravenous fluids
Antibiotics (β-lactamase–resistant penicillin such as oxacillin or nafcillin)

ACQUIRED IMMUNODEFICIENCY SYNDROME (AIDS)

What is the cause and pathophysiology of AIDS?

Caused by the human immunodeficiency virus (HIV)
HIV attacks CD4+ T-lymphocytes.
Opportunistic infections occur when the CD4+ count drops below 200.

What are the clinical presentations of AIDS?

Community-acquired pneumonias and gastroenteritis
Pneumocystis carinii pneumonia
TB
Cryptococcus infection
Candidiasis
Toxoplasmosis
Cytomegalovirus infection
HSV infection

Which presentations are most common in women?

Candidiasis and HSV infections

How is a diagnosis of AIDS made?

Two tests:
1. Enzyme-linked immunosorbent assay test for antibodies against HIV; has a high rate of false-positive results.
2. Western blot identifies antibodies to an HIV-specific protein.

What is the incidence of AIDS in women?

Approximately 11% of people with AIDS are women.
Fastest growing population

28

Leiomyomas

What is a leiomyoma?

Also known as a fibroid

Benign smooth muscle tumor of the uterus

Most common neoplasm in the female pelvis

What causes leiomyomas?

Thought to arise through somatic mutations of smooth muscle cells

Possible mutations include translocations and deletions most commonly involving chromosome 12.

Individual leiomyomas in the same uterus arise through different mutations.

What receptors are present in leiomyomas?

Estrogen and progesterone receptors

Which has a greater concentration of receptors: a leiomyoma, endometrium, ormyometrium?

Leiomyomas have greater concentrations of receptors than endometrium or myometrium.

How do leiomyoma receptor concentrations vary?

With the menstrual cycle

Greater concentrations in the first 18 days of the cycle

What are the locations of leiomyomas?

Intramural: within the myometrial wall

Submucosal: grow from myometrium toward and into the endometrial cavity

Subserosal: grow from myometrium toward and into the abdominal cavity

Interligamentary: grow from myometrium into the broad ligament

Parasitic: grow into abdominal cavity, achieve secondary blood supply from mesenteric arteries, and detach from initial blood supply of myometrial arteries to become autonomous tumors on bowel or mesentery

Pedunculated: Connected to myometrium by a narrow stalk and "float" in the abdominal cavity, endometrial cavity, or even through the cervical os in the vagina

Which type is most symptomatic?

Submucosal

What is the incidence of leiomyomas?

Present in 20% of women of reproductive age

3x more common in African-American women

What is the surgical impact of leiomyomas?

Account for approximately one-third of all hysterectomies (most common indication for hysterectomy)

Account for a significant number of other surgical procedures, including dilation and curettage; diagnostic and operative hysteroscopy; laparoscopy and myomectomy

What are the symptoms?

Many are asymptomatic

Symptoms are associated with size, number, and location

Abnormal uterine bleeding: most common symptom associated with leiomyomas and usually manifests as menorrhagia

Pelvic pain

Pressure from a leiomyoma on bladder or rectum can result in urinary frequency, urgency, incontinence, and the sensation of rectal pressure

Why do leiomyomas cause abnormal uterine bleeding?

Theories:

Increased surface area of endometrial cavity mucosa leading to increased bleeding

Vascular alteration of the endometrial surface

Mechanical interference from leiomyomas on normal myometrial contractions during menses preventing blood loss

Compression of endometrial venules by intramural leiomyomas, causing venular dilatation and increased venous blood loss

Why do leiomyomas cause pain?

Theories:

Carneous (red) degeneration:

Hemorrhagic degeneration of leiomyoma causing acute pelvic pain, low-grade fever, mild peritoneal signs, and occasionally leukocytosis

Often difficult to distinguish from other causes of acute abdominal pain (including placental abruption in pregnancy)

How are they diagnosed?

Physical exam, ultrasound, hysterogram, saline sonohysterography, hysteroscopy

How do leiomyomas interfere with the ability to achieve a term pregnancy?

Theories:

Prevention of conception (infertility):

Bilateral cornual obstruction secondary to cornual leiomyomas leading to complete bilateral tubal occlusion

Other mechanisms

Prevention of implantation or growth of the developing embryo (recurrent pregnancy loss): Conception occurs but submucosal leiomyomas interfere with implantation, placentation, or continued adherence to myometrial wall.

Prevention of progression to term (preterm labor): Leiomyomas cause myometrial irritation, which stimulates the onset of premature uterine activity and premature contractions.

How are the above-stated effects on pregnancy remedied?

Interference with the ability to achieve or maintain pregnancy: correction of the structural abnormality imposed by leiomyoma with myomectomy (using laparotomy, hysteroscopy, or laparoscopy)

Myomectomy during pregnancy:

Has been accomplished when the size or location may interfere with the ability to carry the pregnancy to term or lead to other complications in pregnancy

Is best performed in the nonpregnant state

What other complications in pregnancy are related to leiomyomas?

Dystocia:

Can prevent vaginal delivery

Accounts for the increased cesarean section rate in women with leiomyomas

Increased risk of uterine inversion with submucosal leiomyomas

Red (carneous) degeneration occurs more frequently in pregnancy.

Preterm labor

How does pregnancy affect preexisting leiomyomas?

Recent studies suggest that whereas some leiomyomas grow during pregnancy, the majority do not and most shrink in the third trimester.

What condition could rapid growth of leiomyomas indicate?

Leiomyosarcoma, a malignant sarcoma that can mimic benign leiomyomas, is characterized by rapid uterine enlargement.

What is the incidence of leiomyosarcoma?

Approximately 0.1% to 1% of all pathologic specimens submitted as leiomyomas are actually leiomyosarcoma.

Leiomyosarcoma is more prevalent in the fifth and sixth decades of life.

What is the prognosis of leiomyosarcoma?

Poor prognosis if discovered after menopause

More favorable prognosis in early stages (I or II) in younger women

What is the management/ treatment of asymptomatic leiomyomas?

Serial examinations to determine rate of growth and careful history to detect new symptomatology

Rapid enlargement is of concern.

If leiomyomas are not enlarging rapidly, annual examinations are sufficient.

Nonsteroidal anti-inflammatory drugs: decrease blood loss associated with menses

What is the management treatment of symptomatic leiomyomas?

Surgery is the preferred treatment option but medical options include GnRN analogs, & RU 486.

What are gonadotropin- releasing hormone (GnRH) agonists?

Synthetic derivatives of GnRH created by substitutions of amino acids at the sixth and sometimes tenth amino acid residues

Confer a longer half-life and better binding of GnRH to the GnRH receptor

How do GnRH agonists affect the size of leiomyomas?

Inhibit GnRH secretion by downregulation after 2 weeks of use, leading to a decrease in gonadotropin secretion and, thus, a decrease in ovarian estrogen synthesis and a hypoestrogenic state

Decrease leiomyoma size approximately 50%, with maximal effect after 12 weeks of use and no decrease in size after that time; temporary effect

What are the indications for use of GnRH agonists in the management of leiomyomas?

American College of Obstetrics and Gynecology (ACOG) recommendations:

  For treatment of large submucous leiomyomas prior to hysteroscopic resection to facilitate resection and decrease blood loss

  For treatment of leiomyomas while awaiting menopause (a hypo-estrogenic state that leads to shrinkage of leiomyomas) in a perimenopausal woman

  For treatment preoperatively while awaiting work-up of medical problems or when other considerations prohibit immediate surgery

How long should GnRH agonist therapy last?

Use is generally limited to less than 6 months to limit side effects.

What are the purported benefits of GnRH agonist therapy?

Reduction in menstrual blood loss
Improvement in anemia prior to surgery
Allowance of time for autologous blood donation
Reduction of operative blood loss
Decrease in the need for hysterectomy
Improvement in chance that a hysterectomy can be done vaginally instead of abdominally

What are the side effects of GnRH agonists?

Similar to menopausal symptoms

What surgical treatments are available?

Myomectomy
Hysterectomy
Dependent on patient's desire for future fertility, severity of symptoms, and size of myomata

What is the definition of myomectomy?

Removal of individual leiomyomas from an intact uterus

What are the indications for myomectomy in the treatment of leiomyomas?

Usually performed when preservation of fertility is an issue

ACOG recommendation: when the leiomyoma is a probable factor in failure to conceive or in recurrent pregnancy loss

What are the benefits of myomectomy?

Approximately 80% of women who have a myomectomy have improvement in hypermenorrhea, pelvic pain, or pressure but recurrence is common.

How is myomectomy performed?

Laparotomy or via hysteroscopy for submucosal tumors

Laparoscopic myomectomies have been performed.

What are the indications for hysterectomy in the treatment of leiomyomas?

Controversial

General guidelines:

For treatment of asymptomatic leiomyomas that are palpable abdominally and of concern to the patient

For treatment of excessive bleeding with either flooding and/or clots for greater than 8 days, or for acute or chronic blood loss

For treatment of pelvic discomfort when the pain is either acute or severe, causes chronic lower abdominal or back pain, or causes bladder pressure with urinary frequency

Other Treatments?

Uterine artery embolization

Laparoscopic BSO

29

Pelvic Relaxation

What is the pelvic floor?

Paired levator ani muscles are fused to the bony pelvis anteriorly and posteriorly and attached laterally to the white line (the arcus tendineus fasciae pelvis) which overlies the obturator internus muscles.

The normal tone of the levator ani muscles supports the pelvic organs from below and contributes to urinary and fecal continence.

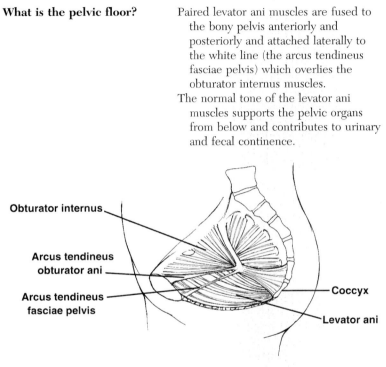

Obturator internus

Arcus tendineus obturator ani

Arcus tendineus fasciae pelvis

Coccyx

Levator ani

Figure 29.1

What is the levator hiatus?

The anterior separation through which the urethra, vagina, and rectum pass

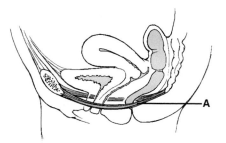

Figure 29.2. The vaginal axis of the erect or standing living female is shown. Notice the almost horizontal upper vagina and rectum lying on and parallel to the levator plate. The latter is formed by fusion of the pubococcygei muscles *(A)* posterior to the rectum. The anterior limit of the point of fusion is the margin of the genital hiatus immediately posterior to the rectum. (From Nichols DH, Milley PS: Clinical anatomy of the vulva, vagina, lower pelvis, and perineum. In Sciarra (ed): *Gynecology and Obstetrics*, 1977; reproduced with permission of Harper & Row.)

What is endopelvic fascia? Visceral fascia investing the pelvic organs that form bilateral condensations known as ligaments. For example:
To maintain support of the bladder, pubocervical fascia is plicated in the midline when repairing a cystocele.
Likewise, to support the rectum, perirectal fascia is plicated to repair a rectocele.

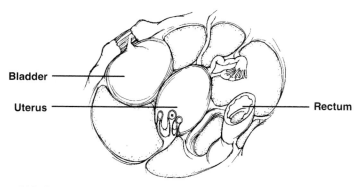

Figure 29.3. Stereograph shows the connective tissue septae and paravaginal spaces in relation to the bladder, uterus, and rectum. The spaces permit these three organs to function independently of one another.

What are the important ligaments of pelvic support?

In general, all pelvic ligaments attach organs to the pelvic sidewall and/or bony pelvis.

From caudad to cephalad for the uterus:
Uterosacral
Cardinal
Round

For the bladder and urethra:
pubourethral

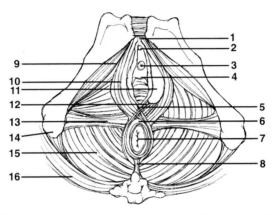

Figure 29.4. Normal anatomy of layers of pelvic supports (vaginal view): Superficial skin and adipose tissue have been removed to expose the *numbered* structural layers. 1, suspensory L. clitoris; 2, clitoris; 3, urethral meatus; 4, hymen; 5, perineal body; 6, anal sphincter; 7, anus; 8, anococcygeal body; 9, ischiocavernosus muscle; 10, bulbocavernosus muscle; 11, vestibular bulb; 12, Bartholin gland; 13, superficial perineal muscle; 14, ischial tuberosity; 15, levator ani muscle; 16, gluteus maximus muscle.

How does the perineal body help maintain pelvic support?

It is the central point for attachment of the perineal musculature.

It is inferior to, and serves to support, the urogenital diaphragm. It also supports the distal vagina and rectum.

What is pelvic relaxation?

Loss of support for the female urogenital organs

Can include the uterus, vagina, rectum, or small bowel

Primarily occurs in adult women as a result of direct or indirect damage to the vagina, its support systems, or both

What factors contribute to pelvic relaxation?

Childbirth: detachments, lacerations, denervations from parturition

Iatrogenic: failed episiotomy repairs, prior surgical repairs

Medical: chronic obstructive pulmonary disease, obesity, strenuous physical activity, ascites, or other situations resulting in chronic increased intra-abdominal pressure

Inherent: hypoestrogenic atrophy of tissues; inherent connective tissue characteristics

What are the signs and symptoms of pelvic relaxation?

Generally visceral, sexual, and hernia related

Protrusion of organs; ulceration or bleeding in severe cases (or with procidentia); low back pain; pressure; and heaviness, especially at the end of the day.

Dyspareunia or a complete inability to have intercourse

Bladder: incontinence, inability to void, frequent urinary tract infections

GI: constipation, need to splint the vagina for defecation

What questions should be asked in taking the patient history?

In addition to the previously mentioned, ask about:

Prior vaginal/abdominal surgeries

Parity: birth weights, use of forceps, difficult labors, etc.

Interest in future fertility

Hormone replacement

Occupation and activities involving lifting or straining

Cardiac and respiratory problems or obesity in medical history

What should be included in the physical examination?

Examination of patient in both lithotomy AND standing positions

Inspection of the genital hiatus: Protruding tissues?

Is the uterus present or absent?
Does the cervix or vaginal apex
  descend?
Instruct the patient to bear down
  (Valsalva) and note any change.
Be as SITE-SPECIFIC as possible.

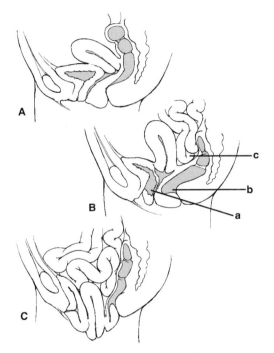

Figure 29.5. Types of genital prolapse are diagrammatically shown. A, Sagittal section of a normally supported pelvis. B, Incomplete uterine prolapse is noted along with specific types of herniation, (a) cystocele, (b) rectocele, and (c) enterocele. C, Complete uterine prolapse (procidentia) is shown.

What is a cystocele?   Relaxation and/or descent of the bladder
                                          anteriorly into the vagina

What is a rectocele?   Relaxation and/or descent of the rectum
                                          posteriorly into the vagina

What is an enterocele?   Herniation of the small bowel into the
                                          cul-de-sac (or pouch of Douglas)

How is pelvic organ prolapse graded?

One common grading system is as follows:

Grade 0: no descent (organs well supported and above the level of the ischial spines)

Grade 1: descent halfway down to the introitus

Grade 2: descent to the introitus

Grade 3: descent halfway out of the introitus

What is uterine procidentia?

Grade 4: descent completely outside of the introitus

What are the nonsurgical treatment options?

Correction of reversible medical conditions such as obesity, smoking, and asthma

Modification of strenuous activities such as heavy lifting

Estrogen therapy to assist with tissue integrity

Kegels

Pessaries

What are Kegel exercises?

Pelvic muscle exercises (daily repetitions of pubococcygeus muscle contractions) to strengthen the pelvic floor

What are pessaries?

Devices placed in the vagina that press against the vaginal sidewalls to support the pelvic organs within the vagina (various shapes and names)

What is their use in treatment of pelvic relaxation?

Generally used for the nonsurgical patient; can be used for years

What problems are associated with pessaries?

Vaginal irritation and ulceration

Work best in well-estrogenized tissue

Require periodic removal and cleaning

What are the goals of surgery in the treatment of pelvic organ prolapse?

Relieve symptoms
Restore normal anatomy
Restore normal visceral function
Allow satisfactory coital function
Obtain a durable result

What are the considerations in choosing a particular surgical treatment?

Type of surgery depends on the patient's particular constellation of symptoms and physical findings, along with her interest in future fertility, if any.

What are some commonly performed vaginal procedures?

Vaginal hysterectomy, enterocoele plication, anterior and posterior colporrhaphy
Vaginal hysterectomy:
For patients who have completed childbearing, especially if they have other pelvic defects.
Will not correct uterovaginal prolapse; proper suspension of the vaginal apex is needed.

What are the key principles in the repair of an enterocele?

Same as with repair of any hernia: completely identify the sac, reduce any small bowel found in the sac; perform high ligation and then excision of the distal portion of the sac.

What is an anterior colporrhaphy (or an anterior repair)?

Indication: repair of a cystocele
Basic technique: interrupted horizontal sutures to plicate the endopelvic (or pubocervical) fascia in order to elevate and support the urethrovesical junction and the bladder

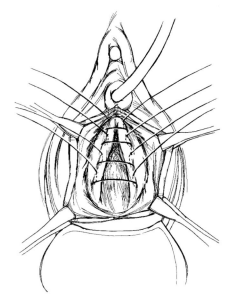

Figure 29.6. A specific supporting suture or two is placed at the level of the urethrovesical junction and anchored to the fibromuscular tissue of the underside of the pubic ramus bilaterally. The bladder neck is elevated when these sutures are tied. The cystocele is then reduced by placement of a series of plicating sutures along the bladder base.

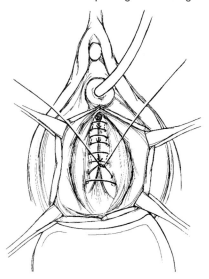

Figure 29.7. The pubovesical fascia is plicated to the midline, reducing the cystocele.

What is a posterior colporrhaphy (or a posterior repair)?

Indication: repair of a rectocele

Basic technique: dissection of the rectovaginal septum up to the vaginal apex, then interrupted horizontal sutures to plicate the perirectal fascia over the rectum

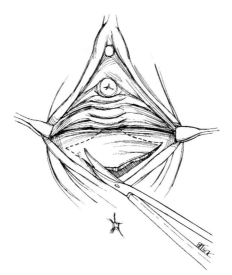

Figure 29.8. The rectocele repair is initiated by incising the skin of the perineal body along the mucocutaneous junction.

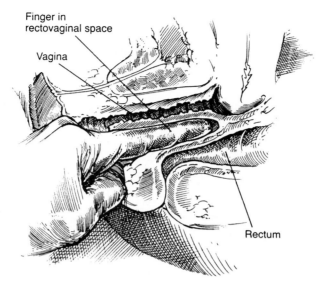

Figure 29.9. The rectovaginal space is bluntly developed once any scar tissue has been incised. The space is developed to a point above the site of the rectocele.

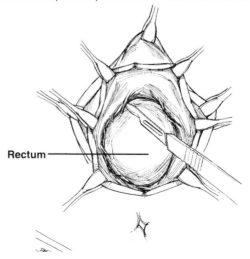

Figure 29.10. The posterior vaginal wall and rectovaginal septum are incised and reflected. The underlying rectum and perirectal fascia are exposed.

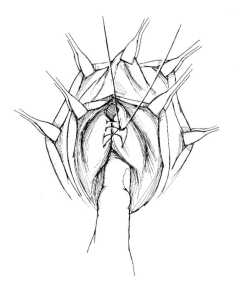

Figure 29.11. The rectocele is reduced by plicating the perirectal fascia to the midline. As the distal vagina is reached, the medial bodies of the levator ani are incorporated into the plicated tissues for additional support.

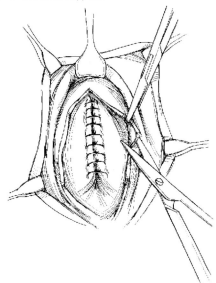

Figure 29.12. Excess vaginal mucosa is excised from the posterior vagina, and the vaginal incision is closed.

What are the choices for correction of prolapse of a post-hysterectomy vaginal vault prolapse?

Vaginal approaches:

McCall's culdoplasty, which incorporates the strong uterosacral ligaments to the vaginal mucosa

Sacrospinous ligament fixation, which tacks the vaginal apex to the sacrospinous ligament

Abdominal approaches: *sacro-colpopexy*, which uses synthetic mesh to connect the vaginal apex to the sacral promontory

What other abdominal procedures can be performed to address pelvic organ prolapse?

Abdominal hysterectomy, if indicated, with particular attention given to reattachment of the cut ends of the cardinal and uterosacral ligaments to the vaginal apex

What is a Moschcowitz procedure?

An abdominal procedure used to obliterate the cul-de-sac to prevent an enterocele

Permanent suture is used in a circumferential manner.

What is a Halban procedure?

Same as a Moschcowitz procedure, but performed in a vertical fashion

What is a paravaginal repair?

Procedure of choice if a cystocele exists as a result of loss of LATERAL support

Can be accomplished from either a vaginal or an abdominal approach

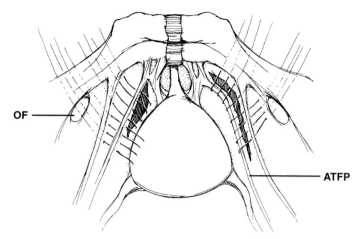

Figure 29.13. The reparative phase of paravaginal repair. ATFP, arcus tendineus fasciae pelvis; OF, obturator foramen. Defects and suture placement are shown on right and left sides.

The basic technique involves reattaching the lateral fascia of the anterior superior vagina to the "white line," or fascia of arcus tendineus levator ani.

What are the potential surgical complications from pelvic reconstructive surgery?

Failure of the procedure, especially if all defects are not addressed or if the patient does not address concomitant medical conditions

Gastrointestinal: small or large bowel injury

Genitourinary: postoperative voiding dysfunction from temporary bladder denervation or edema, urinary retention or incontinence, ureteral injury, unintentional cystotomy

Sexual: vaginal stenosis or shortening of the vagina if too many sutures are placed or if too much vaginal mucosa is excised

Bleeding: pudendal vessel injury with sacrospinous ligament fixation, presacral vessel injury with abdominal sacrocolpopexy

Nerve damage: peroneal damage from improper lithotomy positioning (recall the nerve that runs lateral to the head of the fibula); sciatica from needle penetration with sacrospinous ligament fixation

What is the LeFort procedure?

A technique of vaginal obliteration, mainly used in older, infirm patients who are not sexually active

It is important to leave a tunnel between the cervix and vagina for exit of abnormal discharge or bleeding.

What are the options for women who have not completed childbearing?

Usually it is better to delay treatment until childbearing is complete.

Nonsurgical methods such as Kegel exercises or pessaries

Ventral suspensions of the uterine fundus are points of historical interest only.

30

Pelvic Pain

What are the differences among nociception, pain, suffering, and pain behavior?

Nociception refers to the origination and detection of a neurologic signal based on a noxious event.

Pain is the recognition of the signal or event.

Suffering is the affective response to the event.

Pain behavior involves adaptive behavioral changes made as a result of pain.

What noxious events can lead to pain?

Thermal stimuli: Heat or cold

Mechanical stimuli: Stretch, distention, muscular contraction

Chemical stimuli: Various biologic pain mediators, neurotransmitters, and ions

How does the character of pain mediated by slow versus fast pain fibers vary?

Slow pain fibers characteristically mediate visceral pain, which is usually described as a diffuse burning or aching and is usually the result of inflammation or ischemia (e.g., the referred periumbilical aching in appendicitis).

Fast pain fibers characteristically mediate parietal peritoneal pain, which is usually described as a well-localized, sharp pain (e.g., the sharp pain over the right lower quadrant in appendicitis).

What are the three main models of pain perception?

1. Medical Model: Pain perception is the result of anatomic or physiologic abnormalities of tissues that, if corrected, result in the amelioration of pain.
2. Gate Control Model: Pain perception is the result of a complex interaction

between peripheral stimuli and cortical variables (mood, anxiety). Amelioration of pain must target both somatic and psychogenic precipitants.

3. Biopsychosocial Model: Pain perception is the result of nociceptive stimuli, psychological factors, and social determinants. Elimination of nociceptive stimuli leads to symptom shifting, which results in disabling symptoms elsewhere.

What is pelvic pain?
A general term that refers to pain of gynecologic or nongynecologic origin perceived by the patient as originating from the female pelvis. Chronic pelvic pain refers to symptoms lasting greater than six months.

Where is pelvic pain localized?
Right lower quadrant, left lower quadrant, infraumbilical, deep pelvic, or cervicovaginal

What percentage of office visits are for pelvic pain?
The presenting complaint in approximately 10% of gynecologic office visits and comprises a significant percentage of emergency room visits

What are some common extrauterine gynecologic causes of pelvic pain?
Adhesions, ectopic pregnancy, pelvic inflammatory disease, endometriosis, ovarian cysts or masses, ovarian torsion, and pelvic residual ovary syndrome, congestion syndrome.

What are some common uterine causes of pelvic pain?
Adenomyosis, leiomyomas, intrauterine device, pelvic support defects, endometritis, primary dysmenorrhea, cervical stenosis

What are some common urologic causes of pelvic pain?
Urinary tract infection, interstitial cystitis, chronic urethral syndrome, nephrolithiasis, urethral diverticulitis, detrusor overactivity, and urethritis

What are some common gastrointestinal causes of pelvic pain?

Cholelithiasis, appendicitis, constipation, diverticular disease, inflammatory bowel disease, irritable bowel syndrome, gastrointestinal neoplasm, hernias, chronic pancreatitis, peptic ulcer disease intussusception, volvulus

What are some common musculoskeletal causes of pelvic pain?

Gait disorders, postural dysfunction, intervertebral disc disease, degenerative joint disease, fibromyositis, pelvic floor spasm (levator ani or obturator), myofascial pain, rectus abdominus spasm, nerve entrapment syndromes, strains and sprains, and coccydynia

What are some other causes of pelvic pain?

History of or current physical or sexual abuse, heavy metal poisoning, porphyria, psychiatric disorders (depression, bipolar disorder, personality disorders), psychosocial stressors, somatiform disorders, sickle cell disease, sleep disturbances, fibromyalgia, aneurysm, herpes zoster

What is chronic pelvic pain?

Pelvic pain that lasts more than 6 months, as opposed to subacute (3–6 months) or acute (less than 3 months)

What is the general approach in the evaluation of pelvic pain?

Initially, a determination of the acuity and duration of pain should be made to determine if the pain requires emergent treatment (i.e., it is potentially life-threatening, subacute, or long-standing in nature).

History and physical examination are particularly important in determining the cause of pelvic pain given the extensive differential diagnosis.

Once acute causes of pelvic pain have been ruled out or appropriately treated, diagnosing the cause of chronic pelvic pain may require numerous office visits and varied treatments.

Assessment of pelvic pain requires an integrated multidisciplinary approach that addresses medical, psychological, and social issues.

What important questions should be asked when evaluating the patient with chronic pelvic pain?

The character, intensity (often graded subjectively on a scale of 1 to 10), location, and radiation of the pain

Temporal aspects (typical pattern throughout the day/week/month, cyclicity, duration) and exacerbating or relieving factors

Menstrual symptoms, including menorrhagia, colicky dysmenorrhea, and the relation of the menstrual complaints to pelvic pain

Sexual history, including contraceptive history, dyspareunia (if present), and vaginal symptoms (if present)

Gastrointestinal symptoms, including changes in bowel habits (constipation or diarrhea), anorexia, nausea, vomiting, bloating, and hematochezia

Urologic symptoms, including dysuria, hematuria, changes in urinary habits, nocturia, and incontinence

Musculoskeletal symptoms, including low back pain, hip pain

History of prior surgeries and gynecologic or obstetric problems, including PID

Psychological history, including history of depression, somatization, anxiety disorders, sexual or physical abuse, marital or relationship discord, substance abuse, sleep disturbances, or other stressors

What aspects of the physical examination are important in the evaluation of chronic pelvic pain?

Thorough abdominal examination, including inspection for deformity, scars, hernias, distention; auscultation for bowel sounds; and palpation of the epigastrium, flanks, back, and inguinal regions for tenderness and masses

Special attention to pain reproduction during pelvic and rectovaginal examination, with an attempt to determine adnexal or uterine tenderness and uterosacral ligament or cul-de-sac nodularity or tenderness

Evaluation for rectal masses or tenderness, cystocele, pelvic relaxation, and tenderness or thickening in the bladder or urethra

Evaluation for spinal and musculoskeletal anomalies, including scoliosis, leg asymmetry or motion restriction, gait dysfunction, and neurologic examination

Elucidation of trigger points, including myofascial (especially in the levator ani and obturator internus), musculoskeletal, and abdominal (lateral edges of rectus abdominus)

What laboratory studies are important in the evaluation of chronic pelvic pain?

Complete blood count to evaluate for infection or hemorrhage

Human chorionic gonadotropin assay to evaluate for intrauterine, ectopic or molar pregnancy

Cervical cultures and wet preparation (saline and KOH) to evaluate for the presence of infection or inflammation

Urinalysis and culture to evaluate for kidney stones, cystitis or pyelonephritis

Hepatic transaminases, bilirubin, and lipase and amylase to evaluate hepatobiliary obstruction, hepatitis, or pancreatitis

Erythrocyte sedimentation rate and C-reactive protein to evaluate chronic disease states

What imaging modalities may be useful in the evaluation of pelvic pain?

Ultrasound (see below), CT scan (especially acute causes of pain such as kidney stones and appendicitis), MRI (adenomyosis and other uterine anomalies)

How can ultrasound be helpful in the evaluation of pelvic pain?

Pelvic ultrasound can supplement an inconclusive or limited (usually secondary to obesity) pelvic examination.

Structural anomalies such as ovarian cysts or masses, uterine fibroids, and tubal pathology (including hydrosalpinx, tubo-ovarian abscess, or ectopic pregnancy) may be seen.

How is diagnostic laparoscopy helpful in the evaluation of pelvic pain?

Laparoscopy can be useful in the evaluation of acute pelvic pain by identifying endometriosis, adhesions, hydrosalpinx, tubo-ovarian abscess, pelvic inflammatory disease (PID), ectopic pregnancy, and appendiceal or intestinal pathology.

Chronic pelvic pain is the indication for about 25% of all laparoscopies performed in the United States annually.

What are the two most common gynecologic problems encountered in women undergoing laparoscopic evaluation for pelvic pain?

Endometriosis is the most common abnormality encountered, and one large study suggested that one in three women undergoing laparoscopy have endometriosis present, although the severity of pain does not seem to correlate with the severity of the lesions present.

Adhesions are the second most common finding. The same study found adhesions in about one in five women undergoing laparoscopic evaluation for chronic pelvic pain, although the role of adhesions in the cause of pelvic pain is controversial.

What is the role of PID in chronic pelvic pain?

Chronic pelvic pain is one of the sequelae of PID, along with infertility and ectopic pregnancy.

Some authors have estimated that chronic pelvic pain develops in one in four women with PID.

What is the most common gastrointestinal diagnosis made in the workup of chronic pelvic pain, and what are the associated symptoms?

Irritable bowel syndrome (IBS) may be diagnosed in up to half of all patients undergoing workup for chronic pelvic pain.

Pain is often colicky, with a sensation of rectal fullness relieved with bowel movements and intensified with meals.

Pain may be worse during menstruation and associated with dyspareunia.

Associated symptoms include alternating constipation and diarrhea.

What is the association of physical or sexual abuse and chronic pelvic pain?

Studies have shown that up to 60% of women with chronic pelvic pain have a history of sexual abuse, and that there is also a significant association between physical abuse and chronic pelvic pain.

What medications are commonly used to treat chronic pelvic pain?

Mild pain relievers such as aspirin, nonsteroidal anti-inflammatory drugs, and acetaminophen can be used to treat mild pain.

Stronger agents, including narcotics such as codeine, oxycodone, propoxyphene, pentazocine, and hydromorphone, can be used for relief of more severe pain. Tolerance and physical dependence can develop with opioid use, and thus use of narcotics should be for a defined period of time.

Agents classically used as antidepressants, such as SSRIs, and tricyclic antidepressants, have been found to have a profound response on peripheral as well as central pain receptors, and are a useful adjunct or replacement to pain relievers. Antiepilectic agents such as gabapentin are also used.

Standing medications usually are more helpful than prn medications. IBS may respond to bulk-forming agents, anxiolytics, and low doses of antidepressants.

Occasionally, empiric antibiotic treatment for PID is used in the absence of culture-proven infection.

Oral contraceptives can be used to suppress ovulation and regulate the menstrual cycle in cases where dysmenorrhea or ovulatory pain appears to be a significant component of pain. Either cyclic or continuous OCP regimens may be employed.

Danazol or leuprolide acetate can be used to suppress endometriosis.

What considerations should be taken into account before surgical treatment of pelvic pain?

Identifiable causes of pelvic pain should be treated as indicated surgically, but the patient must be informed that removal of the suspected problem does not guarantee relief of the pain.

Patients with a history of unsuccessful attempts to treat pelvic pain surgically have a much higher risk of having persistent pain after another operation.

What are surgical options for treatment of chronic pelvic pain?

Ablation of endometriotic lesions can be accomplished with laser fulguration, coagulation, or excision.

Lysis of adhesions can be accomplished with laser or sharp dissection.

Laparoscopic uterosacral nerve ablation and presacral neurectomy interrupt the pathways of nerves responsible for pain transmission.

Hysterectomy is an option provided the patient has had gastrointestinal and urologic sources of pain ruled out and has failed medical management for greater than 6 months. If endometriosis is the cause of pain, hysterectomy and BSO is often required.

How successful is hysterectomy in curing chronic pelvic pain?

Traditionally, chronic pelvic pain is not thought to respond well to hysterectomy, although recent studies suggest that up to three in four women undergoing hysterectomy for chronic pelvic pain may have complete resolution of pain.

What are the predictors for persistent pain after hysterectomy?

Age < 30 years, history of PID, no identified pelvic disease, or having a history of at least two pregnancies

What conditions are associated with resolution of pain after hysterectomy?

Resolution occurred in 84%, 77%, and 81%, respectively, with adenomyosis, leiomyomas, or endometriosis.

What modalities of treatment other than conventional surgical and medical methods are used in the multidisciplinary approach to chronic pelvic pain treatment?

Addressing and treating the physical, psychological, and social factors involved in chronic pelvic pain has proved to be effective.

Techniques include teaching methods for coping or relaxing, biofeedback, pelvic pain physical therapy, depression therapy, psychotherapy, marital and sexual counseling, nerve blocks, exercise programs, transcutaneous electrical nerve stimulation (TENS units), and hypnosis.

31

Endometriosis

What is endometriosis?

Ectopic occurrence of hormonally responsive endometrial tissue

Where is endometriosis most commonly found?

In or on the ovaries, posterior cul-de-sac, uterosacral ligaments, broad ligament, and anterior cul-de-sac

Can involve the uterine serosa, rectovaginal septum, cervix, vagina, rectosigmoid, ileum, appendix, cecum, bladder, and ureter

Rarely involves the umbilicus, laparotomy or episiotomy scars, lungs, or distant organs

What problems do endometriosis implants cause?

Bleeding, inflammation, and adhesions leading to pelvic pain, dyspareunia, and infertility

How does endometriosis cause infertility?

Unknown, but proposed mechanisms include:

Adhesion formation:

Leads to distorted anatomy, increased distance from the ovary to the fimbriae, encasement of the ovary by adhesions, and destruction of ovarian and tubal tissue

All can disrupt ovulation and ovum transport.

Altered peritoneal fluid constituents (including hormones, prostaglandins, and immune substances) leading to alterations in ovulation, ovum "pickup" by the tube, tubal function, nidation, and luteal phase adequacy

Interference with ovulation and menstrual cyclicity

Luteinized unruptured follicle syndrome: A condition in which there is objective evidence of ovulation but the oocyte is not released by the ovary

Increased incidence in women with endometriosis

What are endometriomas?

Invasive endometriotic lesions found in the ovary

Also called "chocolate cysts" because of the chocolate-colored blood inside the lesions

Can cause extensive pelvic adhesions, especially periovarian, when repeated leakage results in dense, fibrotic tissue formation

What are the ultrasound findings suggestive of endometriomas?

Large cysts with homogenous, low-level internal echoes

What is the incidence of endometriosis?

Occurs in 3%–10% of women of reproductive age and 25%–35% of infertile women

What three mechanisms have been proposed to cause endometriosis?

Retrograde menstruation:

Menstrual material flows retrograde through fallopian tubes and implants on pelvic and abdominal structures.

Reinforced by studies that showed that monkeys with cervices surgically altered to empty into peritoneal cavity developed endometriosis.

Coelomic metaplasia:

Peritoneal coelomic epithelium undergoes metaplastic changes to assume characteristics of endometrial tissue.

Reinforced by the finding of endometriosis in prepubertal girls and women who have never menstruated

Hematogenous/lymphatic spread: Endometrial tissue "metastasizes" by vascular and lymphatic pathways to implant on various pelvic, abdominal, and distant organs.

Explains extrapelvic and pulmonary endometriosis

Is there a genetic predisposition to development of endometriosis?

Genetic or immunologic factors may play a role in endometriosis.

Seven percent of first-degree relatives of women with endometriosis have the disease, compared to one percent of control group, in one study.

A polygenic/multifactorial mechanism of heredity has been proposed.

What are the risk factors for endometriosis?

Nulliparity
Infertility
Reproductive age (usually, late teens to forties)
A first-degree relative with endometriosis
Regular menstrual cycles less than 27 days
Prolonged menses of 8 or more days

What is the most common endometriosis symptom?

Pelvic pain; can manifest as secondary dysmenorrhea, deep dyspareunia (pain on deep penetration), low sacral backache (especially premenstrually), or constant diffuse pelvic pain

Disease severity does not predict the degree of pain.

How does endometriosis affect organs adjacent to the uterus?

Rectosigmoid involvement can lead to perimenstrual tenesmus or diarrhea.

Bladder involvement can result in dysuria or hematuria.

What physical examination findings are suggestive of endometriosis?

Tenderness on bimanual examination
Tenderness or nodularity on the posterior vaginal fornix
Uterosacral ligament tenderness or nodularity
Cystic ovarian enlargement
Fixation of adnexal structures
Retroflexed uterus
Episiotomy or cesarean section scar implants

Is an OCA-125 level helpful in diagnosing endometriosis?

OCA-125 is elevated (> 35 U/ml) in approximately one-third of women with advanced endometriosis.
Elevated OCA-125 level is neither diagnostic nor an accurate screening test.

Are radiologic studies useful in making the diagnosis?

Ultrasound or magnetic resonance imaging may reveal endometriomas, but otherwise are not useful in the diagnosis of endometriosis.

Is endometriosis a clinical diagnosis?

Endometriosis is **not** a clinical diagnosis!
Definitive diagnosis of endometriosis can be made **only** by direct visualization of endometriotic lesions at time of laparoscopy or laparotomy **or** tissue diagnosis by pathologist revealing endometrial stroma & glands.

What do endometriosis lesions look like?

"Classic" endometriosis lesions are red, dark brown, dark blue, or black peritoneal implants or "chocolate cysts" of the ovary, but endometriotic lesion appearance varies as follows:
"Powder burn" implants from thickened or scarred perilesional peritoneum
Clear vesicles
White or yellow spots or nodules
Normal-appearing peritoneum (microscopic disease)

How is endometriosis classified?

The American Fertility Society classification system is based on findings at time of laparoscopy or laparotomy to determine severity of disease.
Numeric values are assigned to various findings, with higher numbers implying more severe disease.

How is endometriosis staged?

Stages are determined by the total point assignment for the constellation of findings in a given patient.

Stage I: Minimal
Stage II: Mild
Stage III: Moderate
Stage IV: Severe

What are some examples of point assignment for various findings at the time of laparoscopy or laparotomy?

1: Filmy adhesions enclosing less than one-third of the ovary *or* filmy adhesions enclosing less than one-third of the tube *or* superficial ovarian endometriotic implants < 1 cm in size
2: Superficial peritoneal endometriosis 1–3 cm in size
4: Partial cul-de-sac obliteration or superficial peritoneal endometriosis ≥ 3 cm in size
6: Deep peritoneal endometriosis ≥ 3 cm in size
8: Dense tubal adhesions with less than one-third enclosure
16: Deep ovarian implants 1–3 cm in size *or* dense tubal adhesions with more than two-thirds enclosure
40: Complete cul-de-sac obliteration

How useful is classification of endometriosis?

High intraobserver and interobserver variability limits utility, but classification is helpful in operative report summaries.

What are the goals of management/treatment of endometriosis?

Control of symptoms
Treatment of infertility
The disease is progressive and difficult (or impossible) to "cure."

What are the types of management/treatment of endometriosis?

Medical (hormonal)
Surgical (conservative or definitive)
Combination of medical and surgical

How is the choice of management/treatment determined?

By severity of disease, reproductive considerations, and physician/patient preference

What medications are used in the treatment of endometriosis?

Medications suppress estrogenic stimulation of ectopic endometrial tissue:
Combined estrogen–progestin
Progestins
Danazol
Gonadotropin-releasing hormone (GnRH) agonists

Indications for medical therapy?

Used only after surgery confirms the presence of endometriosis through viewing classic endometriotic lesions, or a tissue diagnosis is made

What is danazol, how does it work, and what are its side effects?

Danazol (Danacrine) is a weak synthetic androgen.
Mechanism of action: Suppresses luteinizing hormone (LH) and follicle-stimulating hormone (FSH) secretion, leading to decreased ovarian steroidogenesis, and directly inhibits endometrial cells (by androgen receptors), creating a high-androgen/low-estrogen environment
Side effects: Increased liver enzymes, increased low-density lipoproteins, decreased high-density lipoproteins, weight gain, edema, decreased breast size, oily skin, acne, hirsutism, and, rarely, permanent voice deepening

What are GnRH agonists, how do they work, and what are their side effects?

GnRH agonists are novel peptides synthesized by substituting the sixth amino acid residue (and sometimes the tenth) of the native GnRH molecule to achieve a longer half-life and better binding to the GnRH receptor. No evidence to suggest that they improve fertility.
Mechanism of action:
Initially cause an increase in gonadotropin release from the anterior pituitary (the "flare effect")

After 2 weeks, acts in downregulating the pituitary, leading to a decrease in FSH and LH secretion and thus decreased ovarian estrogen synthesis (hypoestrogenic state), which causes shrinkage of endometrial implants

Side effects:

"Pseudomenopause"

Include hot flashes, sweating, vaginal dryness/vaginitis, headache, decreased libido, depression, emotional lability, and, eventually, bone loss

What is the effect of oral contraceptive pills (OCPs) and progestins on endometriosis?

Create a "pseudopregnancy"

OCPs suppress FSH and LH secretion and endogenous estrogen production **and** reduce menstrual volume, which may lead to decreased reflux of menstrual products and decreased formation of new endometriosis lesions.

Progestins (Provera) have similar effects on FSH/LH secretion and estrogen synthesis, but also induce decidual change in endometriosis implants.

What is the treatment for infertility in a woman with endometriosis?

Laparoscopic ablation of endometrial implants with or without medical treatment

What are the goals of conservative surgery (with laparoscopy or laparotomy) for endometriosis?

Destruction of implants

Drainage and excision of endometriomas

Lysis of adhesions

Relief of pelvic pain through uterosacral ligament ablation or presacral neurectomy

How do postoperative pregnancy rates after laparoscopy or laparotomy compare in severe endometriosis?

Fifteen nonrandomized, retrospective studies of 206 patients with severe endometriosis after laparoscopic treatment revealed a mean crude postoperative pregnancy rate of 47.6%.

Fourteen nonrandomized, retrospective studies of 591 patients after treatment with laparotomy revealed a mean crude postoperative pregnancy rate of 38.2%.

What is the goal of definitive surgery for endometriosis?

Removal of any potential sites of origin or implantation of endometriosis

What are the potential sites of origin or implantation of endometriosis?

Uterus
Treated with hysterectomy
Leaving nondiseased ovaries intact is also an option if ovarian function is important.
Ovaries (treated with bilateral oophorectomy)
Cul-de-sac (treated with obliteration)
Bowel (treated with resection of bowel lesions)

Indications for subtotal hysterectomy?

Extensive fibrosis and pelvic adhesions, to avoid complications from difficult dissection

How are medical and surgical therapy used together in endometriosis treatment?

After surgery, medical therapy can be used to treat severe or extensive endometriosis.

Options for postoperative medical therapy?

GnRH agonist
Danazol
Postoperative oral contraceptives

What is the incidence of recurrence of endometriosis after medical treatment? After surgical treatment?

Medical therapy: Recurs in 30%–50% of patients treated
Conservative surgical treatment: Recurs in 14%–40% of patients
The more radical the surgery (oophorectomy, hysterectomy), the less likely a recurrence.
In reality, endometriosis is probably never "cured" until the hypoestrogenic postmenopausal state ensues.

32

Contraception

What are the three general types of reversible contraception?

Barrier methods (with or without spermicide)
Intrauterine devices (IUDs)
Hormonal agents

What are the failure rates for the commonly used contraceptives?

Table 32-1.

Contraceptive Method	Annual Pregnancy Rate
No contraceptive action	85%
Withdrawal	14.7%
Condom	9.8%
Diaphragm	12.0%
Sponge	16.0%
IUD	2.5%
Pill	3.8%
Implants	0.8%
Injectables	0.4%
Tubal sterilization	0.5%

BARRIER METHODS

What are the most commonly used barrier methods for contraception?

Condoms, diaphragms, and sponges
All may be used in conjunction with spermicidal compounds.

CONDOM

What are the advantages and disadvantages of the condom?

Advantages: No danger to health; rare side effects; instant reversibility; and protection against human immunodeficiency virus (HIV), other sexually transmitted diseases (STDs), and cervical intraepithelial neoplasia

Disadvantages: Interference with flow of sexual activity, need for availability, and risk of the condom breaking or slipping off

How effective is the condom in preventing HIV and other STDs?

One study found a zero HIV transmission rate for couples in which one partner was HIV positive and condoms were consistently used.

Condoms may be less effective in preventing transmission of HPV and HSV when uncovered skin lesions are present.

DIAPHRAGM

What is it?

A dome-shaped device made of latex rubber; the shape is maintained by a metal spring within the latex rim

How are diaphragms classified?

By the shape of the spring and rim

What are the different types of diaphragms?

Arcing spring
Coil spring
Flat spring
Wide seal rim

How does the diaphragm prevent conception?

Acts as a physical barrier to sperm and serves as a reservoir for spermicide (nonoxynol-9) at the cervix.

How does the diaphragm prevent transmission of STDs?

The combination of chemical and physical barriers is thought to be involved in the prevention of STDs.

What is the proper placement of a diaphragm?

A properly placed diaphragm rests posterior to the pubic symphysis and extends backward to the posterior fornix, thereby covering the cervix.

How long before and how long after coitus should the diaphragm be left in place in order to prevent conception effectively?

The diaphragm containing spermicide on the cervical side should be inserted no more than 6 hours before intercourse, and additional spermicide should be applied if coitus occurs again.

The diaphragm should remain in place for 6–8 hours after the last act of coitus.

What are the advantages and disadvantages of the diaphragm?

Advantages: Self-managed method and protection against STDs and cervical neoplasia

Disadvantages: Increased risk of urinary tract infections secondary to alteration of vaginal flora by spermicide, lack of protection of the entire genital tract against pathogens, must be fitted by trained personnel, small risk of toxic shock syndrome

What are the contraindications for diaphragm use?

Anatomic abnormalities that impair adequate fit such as vaginal septum, uterine prolapse, vesicovaginal fistulas, severe cystocele or rectocele, and poor vaginal muscle tone

Allergy to rubber, latex, or spermicide

History of toxic shock syndrome

Recurrent cystitis associated with diaphragm use

Inability or unwillingness of the user correctly to use or care for the diaphragm

Lack of trained personnel to fit the diaphragm

CONTRACEPTIVE SPONGE

What is it?

A cup-shaped sponge made of polyurethane foam, impregnated with nonoxynol-9, and inserted into the vagina

How long before intercourse can the sponge be inserted?

Up to 24 hours

What are the advantages and disadvantages of the contraceptive sponge?

Advantages: Absence of serious side effects, universal size eliminates the need for fitting, available over-the-counter, allows user to engage in multiple acts of coitus without additional preparation, no need to wait after insertion, can be inserted hours in advance of intercourse, and disposability

Disadvantages: Availability (currently, the only manufacturer stopped the production of the contraceptive sponge secondary to bacterial contamination problems); toxic shock syndrome

Can be purchased in Canada; and is available on www.birthcontrol.com

INTRAUTERINE DEVICES

What are IUDs?

The currently available IUDs are T-shaped devices bearing either copper or a slow-release progestin agent.

An IUD is placed by the physician high in the uterine fundus and is thought to interfere with fertilization by altering sperm function or implantation.

IUDs have a nylon thread "tail" for the purposes of detection and future removal.

What is the mechanism of action of copper-containing IUDs?

Prevent fertilization of the egg within the fallopian tube by reducing the number of sperm in the tube and possibly by an additional effect of copper on fertility of the egg

What is the mechanism of action of progestin-containing IUDs?

Act mainly by rendering the endometrium atrophic and thereby interfering with implantation of the fertilized egg

Also, in 50% of women using this type of IUD for at least a year, ovulation is prevented.

What is the effect on menstruation of progestin-containing IUDs?

Tend to cause a gradual decrease in menstrual blood loss

May lead to partial or total amenorrhea

Which patients are good candidates for an IUD?

Patients should have a monogamous sexual relationship.

Both the patient and her partner should be free of any STDs.

IUDs may be the contraceptive method of choice for women 35 years of age or older involved in a monogamous relationship, who smoke, and who are therefore not candidates for oral contraceptives.

Do IUDs cause pelvic infections?

The risk of infection associated with IUDs was overstated in the 1970s and 1980s.

The IUD does not itself cause infection, but contraction of gonococcal and chlamydial infections in an IUD user may lead to a more severe course of infection.

Nonmonogamous women are at greater risk for contracting these illnesses and are therefore not candidates for IUD use.

What is the only pelvic infection that is unequivocally related to the use of an IUD?

Actinomycosis

Actinomycosis PID has only been documented in IUD users.

What is the treatment for Actinomycosis?

Penicillin derivative

What are the contraindications for the use of IUDs?

Absolute contraindications: Pregnancy, known or suspected pelvic malignancy, and current or chronic pelvic infection

Relative contraindications: History of ectopic pregnancy or pelvic inflammatory disease (PID), debilitating dysmenorrhea, congenital anomalies of the genital tract, and sickle cell anemia (because of increased susceptibility to infection)

Some authorities consider valvular heart disease a contraindication to use of IUDs.

When during the menstrual cycle should the IUD be inserted?

During menses so that the spotting and cramping associated with insertion become less noticeable and important to the patient; also, so that the physician can be more confident that the patient is not pregnant.

What are the possible complications of IUD use?

Expulsion of the IUD (partial or complete)

Uterine perforation

Dysmenorrhea

Pregnancy (both ectopic and intrauterine)

What is the significance of the patient not being able to feel the tail of her IUD?

The IUD may have been expelled from the uterine cavity, especially if the patient cannot feel the tail after a menstrual period.

The patient should see her physician promptly and use a different method of contraception until then.

What is the significance of elongation or shortening of the IUD tail?

Elongation of the tail may represent partial expulsion; may indicate that the device has lost its contraceptive effect and pregnancy must be ruled out.

Shortening of the tail may be due to the gradual migration of the IUD out of the uterine cavity; may represent perforation of the uterine wall.

HORMONAL AGENTS

ORAL CONTRACEPTIVE PILLS (OCPS)

What are the two types of OCPs currently available?

Combination estrogen and progesterone pill (either ethinyl estradiol or mestranol as the estrogenic compound and one of a variety of different progestins as the progestational agent)
Progesterone-only pill

How do OCPs prevent conception?

Mainly by suppressing the pituitary–gonadal axis and reducing the secretion of gonadotropins
Also by thickening of the cervical mucus and inhibition of endometrial proliferation, making fertilization and implantation less likely

What are the contraindications to OCP use?

Absolute contraindications: Past or present thrombophlebitis, inherited susceptibility to thrombosis, history of thromboembolism; smoker and 35 years of age or older; cerebrovascular or coronary artery disease; current or past breast or endometrial cancer or other estrogen-dependent tumor; impaired liver function; cholestasis of pregnancy, or jaundice before pill use
Pregnancy; Undiagnosed abnormal vaginal bleeding
Relative contraindications: Vascular or migraine headaches, especially with concomitant cigarette use; hypertension (blood pressure ≥ 160/ 100 mm Hg); gallbladder disease; lactation
Elective surgery

Can women 35 years of age and older who do not smoke use the OCP?

Yes, provided that they do not have any other significant cardiovascular risk factors (e.g., high-risk lipid profile)

How is OCP therapy managed in patients undergoing surgery?

Combination OCPs should not be taken during surgery or any hospitalization involving long periods of immobilization because of the four- to sixfold increased risk of thromboembolic complications.

Patients scheduled for elective surgical procedures that may place them at increased risk for thromboembolic disease should stop using combination OCPs a month before date of surgery and use a different method of birth control during this time.

Progestin-only OCPs pose no increased health risks during surgery and patients can continue taking them.

What are the beneficial effects of OCPs?

Decrease the prevalence of menorrhagia, dysmenorrhea, and premenstrual tension

OCP users have lower incidences of benign cystic breast disease (fibroadenoma and chronic cystic disease), ovarian and endometrial cancer, and PID.

What is the association between OCPs and thromboembolic disease?

OCPs are associated with an increased incidence of thromboembolism because of estrogen-induced increase in blood levels of clotting factors VII and X and decrease in levels of antithrombin III. Progesterone's fibrinolytic effects oppose, at least in part, the hypercoagulable state produced by estrogen.

The risk of thromboembolism due to OCP use is synergistic with other risk factors such as hyperlipidemia and smoking.

It is believed that the risk of thromboembolic disease outweighs the benefits of OCPs only in predisposed patients (i.e., those with prior history)

and in those with multiple risk factors (e.g., women 35 years of age or older who smoke).

What is the risk of venous thromboembolism for any reproductive age woman without significant risk factors?

4–5 per 100,000 per year

What is the risk of venous thromboembolism for young women taking OCPs?

12–20 per 100,000 per year

What is the association between OCP use and incidence of myocardial infarction (MI)?

OCP-associated increases in the risk for MI of zero to fourfold have been reported.

The larger relative risks were reported in studies of OCPs with higher estrogen content than commonly used today.

As in thromboembolic disease, this risk increases synergistically with other risk factors such as smoking, diabetes, and hypercholesterolemia.

It is believed that smoking represents the major risk factor for MI in OCP users.

What is the association between OCP use and cerebrovascular disease?

The major cerebrovascular risk associated with OCP use is that of subarachnoid hemorrhage, which is about six times the risk of nonusers.

Women who smoke and use OCPs have a 22 times greater chance of having a subarachnoid hemorrhage than the control group.

Strokes seem to be limited to older ($\geq$ 35 years of age) women who smoke or have other risk factors.

What effects do OCPs have on blood pressure?

About 1%–5% of OCP users have mild to moderate hypertension with elevations of 20–40 and 10–20 mm Hg in the systolic and diastolic pressures, respectively.

Cause of OCP-associated hypertension is thought to involve abnormalities of the renin–angiotensin system, leading to increased aldosterone production and sodium retention.

Incidence increases with age, parity, and obesity.

Hypertension resolves after discontinuation of the pill in the absence of other contributing causes.

What is the relationship between OCPs and diabetes mellitus?

Studies have shown that some OCPs can cause a decrease in glucose tolerance that appears to be associated with the progestin component of OCPs.

Incidence of diabetes mellitus is not increased by OCP use.

In predisposed patients, insulin dependence may occur sooner if certain OCPs are used.

In diabetic women with vascular complications of the disease (retinopathy, nephropathy), there may be an increased risk of thrombus formation secondary to OCP use.

In patients at risk, the progestin of choice is low-dose norethindrone or one of the newer progestins (levonorgestrel, gestodene, desogestrel, or norgestimate).

How is thyroid function affected by OCP use?

Induces increased production of thyroid-binding globulin, and increases thyroxine levels

Triiodothyronine RU declines, and thyroid index is normal. Patients remain euthyroid.

What liver disease is associated with OCP use?

Hepatocellular adenoma, a benign liver neoplasm, is associated with long-term OCP and other exogenous steroid use.

Presents as right upper quadrant pain or a palpable mass

If ruptured, can present as acute abdomen with hemodynamic instability

What is the management of hepatocellular adenoma?

Discontinuation of OCP leads to regression of the tumor and is the treatment of choice in most patients.

Pregnancy should be avoided in patients with hepatocellular adenoma because of the associated hyperestrogenic state, which can lead to enlargement and potential rupture of the adenoma.

If pregnancy is desired, patients should first undergo surgery to remove the adenoma.

What is meant by "breakthrough bleeding" in OCP users?

Bleeding that occurs at an inappropriate time during the cycle

What causes it?

Usually an imbalance between estrogen and progestin levels

What increases the likelihood that a patient will have breakthrough bleeding?

Smoking
Improper pill use

How is it managed?

If it occurs early during OCP use (first 3 months), it usually resolves spontaneously; reassurance and counseling are usually sufficient.

Pathologic causes such as spontaneous abortion, neoplasia, ectopic pregnancy, PID, and benign uterine pathology should be considered.

If bleeding continues after the first 3–4 months of use, switching to a formulation with a higher estrogen dose or a less potent progestin is advisable.

How is the initial OCP selected?	General evaluation for risks and contraindications to OCP use is done. Low-dose estrogen pills usually are appropriate. Menstrual characteristics and hormonal sensitivity should be noted.
What signs and symptoms may be present in estrogen-hypersensitive/ progesterone-deficient patients?	Severe nausea or edema during pregnancy or at mid-cycle Prolonged and heavy menses with severe cramps Severe and prolonged premenstrual symptoms beginning 7–12 days before menses
What signs and symptoms may be present in progesterone-hypersensitive/estrogen-deficient patients?	Scant menses Mid-cycle spotting
What signs and symptoms are indicative of androgen excess?	Very oily skin Acne Male-pattern hair loss or hair growth on face and chest Oligomenorrhea Amenorrhea
How do OCP hormones affect acne?	Progestins increase sebum production (androgenic side effect) and hence cause a worsening of acne; estrogens have the opposite effect. OCP's increase sex-steroid binding hormone and reduce levels of circulating free androgens
What causes the androgenic side effects associated with OCPs?	Related to the quantity and quality of the progestin agent in the pill Include hirsutism and hair loss in addition to acne Can be treated by using a less androgenic progestin or, if problems persist, increasing the estrogen dosage

What are the relative androgenic activities of the commonly used progestins?

The androgenic activities of the common progestins, from highest to lowest, are: Levonorgestrel > norgestrel > desogestrel > norgestimate > norethindrone acetate > norethindrone > ethynodiol diacetate > megestrol acetate = medroxyprogesterone acetate.

What are examples of the appropriate initial choice of OCP for each of the listed types of patients?

Patients with normal menses

Ethinyl estradiol 35 μg–desogestrel 0.15 mg (e.g., Ortho-Cept, Desogen) or the equivalent

Patients with menses-associated headaches

Continuous oral contraceptives (without placebo week)

Biphasic oral contraceptive with estrogen supplemented placebo week pills (Mircette)

Estrogen-hypersensitive/progesterone-deficient patients

Require lower estrogenic activity (20–30 μg of ethinyl estradiol)

Examples: Ethinyl estradiol 20 μg–norethindrone acetate 1.0 mg (Lo Estrin), ethinyl estradiol 30 μg–norgestrel 0.3 mg (Lo/Ovral) or the equivalent

Progesterone-hypersensitive/estrogen-deficient patients

Require low progesterone dose and progestational activity and slightly higher estrogen dose

Examples: Ethinyl estradiol 35 μg–norgestimate 0.25 mg (Ortho-Cyclen), ethinyl estradiol 35 μg–norethindrone 0.5 mg (Brevicon, Modicon) or the equivalent

Androgen-hypersensitive patients/patients with polycystic ovary disease

Pills with high progestational and low androgenic activity are best suited for this group. Examples: Ethinyl estradiol

30 μg–desogestrel 0.15 mg (Desogen, Ortho-Cept) or ethinyl estradiol 35 μg–ethynodiol diacetate 1.0 mg (Demulen 1/35) or the equivalent or Ethinyl estradiol 30 μg - Drospirenone 3 mg (Yasmin).

What should the patient do if she forgets to take one or more of her OCPs?

Use additional contraceptive measures for the remainder of that cycle.

Missed single pill: Take the missed dose immediately and the next dose at the regular time.

Missed two pills: Take two pills immediately and two the following day.

Missed three or more pills: Discard the old packet of pills and start a new packet on that day.

If menstruation does not occur at the regular time, a pregnancy test must be performed.

What is postpill amenorrhea?

Failure to resume menses by 6 months after termination of OCP use

What is its incidence?

One percent of patients

Almost half of these patients have a history of oligomenorrhea before pill use.

What is the management of postpill amenorrhea?

Most cases spontaneously resolve within 6 months of the discontinuation of OCPs.

An endocrinologic workup is not needed until amenorrhea continues for 6 months unless galactorrhea is also present; in this case, workup should occur at 3 months after discontinuation of the OCP.

Workup should:

Rule out pregnancy because it may occur before resumption of menses

Rule out other causes of amenorrhea such as strenuous exercise and anorexia nervosa
Include progestin challenge test

What is a progestin challenge test?

Helpful in assessing the status of the hypothalamic–pituitary–ovarian axis.
Provera (medroxyprogesterone acetate) 10 mg can be given for 5–10 days.
Presence of bleeding signifies anovulatory dysfunction.
Absence of bleeding indicates absence of estrogen or a nonfunctional endometrium.

How is anovulatory dysfunction managed?

With ovulation-inducing agents such as clomiphene, oral contraceptives, or cyclic progesterone

How is absence of estrogen or nonfunctional endometrium managed?

Requires further evaluation for pituitary, hypothalamic, and endometrial disorders

What drugs can interfere with OCP action?

Those that are strong inducers of the liver cytochrome P_{450} system
Include anticonvulsants (e.g., phenobarbital, carbamazepine, phenytoin, primidone) and some antibiotics (e.g., rifampin, isoniazid, neomycin, ampicillin, penicillin V, tetracycline)

What are signs and symptoms of drug interaction with OCP?

Breakthrough bleeding
Absence of withdrawal menses (due to pregnancy)

How is drug interaction managed?

Short-term use of interfering drug (e.g., a course of antibiotics): Backup method for contraception
Long-term use (e.g., seizure prophylaxis): Another method of birth control may be advisable, or consideration of a higher estrogen content pill.

Do OCPs cause weight gain?	An equal number of people lose and gain weight on OCPs; however, both estrogens and progestins are capable of causing weight gain.
How can weight gain be minimized?	By using the lowest effective estrogen–progestin combination with the lowest potency progestin and maintaining a sensible diet and exercise program

PROGESTIN-ONLY PILL

How does the progestin-only pill prevent conception?	Creates a poor endometrial environment for implantation Thickens cervical mucous Gonadotropins are not consistently suppressed
What is the failure rate of the progestin-only pill?	1.1–9.6 per 100 women will become pregnant in the first year of use. The pill must be taken at the same time every day because the effects of the pill no longer exist after 24 hours.
Who are the ideal candidates for progestin-only pill contraception?	Lactating women Women over 40
Which patients should not utilize the progestin-only pill?	Latina women with a prior history of gestational diabetes have a 3-fold increased risk of developing NIDDM on the progestin-only pill.

INJECTABLE MEDROXYPROGESTERONE ACETATE

What is injectable medroxyprogesterone acetate?	Also known as DMPA and Depo Provera Similar to naturally occurring progesterone Available in the form of microcrystals in an aqueous suspension

How is medroxyprogesterone acetate absorbed?

After intramuscular injection, medroxyprogesterone acetate is slowly absorbed over the following 3–4 months.

What is the dosing schedule for medroxyprogesterone acetate?

150 mg every 3 months

What is the mode of action of medroxyprogesterone acetate?

Inhibits ovulation through the suppression of the pituitary–gonadal axis, decreasing luteinizing hormone and follicle-stimulating hormone, and preventing luteinizing hormone surges

What are the advantages and disadvantages of medroxyprogesterone acetate?

Advantages: Effective, easy-to-use contraceptive method; decrease in menses and menstrual blood loss (in most patients); decreased incidence of PID, candidal infections, and endometrial cancer; retains efficacy in presence of anticonvulsant medications; and does not affect infant nutrition in women who are breast-feeding
Disadvantages: Menstrual changes (number one cause of discontinuation); slight weight gain (1–3 kg); slightly slower return to fertility after discontinuation; minor complaints such as headaches, dizziness, and hair loss in some patients

What menstrual changes are associated with use of medroxyprogesterone acetate?

From amenorrhea to heavy bleeding Amenorrhea is more common with continued use.

What is the incidence of conception after discontinuation of medroxyprogesterone acetate?

Respectively, 70% and 90% of patients conceive within 1 and 2 years after discontinuation of medroxyprogesterone acetate.

In what conditions is medroxyprogesterone acetate especially useful?

Postpartum/lactation

Conditions contraindicating use of estrogen-containing contraceptives (e.g., women 35 years of age or older who smoke)

Conditions that may benefit from a reduction in menstrual blood loss (e.g., menorrhagia, fibroids, hemoglobinopathies)

Concomitant use of drugs that may interact with oral or implantable contraceptives, such as carbamazepine, rifampin, and phenytoin

Conditions associated with poor compliance with other contraceptive methods

Conditions in which pregnancy has catastrophic fetal risks, such as use of teratogenic medications (e.g., isotretinoin, valproate)

LEVONORGESTREL IMPLANTS (NORPLANT)

What are levonorgestrel implants?

Six subdermally placed 34 x 2.4 mm Silastic tubes filled with the progestin levonorgestrel

How long are the implants effective?

Recommended period of use is 5 years. As release and plasma levels of levonorgestrel from the implants decrease, the failure rate increases, reaching 2 per 100 users in the sixth year of use.

What effect does the weight of the user have on implant use?

Because plasma levels of levonorgestrel vary inversely with the user's weight and the release rate is independent of weight, higher failure rates have been reported for women who weigh more than 70 kg.

How do levonorgestrel implants prevent pregnancy?

Inhibition of ovulation

Or, less frequent ovulation

In one-third to one-half of women, cyclic

luteal activity and associated menstrual bleeding are observed, indicating lower-than-normal ovulatory progesterone levels. Luteal insufficiency and disruption of oocyte maturation have been hypothesized to prevent fertilization in this subset of users who ovulate.

Implants may also cause cervical mucus changes that are hostile to sperm.

Which medication can interfere with the implant's efficacy?

Anticonvulsants, presumably due to hepatic enzyme induction by many members of this class of drugs

What are the advantages and disadvantages of levonorgestrel implants?

Advantages: Low maintenance, high efficacy

Disadvantages: Need for placement and removal, menstrual irregularities (main reason for discontinuation), headache, and weight gain

What is the effect on fertility after discontinuation of levonorgestrel implants?

No effect; 86% of women achieve pregnancy within 1 year of removal.

POSTCOITAL CONTRACEPTION

Which patients can benefit from postcoital contraception?

Patients with failure of contraception or no contraception <72 hours prior to administration

What regimens are available?

Any combination which allows administration of 100 μg ethinyl estradiol and 1 mg equivalent progestin in 2 doses (2 hours apart or 0.75 mg levonorgestrel 2 doses 12 hours apart)

Examples:

-2 doses of 4 tablets of Lo Oval, Nordette, Levlen, Triphasil 12 hours apart

-Preven
Plan B
2 doses of 10 pills of progestin-only mini
    pill 12 hours apart

**What are the side effects
of postcoital
contraception?**

Nausea and vomiting
Experienced less when progestin only
    regimen is utilized

**What is the mechanism of
contraception?**

Affects endometrium by creating
    unacceptable environment for
    implantation
Delay of ovulation

**How effective is this form
of contraception?**

98% effective
Risk of pregnancy is 8%, which is
    reduced by 75%

33

Sexual Differentiation and Development

NORMAL DEVELOPMENT

How do the ovaries develop?

Three weeks' gestation:

Primitive germ cells (oogonia) in the yolk sac of the fetus migrate to the genital ridge, where they are incorporated into sex cords.

Oogonia undergo mitosis to reach a maximum of about 6 million by week 20; atresia reduces this number to 1 million at birth and 300,000 at puberty.

Between eight and twelve weeks' gestation:

Oogonia begin meiosis and are arrested in prophase of the first meiotic division; they are then called primary oocytes.

The follicles surrounding primary oocytes are called primordial follicles.

Six months of age:

Formation of primary oocytes is complete.

Primary oocytes remain arrested until puberty when the surge of luteinizing hormone (LH) causes ovulation, stimulating some to resume meiosis.

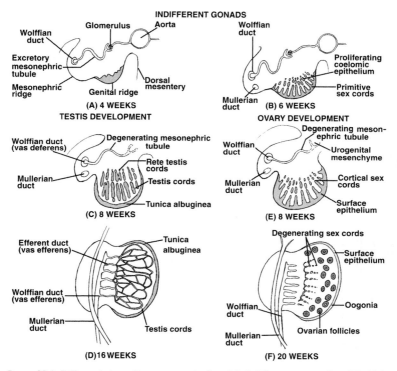

Figure 33.1. Differentiation of human gonads; A and B: Indifferent stages; C and D: Male development showing the primitive sex cords that develop into the testicular ducts; E and F: Female development showing degeneration of the primitive sex cords, which are replaced by secondary sex cords from the surface epithelium. (From Gilben SF: Developmental Biology, 2nd ed. Sunderland, MA: Sinauer Associates, 1988, with permission of the publisher)

What changes occur in the ovary at menarche?

Shortly before ovulation, the primary oocyte completes the first meiotic division to form the secondary oocyte and the first polar body.

First meiotic division is followed by the second meiotic division, which is again arrested (in metaphase) and does not resume meiosis unless fertilization by sperm occurs.

If a sperm cell penetrates the oocyte, meiosis resumes to form the mature oocyte (ovum) and the second polar body.

How do the fallopian tubes, uterus, and vagina develop?

All three structures develop from **müllerian ducts** (paramesonephric ducts):

Develop in both sexes during week six of gestation

In males, androgens and müllerian inhibiting factor (MIF) produced by the developing testes induce resorption of the müllerian ducts.

In females, the absence of MIF and androgens stimulates further müllerian development.

Fallopian tube: Each duct opens into the coelomic cavity cranially and becomes a fallopian tube.

Uterus and upper vagina:
Caudally, the two ducts fuse in the midline at the urogenital septum.
Regression of the septum leads to the development of the uterus and upper vagina.

Lower vagina: formed by the vaginal plate and lengthening of the urogenital sinus.

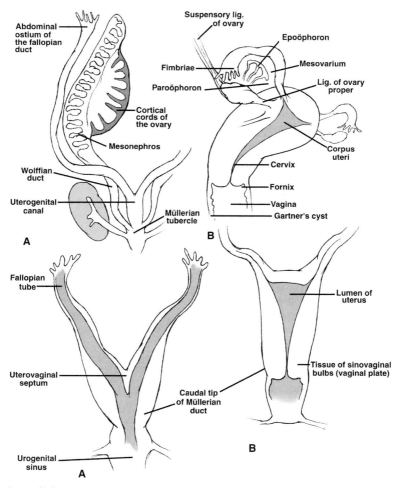

Figure 33.2. A schematic drawing of the genital ducts in the female at the end of the second month of development. **A.** Note the müllerian tubercle and the formation of the uterovaginal canal. **B.** Genital ducts after descent of the ovary. The only parts remaining of the mesonephric system are the epoöphoron, paroöpharon, and Gartner's cyst. Note the suspensory ligament of the ovary, the ligament of the ovary proper, and the round ligament of the uterus.

How do the external genitalia develop?

During the seventh week of gestation, the genital tubercle elongates to form the phallus.

Two sets of folds, the lateral genital folds and the medial urogenital folds, differentiate to form the labia majora and labia minora, respectively.

The urogenital folds also form the prepuce of the clitoris.

Female external genitalia complete during 14th week

What is Tanner staging?

A classification system for the development of secondary sex characteristics (breast and pubic hair development)

List the stages.

Table 33.1 Tanner staging

Stage	Breast	Pubic Hair
1	Preadolescent, elevated papillae	None
2	Breast bud and papillae slightly elevated	Sparse, long, slightly pigmented
3	Further enlargement of breast mound; increased palpable glandular tissue	Darker, coarser, curly
4	Areola and papilla project above breast	Adult-type hair; no spread to medial thigh
5	Papillae projected, mature	Adult-type hair with spread to medial thigh; inverse triangle distribution

In what order do secondary sex characteristics develop?

Breast bud development
Onset of pubic hair
Maximal height achieved
Menarche
Adult breast
Adult pubic hair

CONGENITAL ANOMALIES OF THE REPRODUCTIVE TRACT

What are the main ovarian anomalies?

The many ovarian anomalies are included under the broad term gonadal dysgenesis.

What is the definition of gonadal dysgenesis?

Condition of abnormal gonadal development; denotes the presence of streak gonads regardless of other associated anomalies.

Many chromosomal abnormalities are associated with gonadal dysgenesis.

What is a streak gonad?

Nonfunctioning gonadal tissue consisting of dense fibrous stroma and lack of oocytes or spermatocytes

What are some of the chromosomal abnormalities that cause gonadal dysgenesis?

Turner syndrome
Abnormal X chromosome

What is Turner syndrome?

An abnormality with chromosome count of **45, X**
Chromosome count may also be:
45X/46XX mosaic
45X/46XY mosaic

What is the incidence?

Occurs in 1 per 2000 live births

What is the cause?

In the fetus, oogonia migrate normally to the genital ridge but soon undergo rapid degeneration, resulting in **streak ovaries** (no hormones are produced).

What are the associated clinical findings?

Primary amenorrhea
Short stature
Lack of secondary sexual characteristics
Shield-shaped chest with widely spaced nipples
Webbed neck
Associated with cardiac anomalies (coarctation of the aorta)

Intelligence: usually normal; mental retardation in 10% of patients

Urinary **gonadotropins** (follicle-stimulating hormone [FSH] and LH): markedly **elevated**

Epicanthal folds

High arched palate

Increased risk for hypertension diabetes, and thyroid disease

What is the treatment?

Secondary sex characteristic development can be promoted with exogenous estrogen treatment.

What is a special consideration of 45X/46XY mosaics?

Y chromosome predisposes to **gonadal malignancy**.

Prophylactic surgical removal of the dysgenetic gonads is necessary.

What tumor do persons with dysgenetic gonads develop?

Gonadoblastoma

What is abnormal X chromosome?

Karyotype is **46,XX**, but one of the X chromosomes is **incomplete**.

Deletion of long arm (Xq): streak gonads, sexual infantilism, normal stature, sterility; estrogen replacement therapy necessary for breast development

Deletion of short arm (Xp): phenotypically similar to Turner syndrome

What are some causes of gonadal dysgenesis that have a normal chromosome complement?

Pure gonadal dysgenesis

Gonadal agenesis (male pseudohermaphroditism)

What is pure gonadal dysgenesis?

Condition in which chromosomal complement is normal (46,XX) but streak gonads are present.

What are the etiologic factors?	Occurs when primitive oogonia fail to migrate to genital ridge and ovaries fail to develop May also be the result of nongenetic factors which affect gonadal tissue such as neoplasm or infarction
What are the associated clinical findings?	Primary amenorrhea Infantile secondary sexual characteristics Normal stature No estrogen synthesis (gonads are nonfunctional)
What is gonadal agenesis (male pseudohermaphroditism)?	Also called "vanishing testes syndrome" **Absence of gonads** with normal **male 46,XY** karyotype
What are the associated clinical findings?	Ambiguous external genitalia or normal female external genitalia but **NO internal female** reproductive organs May present at puberty with primary amenorrhea and lack of breast development
What is the theoretic cause?	Sometime in embryonic development testicular tissue was present and MIF suppressed müllerian development. Then, for some unknown reason, the testes disappeared after müllerian inhibition.
What are the etiologic factors of common uterine anomalies?	Malfusion of the müllerian ducts with varying degrees of septation most commonly due to teratogenesis, genetic inheritance, and multifactorial expression. Often do not have clinical manifestations.

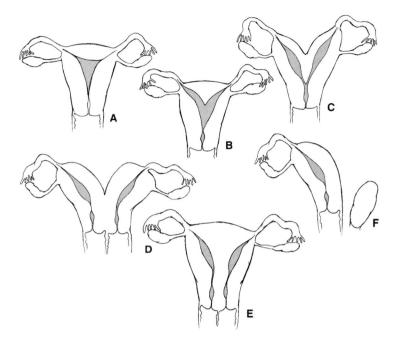

Figure 33.3. Common clinical manifestation of abnormalities of müllerian duct development. **A.** Normal female. **B.** Septate uterus (failure of dissolution of septum). **C.** Bicornuate uterus (failure of fusion of mid müllerian ducts). **D.** Didelphis anomaly (complete failure of fusion). **E.** Septate uterus with duplication of cervix and vagina (combined failure of fusion and dissolution of septum). **F.** Unicornuate uterus failure of formation of one müllerian duct).

What are the different categories of müllerian anomalies?	Bicornuate: 37% of all müllerian anomalies Unicornuate 4.4% Uterus Didelphys 11% Septate 22% Arcuate 15%
What reproductive difficulties might women with müllerian anomalies encounter?	Recurrent miscarriage Preterm labor Nonvertex presentation

What is Mayer-Rokitansky-Küster-Hauser syndrome?

Results in a complete lack of müllerian development (müllerian agenesis).

Usually incomplete development of the fallopian tubes with absence of the uterus, cervix, and most of the vagina.

Occurs in 1 in 4000 female births

What are the common vaginal anomalies?

Vaginal agenesis
Transverse vaginal septum
Longitudinal vaginal septum
Imperforate hymen

What is vaginal agenesis?

Partial or complete absence of vaginal vault

Occurs as part of the Mayer-Rokitansky-Küster-Hauser syndrome, or independently

What are the associated clinical findings?

Since ovaries are present, secondary sex characteristics develop normally.

How is the diagnosis made?

Physical exam confirms absence of vagina

Usually diagnosed in the setting of **delayed menarche**

Pelvic ultrasound to confirm presence or absence of uterus

Intravenous pyelogram is performed to detect urinary tract anomalies (found in 1/3 of patients with müllerian agenesis)

Testosterone level to rule out testicular feminization

Karyotype to confirm patient is 46,XX and to rule out disorders associated with 46,XY (e.g., testicular feminization)

What is the treatment if the uterus is absent?

Treatment is aimed at creating a neovagina to allow satisfactory sexual function (assumes absent uterus).

Nonsurgical: progressive vaginal dilatation if rudimentary vagina present

Surgical: McIndoe procedure—If vaginal atresia is complete, a split-thickness skin graft is used to create a neovagina; graft is placed in the potential space between the bladder and rectum.

Williams vulvovaginoplasty—The labia majora are used to lengthen preexisting rudimentary vagina; does not require skin graft.

What is the treatment if functioning uterus is present?

Immediate treatment is crucial to remove obstruction to menstrual flow.

Surgical treatment: Neovagina is created using a stent with a central opening to allow flow; stent is left in place for 4 to 6 months.

What is a transverse vaginal septum?

A septum composed of vaginal mucosa with or without intervening connective tissue

May be either partial or complete, and can vary in thickness

What are the clinical findings?

Clinical picture varies depending on extent of septation.

Partial septation may present with dysmenorrhea, irregular vaginal spotting, secondary pelvic inflammatory disease (PID) from anaerobic infection, or no clinical symptoms.

Complete septation presents with primary amenorrhea and obstruction; surgical treatment is imperative.

What is the treatment?

Surgery

What is a longitudinal vaginal septum?

Results from improper fusion of the distal müllerian ducts

	May be accompanied by bicornuate uterus with one or two cervices

What are the associated clinical findings?

May present with obstruction to drainage or dyspareunia

What is the treatment?

Necessary only if symptomatic or if childbearing is anticipated

What is an imperforate hymen?

Outlet obstruction which causes build-up of vaginal secretions

What are the associated clinical findings?

Newborns: mucocolpos
Adolescents: hematocolpos; usually diagnosed in setting of primary amenorrhea

What is the treatment?

Surgery at the time of diagnosis

ABNORMAL SEXUAL DIFFERENTIATION

What causes abnormal sexual differentiation?

Many of these disorders are the result of a defect in the steroid hormone biosynthetic pathway.

What is female pseudohermaphroditism?

Masculinization of the female fetus in utero

What is male pseuohermaphroditism?

Feminization of the male fetus in utero

What is congenital adrenal hyperplasia?

Autosomal recessive defect in steroid biosynthesis
Karyotype is **46,XX**
Causes female pseudohermaphroditism
Most frequent cause of ambiguous genitalia in the newborn

What is the incidence?

Occurs in 1 in 5000 live births

What are the etiologic factors?

21-hydroxylase deficiency most common

Also caused by 11-hydroxylase deficiency (associated with hypertension) and 3B-ol-dehydrogenase deficiency (usually fatal due to severe adrenal insufficiency)

Why are only external genitalia affected in CAH?

Internal genitalia differentiation is completed by the 10th week while the adrenal cortex does not begin functioning until the 12th week

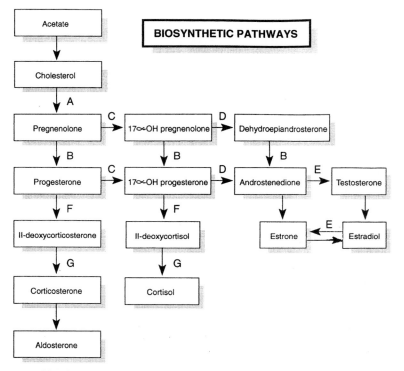

Figure 33.4. Summary of important adrenal and gonadal biosynthetic pathways. Letters designate enzymes required for the appropriate conversions. **A.** 20α-hydroxylase, 22R-hydroxylase, and 20,22-desmolase. **B.** 3β-ol-dehydrogenase. **C.** 17α-hydroxylase. **D.** 17,20-desmolase. **E.** 17-ketosteroid reductase. **F.** 21-hydroxylase. **G.** 11β-hydroxylase. (Simpson JL: Disorders of Sexual Differentiation. Etiology and Clinical Delineation. New York, Academic Press, 1976)

Describe the pathophysiology of congenital adrenal hyperplasia.

Lack of 21-hydroxylase (or others)→**decreased** cortisol→**increased ACTH**→accumulation of intermediate compounds in the pathway prior to the enzyme defect (17-hydroxyprogesterone and 17-hydroxypregnenolone)

These intermediates are converted to the "adrenal androgens" dehydroepiandrosterone (DHEA) and androstenedione, which are then converted peripherally into testosterone.

What are the clinical findings?

Presents as **ambiguous genitalia** in the newborn (clitoromegaly and accentuation of labial folds)

30% Salt wasting

5% Hypertension

Chromosomes, gonads, and internal genitalia are female.

Children will have early development of sexual characteristics and premature closure of epiphyses

How is the diagnosis made?

Increased plasma levels of 17-hydroxyprogesterone or increased urinary levels of 17-ketosteroids (breakdown product of most androgens)

What is the treatment?

Hydrocortisone administered indefinitely

What is 5α-reductase deficiency?

Also called incomplete male pseudohermaphroditism

Autosomal recessive genetic defect **46,XY** karyotype

Describe the pathophysiology of 5α-reductase deficiency.

5α-reductase normally converts testosterone to a more active steroid, dihydrotestosterone (DHT), which is necessary for the androgen target tissues of the urogenital sinus (development of external genitalia).

5α-reductase deficiency leads to **decreased DHT** and **normal testosterone** levels.

What are the associated clinical findings?

Ambiguous genitalia or phenotypic female, with or without palpable labial/inguinal testes

At puberty, testosterone production increases and is converted to DHT, causing virilization with growth of the penis and descent of the testes; pronounced muscle development may also occur.

After puberty, some patients may have penile erection, ejaculation, and fertility.

What is the treatment?

Important to establish diagnosis early, as late diagnosis may have profound psychological impact.

In most circumstances, individual should be raised as a female with gonadectomy and reduction clitoroplasty performed as soon as diagnosis is made.

What is 17α-hydroxylase deficiency?

Karyotype is **46,XX.**

Describe the pathophysiology of 17α-hydroxylase deficiency.

17α-hydroxylase is an enzyme in cortisol and steroid hormone synthesis (androgens and estrogens).

Decreased 17α-hydroxylase results in **increased ACTH** (in effort to produce more cortisol-negative feedback).

Mineralocorticoid pathway (to aldosterone synthesis) does NOT require 17α-hydroxylase, so the increase in ACTH causes **increased aldosterone** production, resulting in sodium retention, hypertension, and low potassium.

What are the associated clinical findings?

Similar to pure gonadal dysgenesis with no estrogen production

What are some disorders of sexual differentiation that are NOT associated with defects of the steroid hormone biosynthetic pathway?

Androgen insensitivity syndrome (testicular feminization)
True hermaphroditism
Female pseudohermaphroditism of maternal origin

What is androgen insensitivity syndrome (testicular feminization)?

X-linked recessive disorder resulting in **46,XY** genotype and **female phenotype** (male pseudohermaphroditism)

Describe the pathophysiology.

Androgen receptors are absent or defective.
Fetal testosterone and MIF production by the testes are normal.
However, because the **receptors** are defective, **male external genitalia do not develop**.
Normal MIF causes müllerian regression; results in absent fallopian tubes, uterus, and upper vagina (vagina ends as a blind pouch).

What are the associated clinical findings?

Secondary sex characteristics:
These patients produce some estrogen; therefore, breast development may be normal. Pubic and axillary hair, however, are sparse or absent (they rely on testosterone).
Presents as primary amenorrhea
The testes are located in the labia or in the inguinal canal (presenting as inguinal hernia) and should be removed after puberty because of increased risk for **gonadal malignancy.**
Patients are often reared as females.

What is true hermaphroditism?

Very rare condition
Dual gonadal development (both male and female gonadal tissue)
Genotype is usually **46,XX**.

What are the associated clinical findings?

External genitalia may appear male, female, or ambiguous; masculinization of the external genitalia depends on the amount of testicular tissue present.

Uterus is usually present

Cryptorchidism is frequent, usually with some degree of labioscrotal fusion.

At puberty, about 75% of patients develop gynecomastia and more than half menstruate.

What is the treatment?

Sex assignment should depend on the dominant appearance of the external genitalia (75% raised as males).

What is female pseudohermaphroditism of maternal origin?

Female pseudohermaphroditism due to exogenous or endogenous androgens

34

Menstrual Cycle and Dysfunction

NORMAL MENSTRUAL CYCLE

What is the mean duration of the menstrual cycle?
Mean: 28 days
Range: 21–35 days

What is the average duration of menses?
Three to seven days

What is the mean age of menarche?
12.8 years

What is the mean age of menopause?
51 years

What is the normal estimated blood loss?
Approximately 30 ml
About 80% of total loss occurs in first 2 days.

When does the menstrual phase occur?
From day 1 to day 4

What uterine changes occur during menses?
Glandular and stromal degradation with sloughing of the functionalis (inner endometrial layer)

What are the hormonal levels during the menstrual phase?
Estradiol and progesterone levels are low from the regressing corpus luteum of the previous cycle.
Follicle-stimulating hormone (FSH) level begins to rise in response to declining estradiol and progesterone levels.
Luteinizing hormone (LH) level rises slowly several days after FSH begins to increase.

What is the follicular phase?
Ovarian phase that begins with menses on day 1 of the menstrual cycle and ends with ovulation
The cumulus oophorus and fluid-filled antrum form.

A cohort of ovarian follicles begins maturation, but only one reaches maturity.

When does ovulation occur in the menstrual cycle?

Usually on day 14 within 30 to 38 hours after the onset of the mid-cycle LH surge

What is the proliferative phase?

Endometrial phase occurring at approximately day 4 to 14

What uterine changes occur during the proliferative phase?

Proliferation of the endometrial glands
Endometrial stromal proliferation
Elongation of spiral arteries

What are the hormonal levels during the proliferative phase?

Estradiol level increases and peaks just before the LH surge and ovulation.
Progesterone level remains low.
FSH peaks at mid-cycle with LH but produces a smaller surge.
LH rapidly peaks at mid-cycle and triggers ovulation.

What is the secretory phase?

Endometrial phase that begins on day 14 and lasts until day 28, approximately

What uterine changes occur during the secretory phase?

Progesterone stimulates the glands to secrete mucus and glycogen.
Glands become tortuous and dilated.
Convoluted spiral arteries extend to the superficial layer of the endometrium.
Stroma becomes edematous.

What is the luteal phase?

Ovarian phase that begins after ovulation
The corpus luteum forms from the granulosa cells of the ruptured follicle.

What is the function of the corpus luteum?

Produces progesterone and estradiol
Maintains pregnancy until placental progesterone production is adequate

What are the normal hormonal levels during the secretory phase?

Estradiol level decreases after ovulation, then begins to rise with production from the corpus luteum, and peaks on day 20 to 21.
Progesterone level begins to rise after ovulation to peak at approximately days 20–21 with production by the corpus luteum.

LH and FSH are at low levels because of negative feedback of the high progesterone and estradiol levels.

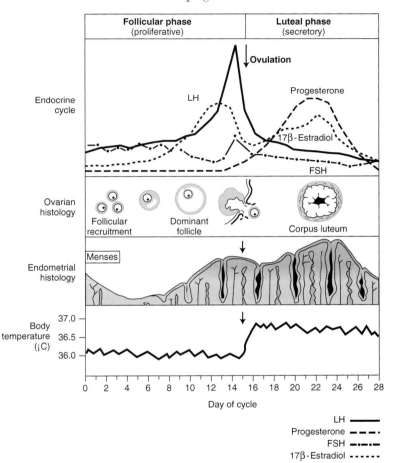

Figure 34.1. Hormone function within the menstrual cycle FSH = follicle-stimulating hormone; LH = luteininzing hormone (Mehta S, Milder EA, Mirarchi AJ, Milder E. Step-Up: A High-Yield, Systems Based Review for the USMLE Step 1 2nd Ed. Philadelphia: Lippincott Williams & Wilkins, 2003:189.)

Does estradiol or progesterone have a higher peak in the secretory phase?

Progesterone

What happens to the following if pregnancy does not occur:

Corpus luteum?

Degenerates into a scar called the corpus albicans

Progesterone level?

Declines as corpus luteum regresses

Estradiol level?

Decreases as corpus luteum regresses

FSH level?

Increases slowly as corpus luteum regresses

Endometrium?

If pregnancy does not occur by day 23, the endometrium begins to degenerate.

What is PMS?

Premenstrual syndrome
Also known as luteal phase dysphoric disorder
Cyclic recurrence of physical, psychological, and behavioral changes that cause distress and interfere with normal daily activities or relationships

When during the menstrual cycle does PMS occur?

Signs and symptoms occur during the luteal phase of the menstrual cycle and remit after the onset of menses.

In whom does it occur?

Most common in women age 25 to 44 years

What is its incidence?

An estimated 5% of women of reproductive age can be diagnosed with PMS by the American Psychiatric Association and National Institute of Mental Health criteria.
About 40% of women report significant problems related to their menstrual cycles, with 2%–10% reporting an impact on work or lifestyle.

What are the American Psychiatric Association

Symptoms are temporally related to the menstrual cycle, starting during the

criteria for PMS/luteal phase dysphoric disorder?

last week of the luteal phase and ending after the onset of menses.

At least five of the following, including one of the first four symptoms:

1. Affective lability (e.g., sudden onset of irritability, anger, sadness)
2. Persistent and marked anger or irritability
3. Marked anxiety or tension
4. Markedly depressed mood, feeling of hopelessness
5. Decreased interest in usual activities
6. Easy fatigability or marked lack of energy
7. Subjective sense of difficulty in concentrating
8. Marked change in appetite, overeating, or food craving
9. Hypersomnia or insomnia
10. Physical symptoms such as breast tenderness, headaches, edema, joint or muscle pain, weight gain

Symptoms interfere with work or usual activities or relationships.

Symptoms are **not** an exacerbation of another psychiatric disorder.

What is the evaluation for PMS?

Examination of patient's daily diary of symptoms over a period of 2–3 months

History and physical examination to rule out other illness (e.g., depression)

What is the treatment of PMS?

Supportive:

Counseling and education

Goal is to provide the patient with greater control over her life.

May include lifestyle changes such as exercise and dietary modifications

Medications:

Fluoxetine (Prozac) and Venlafaxine (Effexor) have been shown to be effective in treating PMS in randomized trials.

Nonsteroidal anti-inflammatory drugs (NSAIDs) such as mefenamic acid may also be of benefit.

Gonadotropin-releasing hormone agonists have been used to treat severe PMS, but have significant side effects associated with the resultant low estrogen level.

What is dysmenorrhea?

Painful menstruation

What is its incidence?

About 50%–75% of women report dysmenorrhea.

What are the two main categories of dysmenorrhea?

Primary dysmenorrhea: Painful menstruation without associated pelvic disease

Secondary dysmenorrhea: Painful menstruation caused by pelvic pathology

Describe the typical pattern of pain in primary dysmenorrhea.
    When?

Usually begins with the onset of menstruation, then gradually decreases.

How long?

Twelve to seventy-two hours

Where?

Lower abdomen; most intense in midline

What type?

Often crampy and colicky

Other symptoms?

Back pain
Nausea
Diarrhea
Fatigue
Headache
Malaise

What is thought to be the cause of primary dysmenorrhea?

Increased prostaglandin release from endometrial cells at the time of menstruation causes uterine smooth muscle contraction, increased intrauterine pressure, and some degree of uterine ischemia.

What is the treatment of primary dysmenorrhea?

NSAIDs are the mainstay of treatment:
Interfere with the cyclooxygenase enzyme pathway
Propionic acid derivatives—ibuprofen, naproxen, ketoprofen
Fenamates—mefenamic acid, meclofenamate, flufenamic acid
Antagonize prostagladin receptors
Oral contraceptives: Inhibit ovulation and decrease endometrial prostaglandin production. If NSAIDs are not effective or are contraindicated and contraception is desired; not as effective as NSAIDs
If NSAIDs and oral contraceptives fail GnRH agonists can be considered (inhibit ovulation)
Follow-up: Consider pathologic cause and secondary dysmenorrhea if there is no improvement with therapy.

What is the pharmacologic mechanism that is responsible for relieving dysmenorrhea for thefollowing drugs:
 NSAIDs?

Inhibit prostaglandin production
The fenamates also have an antagonistic action at the prostaglandin receptors.

 Oral contraceptives?

Decrease prostaglandins through suppression of ovulation and the normal sequence of hormones

What are the side effects of NSAIDs?

Gastric irritation
Nausea

Gastrointestinal ulcer
Increased bleeding time
Nephrotoxicity
Fenamates also associated with blurred
  vision, headaches, and dizziness.

What is the effectiveness of NSAIDs in treating dysmenorrhea?

Relieve dysmenorrhea in about 80% of women

What are the common causes of secondary dysmenorrhea?

Chronic pelvic inflammatory disease
Endometriosis
Adhesions
Müllerian duct abnormalities

What characteristics of secondary dysmenorrhea can help distinguish from primary dysmenorrhea?

Difficult distinction to make
Must look for other signs and symptoms
  to indicate pathology
Secondary dysmenorrhea usually begins
  after age 20 years.
Pelvic pain is often present at times
  other than menstruation.
Patients may have an abnormal pelvic
  exam, although a normal pelvic exam
  does **not** rule out disease.

What other illness is commonly associated with menstruation?

Headache: Tension or vascular type
Migraine headaches may occur only at
  menses or may increase in frequency
  or severity at time of menstruation.

What is the treatment for menstrual migraine?

NSAIDs
Sumatriptan Succinate
Estrogen supplementation during
  menses or continuous oral
  contraceptives

ABNORMAL UTERINE BLEEDING

What is considered excessive blood loss?

> 80 ml

Describe the patterns of abnormal bleeding.

Oligomenorrhea?

Infrequent, irregular bleeding usually at intervals > 40 days

Polymenorrhea?

Frequent but regular bleeding usually occurring at intervals of 21 days or less

Menorrhagia (or hypermenorrhea)?

Excessive bleeding in amount and duration at regular intervals

Metrorrhagia?

Irregular but not excessive uterine bleeding

Menometrorrhagia?

Frequent bleeding that is excessive in amount and duration and occurs at irregular intervals

Hypomenorrhea?

Regular bleeding that is decreased in amount

What is the differential diagnosis for abnormal uterine bleeding?

- Blood dyscrasia
- Inflammatory: Cervicitis, endometritis
- Malignancy: Uterine, cervical, fallopian tube, ovarian, gestational trophoblastic disease
- Benign growth: Leiomyomas, cervical polyps, endometrial polyps
- Anovulation
- Thyroid dysfunction
- Dysfunctional uterine bleeding
- Pregnancy related: Subinvolution of uterus, ectopic pregnancy, spontaneous abortion, postpartum hemorrhage, retained products of conception
- Iatrogenic: Intrauterine device, anticoagulants, progestational agents
- Other sites: Vaginal cancer, vaginal laceration, atrophic vaginitis, urethral or gastrointestinal source, external genitalia lesions

What are the two main causes of abnormal bleeding in an adolescent?

1. Anovulation
2. Blood dyscrasia

What is the most common blood dyscrasia associated with abnormal bleeding?

Von Willebrand's disease affecting 1:1000 individuals

What is desmopressin?

Synthetic analog of vasopressin that can be used to treat abnormal uterine bleeding in patients with von Willebrand's disease

What is the mechanism of desmopressin?

Rapidly increases Coagulation Factor VIII and von Willebrand Factor

What is Halban disease?

Increased bleeding due to persistent corpus luteum
Usually self-limited and not recurrent

What must always be considered in a perimenopausal or postmenopausal woman with abnormal uterine bleeding?

Cancer

What should always be suspected in an ovulatory patient with abnormal bleeding?

A pathologic abnormality such as a polyp

What diagnostic procedures aid in this diagnosis?

Hysteroscopy
Hysterosalpingogram
Biopsy
Saline sonohysterogram

What features help differentiate ovulatory from anovulatory cycles?

Ovulatory cycles tend to be consistent in cycle length, duration of menses, and amount of bleeding.
Also look for associated mid-cycle pain, vaginal discharge, premenstrual breast tenderness, and dysmenorrhea.

What is "dysfunctional uterine bleeding"?

Abnormal uterine bleeding associated with an anovulatory menstrual cycle without the presence of organic disease; a diagnosis of exclusion

What are two theoretical causes of dysfunctional bleeding?

1. **Hormonal theory:** The normal hormonal controls are defective, and therefore the endometrial changes are not synchronous and universal as in normal menstrual cycles. The structural stability of the endometrium is compromised and the fragile tissue is subject to random breakdown. The usual rhythmic vasoconstriction that initiates normal ischemia and endometrial sloughing and the prolonged vasoconstriction that encourages stasis are also defective.
2. **Tissue theory:** The endometrial regeneration is thought to be triggered by endometrial tissue loss, not hormonal changes. Loss of tissue in the presence of excess estrogen is insufficient to restore endometrial structural stability. Curettage may be an effective treatment.

What age groups are typically affected?

About 50% of patients are 40 years of age or older (perimenopausal).
Twenty percent are adolescents, about one or two years past menarche.
Both populations tend to be anovulatory.

What is a commonly associated physical finding?

Obesity

What does the workup include?

History and physical examination
Pap smear
Laboratory studies based on clinical suspicion:
Complete blood count
Human chorionic gonadotropin
Prolactin
Thyroid panel
Serum androgen levels if clinical evidence indicates androgen excess

Head magnetic resonance imaging if hyperprolactinemia or clinical evidence of hypopituitarism

Biopsy and hysteroscopy can be helpful, especially if patient is older or has history of unopposed estrogens.

What are the four main categories of dysfunctional uterine bleeding?

1. **Estrogen withdrawal bleeding:** Low estrogen level
2. **Estrogen breakthrough bleeding:** Chronic estrogen stimulates endometrial proliferation, which outgrows the structural support and leads to endometrial breakdown.
3. **Progesterone withdrawal bleeding:** Low progesterone level; only occurs if the endometrium is first primed to proliferate by estrogen
4. **Progesterone breakthrough bleeding:** High progesterone-to-estrogen ratio

What are the etiologic factors for estrogen withdrawal bleeding?

Bilateral oophorectomy
Radiation of mature follicles
Cessation of exogenous estrogen therapy

What type of bleeding pattern is typically seen in estrogen breakthrough bleeding?

Can only be predicted generally
Relatively **low** levels of estrogen lead to intermittent spotting that is low in flow but prolonged in duration.
High levels of estrogen allow the endometrium to build up beyond the limits of endometrial structural support, leading to prolonged periods of amenorrhea followed by profuse bleeds (oligomenorrhea with bouts of heavy bleeding).

What are two conditions in which estrogen breakthrough bleeding can occur?

Polycystic ovary syndrome and obesity

What is the typical bleeding pattern in progesterone breakthrough bleeding?

Intermittent, low-flow bleeding of variable duration (similar to low estrogen breakthrough bleeding)

What is a common cause of progesterone breakthrough bleeding?

Long-acting progestin-only contraceptives, such as Norplant and Depo-Provera

When does progesterone withdrawal bleeding occur?

Usually after discontinuation of a progestin, such as a contraceptive

What is the usual therapy for dysfunctional uterine bleeding?

Intense estrogen–progestin therapy for 7 days (one low-dose combination monophasic oral contraceptive pill twice a day)

Cyclic low-dose oral contraceptive pill for 3 months (one pill once a day for 3 weeks, then 1 week of withdrawal bleeding)

Contraception wanted: Continue oral contraceptives

Contraception not desired: Medroxyprogesterone acetate 10 mg once a day for 10 days every month

Follow-up: Always needed because recurrent hemorrhage accompanies persistent anovulation and endometrial atypia may occur with unopposed estrogen exposure.

What should you always tell the patient about oral contraceptive therapy for abnormal bleeding?

Expect severe cramping and heavy bleeding for 2–4 days after stopping therapy.

What circumstances warrant initial treatment with estrogens rather than the estrogen–progestin therapy above?

Bleeding has been heavy for several days (need estrogen-stimulated endometrial proliferation).

Biopsy produces minimal tissue.

Patient has been on progestins (endometrium is atrophic).

When follow-up is uncertain: Estrogen therapy stops all types of dysfunctional bleeding temporarily.

What is the estrogen therapy?

Conjugated estrogens (1.25 mg) or estradiol (2.0 mg) daily for 7–10 days; then combine with 10 mg of medroxyprogesterone acetate for 7 days.

If bleeding is acute and moderately heavy, the oral estrogen can be given every 4 hours during the first 24 hours.

If the acute bleeding is very heavy, then conjugated estrogens can be given intravenously every 4 hours until the bleeding stops, followed by estrogen–progestin therapy. If there is no response in 12–24 hours, reevaluate. Patient will likely need dilation and curettage.

What is an alternative therapy if heavy bleeding is thought to be due to estrogen-stimulated proliferation?

Medroxyprogesterone acetate 5 mg for 1 week in each cycle

What is endometrial ablation?

Transvaginal technique to heat and scar endometrial tissue to induce hypomenorrhea or amenorrhea in women with dysfunctional uterine bleeding

What are the types of ablation?

Roller ball
Balloon

What are contraindications to endometrial ablation?

Absolute: Desires fertility
Endometrial atypical hyperplasia or carcinoma
Relative: Presence of uterine fibroids

35

Infertility: The Infertile Couple

GENERAL

What is the definition of infertility?

Inability of a couple of reproductive age to achieve conception after 1 year of sexual intercourse without contraception

What is primary infertility?

Infertility that occurs without any prior pregnancies

What is secondary infertility?

Infertility that occurs after a previous conception

What is the incidence of infertility?

In the United States, occurs in about 28 million couples, or 14% of couples

What are some contributing factors and their incidence in infertility?

Male fertility factor: 35%
Ovulatory factors: 25%
Peritoneal factors: 25%
Cervical factors: 5%
Uterine factors: 5%
Idiopathic: 5%

How are these factors used in evaluation and management of infertility?

Each factor should be considered in the initial evaluation of the infertile couple.
Factors should serve as a guide for further evaluation and management.

What percentage of couples have more than one reason for infertility?

15%

HISTORY

What general questions should be asked during an initial infertility evaluation to elicit information about

Age of each partner?
Previous pregnancies?
Length of time conception has been attempted?

**specific contributing
factors?**

Frequency of intercourse?
Lubricants used? (spermicidal?)
History of impotence or dyspareunia?

**What questions should be
asked of the male partner
during an initial infertility
evaluation?**

Fathered a previous child?
Testicular surgery or injury?
Genitourinary infections (including
    sexually transmitted diseases)?
Postpubertal mumps?
Genital radiation or chemotherapy?
Hypospadias?
Neuropathy associated with nerve
    damage or medical conditions, such as
    diabetes mellitus?
Use of chemotherapeutic drugs,
    Furadantin, or sulfasalazine?
Excessive exposure to heat (hot tubs),
    pesticides, toxins, marijuana, nicotine,
    or alcohol?

**What questions should be
asked of the female
partner during an initial
infertility evaluation to
elicit information about
possible ovulatory factors?**

Detailed menstrual history. Irregularities
    are frequently seen in chronic
    anovulation or oligo-ovulation.
Headaches, visual changes, and
    galactorrhea? Suggests pituitary
    adenoma and resultant
    hyperprolactinemia.
If amenorrhea, primary or secondary?
Excessive exercise? Suggests
    hypothalamic–pituitary failure.
Extreme emotional stress? Suggests
    hypothalamic–pituitary failure.
Excessive hair growth?
Changes in hair texture, weight gain or
    loss, palpitations, heat/cold
    intolerance? Suggest thyroid
    dysfunction.
Hot flashes and vaginal dryness? Suggest
    menopause, perimenopause, or
    premature ovarian failure.
Cycle lengths < 25 days or > 35 days,
    or that vary by > 7 days from cycle to
    cycle? Suggest ovulatory irregularity,

especially if patient has premenstrual symptoms, dysmenorrhea, variation in amount/duration of flow.

Other medical problems

Peritoneal factors?

Pelvic/adnexal surgery (including bilateral tube ligation)?

Pelvic infection [salpingitis/pelvic inflammatory disease (PID)]? PID doubles the incidence of infertility.

Previous ectopic pregnancies?

History of appendicitis, especially ruptured?

Septic abortion?

Previous intrauterine device (IUD) use? IUD use is associated with a fourfold increase in risk for development of pelvic adhesions.

Premenstrual spotting; dysmenorrhea; dyspareunia; and cyclic abdominal or pelvic pain? Suggest endometriosis, which doubles the incidence of infection.

Cervical factors?

A history of the following can cause problems with cervical mucus production or quality, leading to infertility:

Cone biopsy?

Cautery (LEEP)?

Cryosurgery?

Obstetric trauma?

Cervicitis?

Uterine factors?

Leiomyomas?

Diethylstilbestrol (DES) exposure in utero? Can lead to a T-shaped uterus.

Previous dilation and curettage (D & C)?

What are the rates of infertility (percentage) associated with the age of the woman?

20–24 years:7%
25–29 years: 9%
30–35 years: 15%
35–40 years: 22%
40–44 years: 29%

What is the normal rate of conception with unprotected intercourse?	After 1 month: 15%–20% After 6 months: 50%–75% After 1 year: 80%–90%
What is the optimal coital interval for conception?	24–48 hours

PHYSICAL EXAMINATION

What findings in the male physical examination suggest a male infertility factor?	Evidence of congenital abnormalities associated with male infertility, such as lack of body hair; gynecomastia; tall, thin, gynecoid appearance Abnormalities in testicular descent, size, and consistency; presence of varicoceles Varicoceles are compressible globular scrotal distentions that cannot be transilluminated and are caused by a venous abnormality. Associated with increased male infertility Evidence of infection (orchitis, epididymitis) Penile abnormalities

What findings in the female physical examination suggest ovulatory factors?	Signs of androgen excess (as seen in polycystic ovary) including:
	   Clitoriomegaly
	   Enlarged ovaries on pelvic examination
	   Hirsutism
	   Acne
	   Balding
	   Male escutcheon
	 Signs/symptoms of hyperthyroidism:
	   Goiter
	   Tremor
	   Very fine hair
	   Nervousness
	   Exophthalmos
	   Palpitations
	 Signs/symptoms of hypothyroidism
	   Goiter

Bradycardia

Sluggishness

Dry skin

Coarse hair

Myxedema

Obesity

Excess adipose tissue increases extragonadal steroid production.

Increased estrogen production inhibits follicle-stimulating hormone (FSH) secretion from the anterior pituitary and can cause anovulation.

Emaciation leads to hypothalamic dysfunction with loss of pulsatile gonadotropin-releasing hormone (GnRH) secretion.

Galactorrhea

Seen in hyperprolactinemia

High levels of prolactin suppress the pulsatile secretion of GnRH from the hypothalamus, thus preventing cyclic gonadotropin release.

Peritoneal and uterine factors?

Evidence of current infection: Pelvic tenderness or mass or cervical discharge

Nodularity felt on palpation of the uterosacral ligaments suggests endometriosis; best felt on rectovaginal examination.

Fixation of the uterus or ovaries suggests pelvic adhesions or fibrosis from previous pelvic or abdominal infection, surgery, or endometriosis.

Irregularly shaped uterus suggests the presence of leiomyomas or congenital malformation.

Cervical factors?

Discharge, cervical friability, and motion tenderness suggest cervicitis.

Copious amount of cervical mucus suggests impending ovulation or estrogen excess.

Evidence of past surgical procedure or trauma

Signs of DES exposure including:
Vaginal adenosis (glandular appearance
of vaginal wall mucosa)
Cervical "hood" or "coxcomb"
Atrophy consistent with estrogen
deficiency

BASIC INFERTILITY WORKUP

**What is the first test that
should be ordered in the
workup?**

Varies; an infertility workup is unique to
the couple and should be guided by the
information obtained from the history
and physical examination.

**What is the basic workup
to evaluate male factors?**

Semen analysis

Procedure?

Semen sample should be collected after
48 hours of abstinence and examined
within 2 to 3 hours of collection.

Normal values?

Ejaculate volume between 2 and 8 ml
Sperm concentration > 20 million/ml
> 50% motility at 6 hours
> 60% sperm normal morphology
Important value to consider for IVF
success is total motile sperm

Repeat testing?

If any of the values are abnormal, two
additional samples should be
evaluated at 2-week intervals.
Urologic examination if abnormalities
persist

**What is the basic workup
to evaluate ovulatory
factors?**

Documentation of ovulation by:
Basal body temperature (BBT)
Endometrial biopsy
Serum progesterone measurement

**What is the procedure for
BBT?**

Patient measures her temperature before
arising in the morning and records
results on chart.

Normal results?

A biphasic chart characterized by a sustained rise in body temperature of at least 0.4°F (thermogenic effect of progesterone) is typical of ovulation.

Ovulation is thought to occur on the day of lowest temperature; however, ovulation can vary by as much as 2 days, making BBTs a poor method.

What is the procedure for endometrial biopsy?

Biopsy and microscopic examination of endometrial tissue

Why is endometrial biopsy performed in the infertility workup during the luteal phase?

Microscopic examination of the endometrium can be used to "date" the endometrium based on histology.

An endometrial biopsy performed in the luteal phase provides indirect evidence of the presence or absence of ovulation.

Normal results?

No more than a 2-day discrepancy between the date of the endometrium based on histologic findings and the date based on clinical calculation of the menstrual cycle

A discrepancy of 3 or more days suggests a luteal phase defect.

What is the procedure for serum progesterone measurement?

Measurement of progesterone level in serum on days 21–23

Normal values?

A serum progesterone level of 4 ng/ml or three samples (drawn on separate days during the luteal phase) totaling 15 ng/ml indicates that ovulation has occurred.

Because progesterone levels can vary, this test is not as useful as biopsy.

What is a luteal phase defect?

A group of hormonal alterations clinically linked to recurrent abortions and infertility

Diagnosis?

BBT elevations last 10 days or less (short luteal phase) or endometrial biopsy is histologically more than 2 days out of phase with the clinically calculated menstrual cycle.

Incidence in women without infertility?

Found in up to 30% of isolated cycles in normal women

Role in infertility?

Controversial; should be considered as a cause of infertility only if it is documented in at least two consecutive cycles

What is the basic workup to evaluate peritoneal and uterine factors?

Hysterosalpingography (HSG)
Laparoscopy

What is the procedure for HSG?

Oil or water-soluble contrast material is slowly injected through the cervix and into the fallopian tubes to produce fluoroscopic x-ray images of the uterus and fallopian tubes.
Images outline the size, shape, and position of the uterus and also reveal obstruction of the fallopian tubes.
Best performed in the early proliferative phase, after menses, to avoid disturbing a possible pregnancy and to prevent reflux of endometrial tissue (may be a cause of endometriosis).

What abnormalities can be revealed with HSG?

Congenital uterine malformations
T-shaped or hypoplastic uterine cavities associated with in utero DES exposure
Submucous leiomyomas
Intrauterine polyps
Salpingitis isthmica nodosa (SIN)
　Defined as the presence of localized numerous diverticula along the interstitial segment or isthmus of the fallopian tube
　Associated with "healthy" fallopian tubes as well as chronic or healing salpingitis

Associated with a significantly
increased incidence of tubal
pregnancy
Proximal or distal fallopian tube
occlusion
Pelvic adhesions or hydrosalpinx, as
suggested by retained dye on a
delayed abdominal flat-plate
radiograph
Asherman syndrome

**Why does HSG have a high
false-positive rate?**

Thought to be because of transient tubal
blockages caused by smooth muscle
spasm

**What are the
contraindications to HSG?**

Pelvic mass or tenderness (to avoid
exacerbation of an ongoing process)
Allergy to iodine or contrast dye
(relative)
Pelvic infection

**What are the risks of
HSG?**

Dye embolization (rare)
Salpingitis (1%–3%)

**What is the procedure for
laparoscopy?**

Visualization of peritoneal cavity with a
rigid scope

**When should laparoscopy
be performed?**

In general, after the basic minimum
workup is completed
Considered a valuable test for detecting
endometriosis or pelvic adhesions,
which are difficult to evaluate with
HSG alone

**What percentage of
patients undergoing
laparoscopy for infertility
have pelvic pathology?**

Approximately 50%

**What conditions can be
surgically managed with
laparoscopy?**

Adhesions and endometriosis

What does the basic workup to evaluate cervical factors consist of?	Postcoital test
What is the procedure for postcoital test?	Couple is instructed to have intercourse after 24 to 48 hours of abstinence and 2 days before ovulation Cervical mucus and semen interaction are analyzed within 12 hours of intercourse.
How is the cervical mucus analyzed?	For impending ovulation, by spinnbarkeit (ability to be pulled into a string between two surfaces) Glass coverslip is placed on the mucus and slowly drawn from the slide.
Normal results?	Cervical mucus suggesting impending ovulation will stretch 6 to 10 cm
How is semen interaction analyzed?	For the degree of cellularity and the number of sperm
Normal results?	More than 20 sperm/high-power field has been correlated with a statistically significant increase in the percentage of pregnancies.
Abnormal results?	Absence of sperm suggests faulty sperm production or poor coital technique. "Shaking" sperm suggests immunologic infertility.

EVALUATION OF RESULTS AND MANAGEMENT

MALE FACTORS

What is the treatment for low sperm count?	Referral to a urologist for a thorough evaluation, including a complete physical examination, repeat semen analysis, postejaculate urine sample (to look for retrograde ejaculation), and measurement of serum gonadotropin levels

What is the treatment for varicocele?	Varicocele's role in infertility is controversial. Most believe that surgical ligation improves semen quantity in the majority of men. Associated with a 30%–50% pregnancy rate The improved semen quantity is thought to be due to improved blood flow or temperature regulation.
What is intrauterine insemination?	Method by which washed sperm are injected through the cervix around the time of ovulation
Why are sperm washed?	Washing isolates a population of sperm with a higher percentage of motile forms and removes proteins, prostaglandins, and bacteria commonly associated with adverse reactions.
What is the procedure for sperm washing?	Techniques vary. General: Dilution with 7–10 ml of buffer Sample is gently centrifuged. Resultant sperm pellet is resuspended in 0.5-ml buffered solution.
Indications?	Retrograde ejaculation Neurologic impotence High semen volume Isolation of the motile sperm Donor insemination Infertility due to cervical factors

FEMALE FACTORS

Ovulatory factors

What is the rate of conception after treatment in women with anovulation as the cause of infertility?	Women with anovulation alone as the cause of infertility have the highest rate of conception with treatment ($\sim$ 70%).

What factors should therapeutic decisions be based on?

Whether the dysfunction lies within the ovary or elsewhere in the hypothalamic–pituitary–ovarian axis

What are the categories of ovarian dysfunction?

It is helpful to diagnose and manage patients according to the World Health Organization's classification of ovulatory deficiencies.

Group I: Hypothalamic–pituitary failure
Patients have hypogonadotropic hypogonadism with low FSH and estrogen levels, normal prolactin concentrations, and failure to bleed after a progesterone challenge.
Includes hypothalamic amenorrhea, anorexia nervosa, and stress-related amenorrhea

Group II: Hypothalamic–pituitary dysfunction
Patients have anovulation and oligomenorrhea with normal gonadotropin and estrogen levels.
Includes idiopathic anovulation and the classic polycystic ovary syndrome

Group III: Ovarian failure
Patients are hypergonadotropic and hypogonadal with low estrogen levels.
Includes ovarian failure and ovarian resistance
A separate, but important, clinical entity is the hyperprolactinemic patient with ovulatory dysfunction.

What tests should be performed after ovulatory dysfunction is documented?

Measurement of serum thyroid-stimulating hormone (TSH) level
Measurement of serum prolactin level
Progesterone challenge to assess estrogen levels
If the patient fails to bleed after the progesterone challenge, measurement of serum FSH and luteinizing

hormone (LH) to rule out ovarian failure

Why should TSH be measured?

Both hypothyroidism and hyperthyroidism can cause anovulation by altering estrogen metabolism and clearance.

Thyroid disease leads to increased estrogen levels, thus inhibiting FSH secretion and follicular development.

What can the progesterone challenge test reveal?

The presence of estrogen production (the absence of ovarian failure), because only endometrium that has been primed to thicken by the influence of estrogen sloughs when challenged by progesterone withdrawal. Proves hypothalamic–pituitary–ovarian axis is intact.

What is the procedure for progesterone challenge test?

Patient is given medroxyprogesterone acetate 10 mg orally daily for 7 days

Normal result?

Withdrawal bleeding after medroxyprogesterone acetate is discontinued indicates that the hypothalamic–pituitary–ovarian axis is intact.

Abnormal result?

Withdrawal bleeding may be delayed in cases of androgen excess (e.g., polycystic ovary syndrome).

What are additional tests for androgen excess?

Measurement of serum dehydroepiandrosterone sulfate (DHEAS) and testosterone levels

What is DHEAS?

An adrenal androgen that may be overproduced in cases of adrenal hyperplasia (or in some cases of hyperprolactinemia) and can cause an anovulatory hypoestrogenic state by direct inhibition of follicular maturation (as in polycystic ovary syndrome)

What is the treatment for hypothalamic–pituitary failure?

When failure is due to lack of LH and FSH production (hypogonadotropic hypogonadism), ovulation can be induced by replacement of the necessary hormones using human menopausal gonadotropin (hMG).

What is hMG?

A mixture of LH and FSH derived from postmenopausal women

Rate of pregnancy with hMG in patients with hypogonadotropic hypogonadism?

Sixty to 80% of patients achieve pregnancy, most within six cycles.

Risks of hMG therapy?

Increased risks of multiple gestation (10%–15%) and ovarian hyperstimulation syndrome
Because of risks, should be used selectively

What is ovarian hyperstimulation syndrome?

Can be life-threatening if severe
Mild cases: Ovarian enlargement, weight gain, and abdominal distention
Severe cases:
Ovaries > 10 cm
Weight gain of > 20 pounds due to peritoneal, pleural, and pericardial (extravascular) fluid accumulation
Loss of fluid from the intravascular space results in low blood pressure and poor perfusion of tissues, and can cause permanent organ damage or even death.

How is ovarian hyperstimulation syndrome prevented?

Periodic measurement of serum estradiol levels and ultrasonic monitoring of size and number of follicles

What is polycystic ovary syndrome (PCO)?

A hypothalamic–pituitary dysfunction

"Vicious cycle" of hormonal dysfunction:

Increased production of androgens by ovaries, some of which are peripherally converted to estrogen, causes hyperestrogenic and virilizing state.

The high estrogen level increases pituitary production of LH ("pituitary hypersensitivity") but suppresses FSH production by normal feedback inhibition.

The low level of FSH is enough to allow follicle formation, but not maturity and ovulation.

The high LH level stimulates the follicular cells to secrete androgens, and the resulting high ovarian androgen levels further inhibit full maturation of the multiple follicles, and provide substrate for peripheral conversion to estrogen. The anovulatory cycle thus continues.

Their hyperinsulinemic state stimulates ovarian androgen production

What is the treatment of PCO?

Patients with PCO have functional ovaries that produce estrogen and are good candidates for treatment with clomiphene citrate.

Patients with normal renal and hepatic function are good candidates for metformin therapy

What is clomiphene citrate and how does it work?

A nonsteroidal "antiestrogen agent" that causes enhanced release of pituitary gonadotropins by an unknown mechanism

What are the indications for treatment with clomiphene citrate?

PCO (generates follicular maturation and ovulation in anovulatory women who can produce estrogen)

Oligo-ovulation (creates regular cycles)

Luteal phase defect (stimulates follicular development)

Assisted reproduction techniques (produces multiple follicles)

Overproduction of DHEAS by adrenals (stimulates follicular growth and suppresses adrenal DHEAS production when combined with glucocorticoid treatment)

What is the ovulation rate after treatment with clomiphene citrate?

Induces ovulation in 70% of patients

What is the pregnancy rate after treatment with clomiphene citrate?

40% in anovulatory patients

What is the increase in incidence of twin pregnancy after treatment with clomiphene citrate?

5% to 10% increase

What is the risk of developing a persistent ovarian cyst with clomiphene citrate?

10%

What are the side effects of treatment with clomiphene citrate?

Hot flashes

Visual disturbances

Headaches

Nausea

Abdominal bloating

Mood lability

Ovarian enlargement (should be screened for by frequent pelvic examinations)

What is the treatment of ovarian failure?

Anovulation due to menopausal or premature ovarian failure cannot be treated with ovulation induction.

Treatment options include egg donation and adoption.

What is the incidence of elevated prolactin level in ovulation disturbances?

Occurs in about 15% of ovulation disturbances

What conditions should be ruled out in patients with an elevated prolactin level?

Pituitary tumor (macroadenoma) by magnetic resonance imaging
Primary hypothyroidism
   Results in a low level of dopamine, which normally inhibits prolactin production
   Lack of inhibition leads to hyperprolactinemia.
Dopamine depletion due to antihypertensive or neuroleptic drugs

What is the treatment of patients with an elevated prolactin level?

Initial treatment: Bromocriptine
Depending on symptoms, surgical removal of a pituitary tumor may be required after maximal treatment/ tumor shrinkage with bromocriptine.

Peritoneal factors

What factors influence the success of tubal disease treatment?

Success varies widely, and depends on:
The extent of original inflammatory damage
Location of blockage (distal occlusion with hydrosalpinx has a worse prognosis than isthmic block)
The pathogen (surgery is contraindicated if tuberculosis is involved)
Postoperative tube length
State of tubal cilia

What is the treatment of tubal disease?

Endoscopic surgery:
Has largely replaced laparotomy and microsurgery for most cases of obstructive tubal disease.
Laparoscopic salpingostomy is usually performed for distal obstruction.

Tubal cannulation by hysteroscopy is performed for proximal obstruction.
Microsurgery
In vitro fertilization and adoption

What are the goals of microsurgery?

Restore anatomy to its normal appearance
Avoid serosal insults (trauma, ischemia, hemorrhage, infection, foreign body exposure, exposure of raw surfaces), which may lead to adhesions

What techniques are involved in microsurgery?

Removal of talc from gloves
Minimal use of sponges
Bipolar coagulation of bleeding vessels
Use of fine, minimally antigenic sutures to approximate closely tissue planes with minimal tension.
Surgery usually is performed under an operating microscope.
Perioperative antibiotics (usually doxycycline 100 mg twice daily from the night before surgery to 5 days postoperatively) and systemic glucocorticoids may play a role in improved outcome.

What are the risks of microsurgery?

Increased postoperative risk of ectopic pregnancies

Can tubal ligation be reversed?

Yes, but success rates largely depend on the type of sterilization procedure used as well as on the tubal segments anastomosed, postoperative tubal length, and surgical technique.
Banding or ligation procedures create fairly localized damage.
Unipolar electrocautery is associated with the destruction of a large segment of tube.

What is the incidence of endometriosis in infertility?

Generally estimated to be between 10% and 25%
Infertility rates are twice those of women without endometriosis.

What is the treatment of endometriosis?	Most forms can be treated at the time of laparoscopic exploration by electrocoagulation and laser ablation or peritoneal resection.
	Medical treatment
	Most successful in mild to moderate disease; includes leuprolide, danocrine, and low-dose monophasic oral contraceptive pills (OCPs)
What is leuprolide?	A GnRH analog administered in a nonpulsatile manner
How does it work?	Constant level of leuprolide → GnRH inhibition of gonadotropin release → hypoestrogenic state similar to menopause → atrophy of the endometrial implants
What is Danocrine and how does it work?	A drug with a direct androgenic effect that is used to cause an anovulatory, hypoestrogenic state that can result in atrophy of endometrial implants
How do low-dose OCPs work?	Can suppress endometrial implants when used continuously for 6–12 months
What is the pregnancy rate after stopping OCPs in infertile women?	Between 40% and 50%
What are the postoperative pregnancy rates?	Relate directly to stage:
	60% for mild to moderate disease
	35% for severe disease

Cervical factors

What follow-up is indicated for each of the following abnormal results of the postcoital test?	
Few or absent sperm	Repeat test
	Evaluate mucus

Reevaluate male factor

Review coital technique (lubricants, etc.)

Thick, tenacious mucus, with spinnbarkeit < 8 cm

Exclude:

Inaccurate timing of intercourse with ovulation

Inadequate estrogen production

Cervicitis (if lymphocyte count is high) with culture for bacteria, *Ureaplasma urealyticum*, and *Chlamydia trachomatis*

Cervical trauma, surgery

DES syndrome

Nonprogressive ("shaking") sperm

Suggests anti-sperm antibodies in either partner

Treatment involves steroid suppression or intrauterine insemination.

Uterine factors

What kinds of leiomyomas are more commonly associated with infertility?

Submucous or intramural

What is the treatment of leiomyomas?

Surgical removal with or without leuprolide therapy for 3 months before surgery

What is Asherman syndrome?

Partial or complete obliteration of the uterine cavity by intrauterine synechiae (adhesive bands of tissue between opposing uterine walls)

Often associated with menstrual abnormalities (amenorrhea, hypomenorrhea, and dysmenorrhea); recurrent abortion; and infertility

What are its etiologic factors?

Complication of endometritis followed by surgical instrumentation of the uterus (e.g., D & C after term pregnancies or spontaneous or elective abortions)

On what is a diagnosis based?	Filling defect on HSG
What is the treatment for Asherman syndrome?	Hysteroscopically guided lysis of adhesions followed by 14 days of antibiotics and 2 months of oral high-dose estrogen
What are the pregnancy rates after treatment?	As high as 70%
What are the risks of treatment?	Increased risks of spontaneous abortion, placenta previa, placenta accreta, and abruptio placentae
What is DES and how does it cause infertility?	DES is a synthetic estrogen used in the 1950s and 1960s for recurrent abortion. Exposure to DES in utero causes müllerian defects, including: Vaginal adenosis Irregular uterine cavities with adhesions T-shaped uterus with hypoplastic cavity These defects are associated with increased infertility, ectopic pregnancy, spontaneous abortion, and premature labor. Vaginal and cervical clear cell carcinoma Poor outcome is associated with an abnormal HSG.
What is the treatment?	The only treatment available is cervical cerclage for incompetent cervix or drugs for preterm labor.

ASSISTED REPRODUCTIVE TECHNOLOGIES

What are assisted reproductive technologies (ART)?	Techniques involving the direct retrieval of eggs from the ovary Most of these procedures require ovarian stimulation with timed retrieval of oocytes.

What factors influence the success of ART?

Underlying disorder
Number of oocytes/zygotes transferred
Institutional experience

What is in vitro fertilization (IVF)?

Extraction of oocytes (through the vaginal wall under ultrasound guidance), fertilization in the laboratory, and transcervical transfer of the embryos into the uterus 2 days later
Usually requires 100,000 to 200,000 sperm per egg

What are the indications for IVF?

Previously damaged tubes
Immunologic infertility (antisperm antibodies)
Unexplained infertility
Extreme male factor infertility

What is intracytoplasmic sperm injection (ICSI)?

Retrieval of oocytes followed by the injection of a *single* spermatozoon into the egg with a micropipette; embryos are then transferred to the uterus or fallopian tube 2 days later.

Indications for ICSI?

Oligospermia
Sperm motility disorders

36

Amenorrhea

What are the two types of amenorrhea?

Primary and secondary

What are the criteria for primary amenorrhea?

1. No period by age 14 years and no growth or development of secondary sexual characteristics
2. No period by age 16 years regardless of presence of normal development and secondary sexual characteristics

What is secondary amenorrhea?

Cessation of regular menstruation for > 3 cycle intervals or > 6 months total

What is the most common cause of secondary amenorrhea?

Pregnancy

How are the disorders divided into axes?

Menstrual function involves a four-step interrelated system.

Disorders are divided into four axes, depending on the step that fails to function properly.

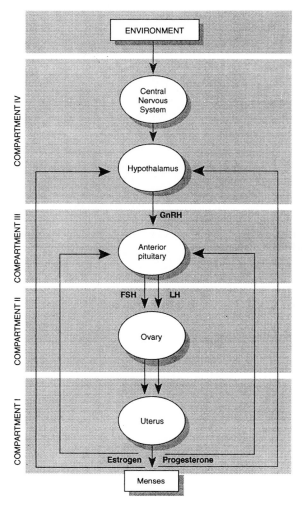

Figure 36.1

What are the four axes?

I. Disorders of the outflow tract—patency and continuity
II. Disorders of the ovary
III. Disorders of the anterior pituitary
IV. Disorders of the central nervous system/hypothalamus

For each axis, what is the corresponding physiologic step in normal menstrual function?

I. Intact outflow tract (vaginal orifice and canal, endocervix, and endometrium)

II. Development of endometrium through influence of estrogen and progesterone; follicle development, ovulation, and corpus luteum function

III. Follicle maturation through gonadotropins from the anterior pituitary [follicle-stimulating hormone (FSH) and luteinizing hormone (LH)]

IV. Anterior pituitary production of FSH and LH through gonadotropin-releasing hormone (GnRH) from the hypothalamus and central nervous system

EVALUATION OF THE AMENORRHEIC PATIENT

What is the first step in evaluating an amenorrheic patient?

History and physical examination:
Discuss psychological dysfunction, emotional stress, eating habits, exercise, and the like, all of which can cause hypothalamic amenorrhea by unknown mechanisms.

Obtain a personal and family history of genetic and endocrine anomalies and whether any other family member has or had similar problems.

Review growth and development if amenorrhea is primary.

Determine pattern of menses before cessation if secondary.

Discuss use of tampons and intercourse activity to delineate anatomic problems.

Laboratory tests:
Pregnancy test
Thyroid-stimulating hormone: Both hypothyroidism and

hyperthyroidism can lead to amenorrhea.
Prolactin: Excess prolactin inhibits gonadotropin secretion.
Progesterone challenge test

What is the procedure for a progesterone challenge test?

Ten milligrams progesterone daily for 5 days
Patient will then either bleed or not bleed.

What does it assess?

Endogenous estrogen and competency of outflow tract

What is the significance of the result if patient bleeds?

Outflow tract is intact and the endometrium has responded to endogenous estrogen.
Anovulation, an axis II disorder, is established.
  Because ovulation has not occurred, no progesterone has been made.
  Menses cannot occur until exogenous progesterone is provided.

What is the significance of the result if patient does not bleed?

Outflow tract or endometrium is inoperative (axis I).
Estrogen proliferation of endometrium did not occur (axis II, III, or IV).
Go to step 2 of evaluation.

What is the second step in evaluating an amenorrheic patient?

Necessary if tests administered in first step are negative
Estrogen and progesterone challenge test

What is the procedure for an estrogen and progesterone challenge test?

1.25 mg estrogen daily for 21 days with the addition of 10 mg progesterone during last 5 days

What is the significance of the result if patient does not bleed?

Axis I disorder: problem with outflow tract

What is the significance of the result if patient bleeds?

Disorder may be axis II, III, or IV.
Go to step 3.

What is the third step in evaluating an amenorrheic patient?

Determine reason for lack of estrogen production.

What are the possible etiologic factors for lack of estrogen production?

Follicle problem (axis II)
Gonadotropin problem (axis III or IV)

What diagnostic procedure is administered to determine the cause of lack of estrogen production?

Serum assay of gonadotropin levels: measure FSH and LH

What are the normal values of FSH and LH?

FSH: 5–30 international units per liter (IU/L)
LH: 5–20 IU/L

What are abnormal values and their significance?

Hypogonadotropic state (axis III or IV):
  FSH < 5 IU/L, LH < 5 IU/L
  Prepubertal state
  Hypothalamic disorder
  Pituitary dysfunction
Hypergonadotropic state (axis II):
  FSH > 30 IU/L, LH > 40 IU/L
  Postmenopausal
  Ovarian failure
Key point: When gonadotropins are low, the problem is at the higher centers (hypothalamus or pituitary). When gonadotropins are high, the problem is at the ovary/follicle (no estrogen = no negative feedback).
Go to Step 4.

What is the fourth step in evaluating an amenorrheic patient?

Determine cause of hypogonadotropic or hypergonadotropic state.

What axes must be differentiated if the patient is hypogonadotropic?	Axis III (pituitary) and axis IV (hypothalamus)
What diagnostic procedure is used to differentiate between the axes?	Imaging of sella turcica (computed tomography or magnetic resonance imaging)
What is the significance of abnormal imaging?	Pituitary tumor (axis III)
What is the significance of normal imaging?	Assume axis IV problem by exclusion.
For a hypergonadotropic patient with primary amenorrhea younger than 30 years of age, what diagnostic procedure should be performed, and why?	Karyotype determination Mosaicism with a Y chromosome requires gonadal excision to eliminate the risk of the testicular component becoming malignant. Thirty percent of women with a Y chromosome do not have virilization, so normal appearance does not preclude karyotyping.

SPECIFIC DISORDERS

What axis I disorders (disorders of the outflow tract) cause primary amenorrhea?	Müllerian anomalies: Imperforate hymen, lack of vaginal orifice, discontinuity by segmental disruptions Müllerian agenesis (Mayer-Rokitansky-Küster-Hauser syndrome): Karyotype is 46XX with normal female phenotype (axillary and pubic hair) but reproductive tract does not develop (see Chapter 29, Sexual Differentiation and Development). Androgen insensitivity (testicular feminization): Patient is phenotypically female with XY karyotype, testes, and normal or slightly elevated male testosterone levels; caused by a defect in testosterone end-organ receptor (see Chapter 29, Sexual Differentiation and Development).

What axis I disorder (disorders of the outflow tract) causes secondary amenorrhea?

Asherman syndrome:
- Caused by destruction of the endometrium from scarring via IUD, dilation and curettage, and the like
- Diagnosed by hysterogram or hysteroscopy
- Treatment involves dilation and curettage to remove adhesions and supplemental estrogen.

What axis II disorders (disorders of the ovary) cause primary amenorrhea?

Disorders under the broad term "gonadal dysgenesis"
Genetic or enzymatic problem that results in abnormal ovarian function

What are some conditions that cause gonadal dysgenesis?

Turner syndrome (see Chapter 29, Sexual Differentiation and Development)
Mosaicism (see Chapter 29, Sexual Differentiation and Development)
17 Hydroxylase deficiency or 17,20 desmolase deficiency: Enzyme deficiency that prevents synthesis of steroid hormones (i.e., estrogen and progesterone); hypertension and hypokalemia are also present in mineralocorticoid deficiencies.
Gonadal agenesis: Ovaries fail to develop; often of unknown etiology

What axis II disorder causes secondary amenorrhea?

Premature ovarian failure: Early menopause (before age 40 years); idiopathic

What co-morbid condition occurs in 20% of premature ovarian failure?

Polyglandular autoimmunity involving hyperparathyroidism, Addison's disease, thyroid disease, diabetes

What axis III disorders (disorders of the pituitary) cause amenorrhea?

Pituitary tumor: May cause additional problems such as prolactinemia, visual changes, acromegaly, hyperthyroidism
Empty sella syndrome: Congenital incompleteness of the sellar

diaphragm, which deforms both the pituitary fossa and gland

Sheehan syndrome: Acute necrosis of the pituitary gland due to shock, often from postpartum hemorrhage

What is the most common pituitary tumor?

Prolactin-secreting adenoma (50%)

How do pituitary tumors cause amenorrhea?

If tumor secretes FSH and LH, it is a continuous release, without regulation by GnRH from the hypothalamus.

Pulsatile release of hormones from both the hypothalamus and pituitary is required for a normal menstrual cycle.

What axis IV disorder (disorders of the central nervous system) causes amenorrhea?

Hypothalamic amenorrhea/ hypogonadotropic hypogonadism: Defect in the pulsatile secretion of GnRH from the hypothalamus; diagnosed by exclusion

What are the etiologic factors of hypothalamic amenorrhea/ hypogonadotropic hypogonadism?

Stress

Weight loss/low body weight: Anorexia

Excessive exercise

Kallmann syndrome: Congenital defect characterized by hypothalamic amenorrhea and anosmia

What long term health concerns affect women with Axis II, III & IV disorders?

Osteoporosis. These women need estrogen replacement therapy

37

Menopause

INTRODUCTION

What is menopause?

Cessation of menses corresponding to the loss of ovarian activity

What is the climacteric?

Transitional period leading to menopause, in which ovarian activity decreases

Includes the perimenopausal and menopausal periods

What percentage of the female population in the United States is currently postmenopausal?

Twenty percent

Why is this percentage increasing?

Life expectancy is also increasing.

What is the median age of the onset of menopause?

Age 50–52 years

What is the age range of the onset of menopause?

Age 48–55 years

What is the approximate length of the perimenopausal period?

Four years

What factors influence the age at which menopause occurs?

Family history, race, parity, or age of menarche **do not** influence the age at which menopause occurs.

Smoking and low weight may decrease the age at which menopause occurs.

EFFECTS OF MENOPAUSE

What hormonal changes occur in perimenopause?

The number of anovulatory cycles increases and cycle length increases.

The level of follicle-stimulating hormone (FSH) increases; the levels of luteinizing hormone (LH) and estradiol remain normal until follicular growth ceases.

The level of LH eventually increases; however, the increase is only 3-fold, compared to a 10- to 20-fold increase in the level of FSH.

With the increased levels of gonadotropins (FSH and LH), the ovarian stroma produces increased levels of testosterone.

Describe sex steroid production.

Estrogen production persists from fat conversion of androstenedione and testosterone to estrogen

What is the correlation between peripheral conversion of estrogen and body weight?

The percentage of peripheral conversion is proportional to body weight—that is, obesity correlates with increased peripheral conversion.

What are the vasomotor symptoms of perimenopause?

So-called "hot flashes"

Typified by a sensation of warmth in the head, neck, and chest with associated sweating

May last from seconds to minutes

Occur more frequently at night, during episodes of stress, and in increased temperatures

How many women experience vasomotor symptoms of perimenopause?

10% to 25%

For how long do vasomotor symptoms continue?

Usually only 1–2 years; at most 5 years

How can vasomotor symptoms be relieved?

Vasomotor symptoms are associated with decreased estrogen levels and may be relieved with hormone (estrogen)

replacement therapy (HRT), progesterone, clonidine, or SSRIs.

What atrophic changes occur in perimenopause?

Genitourinary atrophy, which may cause vaginitis, pruritus, urethritis, vaginal stenosis, and dyspareunia

What is the cause of atrophic changes?

Decreased estrogen levels

How can atrophic changes be relieved?

HRT, orally or topical

What is osteoporosis?

Reduction of the quantity of bone or atrophy of the skeletal tissue

When does bone loss typically begin in women?

In the spine, which is composed of trabecular bone, the onset of bone loss begins at age 20 years.
In the femur, composed of cortical bone, density peaks in the late third decade.

When does bone loss accelerate?

After menopause

What are the rates of bone loss before and after menopause?

After age 40 years, the rate of bone loss is 0.5% per year.
After menopause, the rate of trabecular bone loss is 5% per year; the rate of total bone loss is 1%.

Why does the rate of bone loss accelerate after menopause?

Because of decreased estrogen levels; trabecular bone is the most sensitive to changes in estrogen levels.

What are the risk factors for osteoporosis?

The risk is increased in thin, white, or Asian women; smokers; and women with sedentary lifestyles. All of these factors decrease peak bone density.

What is the incidence of fractures?

Twenty-five percent of women older than age 70 years experience spinal fractures, usually compression fractures.
Twenty percent of all white women experience hip fractures.

Treatment and prevention of osteoporosis?

Weight bearing exercises
Calcium (approx. 1000 mg/day)
Vitamin D (approx. 1000 μ/day)
Medications

What are the 5 medication options?

Table 37–1.

Medication	Best Use	Therapeutic Value	Side Effects
Bisphosphonates (Alendronate, Risedronate)	Women at high risk for, or who already have, osteoporosis	Reduce vertebral and hip fractures by half	GI disturbance including possible esophageal ulcerations
Hormone Replacement (Conjugated estrogen; Estradiol)	Women early in menopause who are at risk, or women with early menopause	Reduces overall fractures by 25%; hip by 34%	Breast tenderness, possible increased risk of breast cancer
Selective Estrogen Receptor Modulations (SERM's) (Raloxifene)	Prevention in postmenopausal women	Reduces vertebral fractures by half	Hot flashes ? increase in DVT's
Calcitonin	Treating osteoporosis	Reduces vertebral fracture risk in patients with previous fractures	Nasal irritation (it's inhaled)
Parathyroid Hormone (Teripratide)	Treating osteoporosis	Stimulates new bone Reduces fractures	Sub-cut injection inconvenient

HORMONE REPLACEMENT THERAPY

Does the type of estrogen prescribed for HRT matter?

Maybe. But the dosage and method of estrogen replacement are the key factors, not the specific type of estrogen.

What are the various estrogen regimens?

The standard oral estrogen dosage is 0.625 mg of conjugated estrogens daily.

> This dosage has been shown to have a beneficial effect on bone density and lipid profile.

> Dosage can be adjusted depending on a particular patient's menopausal symptoms. This dose studied much more than others.

Estradiol in a transdermal system at a dosage of 50 μg twice a week has been shown to be as effective as the standard dosage of conjugated estrogens. Currently, there is no consensus about the long-term effects of bypassing the liver with a transdermal regimen compared with the oral regimen.

Estrogen creams and ointment are also available.

> Studies of these regimens are not as extensive as those of the previously mentioned methods.

What are the combined HRT regimens?

There are two types, sequential and continuous.

Sequential therapy: Estrogen plus a progestational agent such as 10 mg medroxyprogesterone daily for either the first 14 days of the month or the last 10 days (days 16–25) of estrogen therapy

Continuous therapy: estrogen plus 2.5 mg medroxyprogesterone acetate or 0.35 mg norethindrone daily

What percentage of women taking combined sequential HRT experience withdrawal bleeding?

80% to 90%

What percentage of women taking combined continuous HRT experience breakthrough bleeding?

40% to 60%
This incidence decreases to 25% with prolonged use.

For what conditions should a woman taking combined continuous HRT who continues to have breakthrough bleeding be evaluated?

Polyps, fibroids, hyperplasia, and cancer

For what population of women is combined HRT strongly recommended, and why? (as opposed to estrogen alone)

Because of the risk of endometrial hyperplasia and cancer, a combined regimen is strongly recommended in women who have **not** undergone a hysterectomy.

What is an advantage of combined continuous HRT therapy over combined sequential HRT?

Continuous HRT allows the use of lower doses of progestins; therefore, the risk of progestin side effects such as fluid retention, breast tenderness, and depression may decrease.

How should women on HRT be followed?

An endometrial biopsy should be performed before starting HRT if a woman has a history of irregular bleeding, unopposed estrogen use, or endometrial hyperplasia.

The endometrial cavity and the endometrium should be evaluated if a woman experiences breakthrough bleeding once stable on a particular regimen.

Postmenopausal women should have annual pelvic examinations, including Papanicolaou smears.

An annual mammogram should be performed after age 50 years, as recommended by the American Cancer Society.

What are the risks of combination HRT?

Increased risk of thromboembolic disease.

Increased risk of cardiovascular event (7 more heart disease events per 10,000 women per year during first year of HRT use)

Increased risk of breast cancer after 4 years of use (8 more cases of breast cancer per 10,000 women)

What are risks of estrogen-only therapy on women who have had a hysterectomy?

Studies carried out to 5 years of use show no significant increased risk of CV events, thrombolic events, or breast cancer when compared to women who did not use HRT

What is endometrial neoplasia?

Abnormal proliferation of the endometrium, ranging from simple hyperplasia to carcinoma

What is the increase in risk of endometrial neoplasia attributable to HRT?

A 2- to 10-fold increase in risk

What can decrease the risk of endometrial neoplasia in women taking HRT?

Adding progestins to the HRT regimen obviates the increased risk of endometrial neoplasia.

Progestins inhibit the growth of the endometrium; estrogens promote endometrial proliferation.

What dosage of progestin has been shown to decrease the risk of endometrial neoplasia?

Studies have shown that progestins should be given for at least 10 days each month.

Either 10 mg of medroxyprogesterone acetate for days 16–25 each month, or 2.5 mg of medroxyprogesterone acetate every day of the month can reduce the risk of endometrial neoplasia.

Do women taking HRT have an increased risk of gallbladder disease?

No

Do women taking HRT have an increased risk of recurrence of endometriosis?

No

How does HRT affect fibroid tumors of the uterus?

Rarely do fibroid tumors of the uterus increase in size in response to HRT.

When is HRT contraindicated?

Contraindications include liver disease, acute vascular thrombosis, migraine headaches, and possibly seizure disorders.

Can women with a history of endometrial or breast cancer take HRT?

Patients with a history of endometrial or breast cancer must be evaluated on an individual basis.

HRT is contraindicated in patients with a history of endometrial cancer and endometrioid cancer of the ovary. Combination therapy may be instituted 5 years after the cancer has been treated if there is no evidence of recurrent disease.

No long-term studies have been completed that evaluate HRT after breast cancer.

Are herbal or natural remedies/estrogens effective at relieving symptoms of menopause?

Most nutritional supplements have not been studied for safety or effectiveness. Women should be cautioned that these products may contain estrogens that carry the same risks of pharmaceutical-grade estrogens.

38

Preventive Care: Cancer Screening

Not every disease should be screened for in a population. What are the criteria for screening a disease?

The disease should have significant morbidity and mortality.
The disease should be treatable.
The disease should have an identifiable preclinical stage.
Treatment of the disease during the asymptomatic period should be more effective than treatment during the symptomatic period.
The disease should be sufficiently prevalent in the screened population.

What are the criteria for screening tests?

The test should be simple and inexpensive.
The test should be painless, safe, and accurate (i.e., the test must be sufficiently sensitive and specific).

What is sensitivity?

The percentage of positive test results among individuals who have the disease

What is specificity?

The percentage of negative test results among individuals who do not have the disease

What is positive predictive value (PPV)?

The probability that a person with a positive test result will have the disease; for example, a PPV of 10% means that there will be nine false-positive test results for each cancer detected.

What are the potential biases of screening tests?

Selection bias: The screened population does not correspond to the general population.
Lead time bias: Early diagnosis of the disease does not extend the patient's life; only the length of time that the patient has the diagnosis is increased.

Length time bias: The apparent prolongation of life is related more to the intrinsic nature of the disease rather than to its early diagnosis.

What are the American College of Obstetrics and Gynecology (ACOG) guidelines for cervical cancer screening?

Should begin at age 18 years or at onset of sexual activity

Annual examinations throughout a woman's life. Low risk patients may decrease frequency of pap smears after 3 or more consecutive, satisfactory, normal cytologic exams

What are the National Cancer Institute (NCI) guidelines for cervical cancer screening?

Should begin 3 years after onset of sexual activity, but no later than age 21

Screening at least once every 3 years

Women >65 years with at least 3 normal paps and no abnormal paps in past 10 years may elect to stop screening

Women who have had a hysterectomy for reasons other than cancer or precancer may stop screening

What test is used to screen for cervical cancer?

The Papanicolaou smear test (Pap test)

Is the Pap test simple, safe, inexpensive, and acceptable to patient and provider?

Yes

What is the sensitivity of a Pap test?

Sixty-seven percent

What is the specificity?

Sixty percent

What are the implications of the Pap test's overall low specificity?

The Pap test has a high false-positive rate and a low PPV. However, because of the characteristics of this screening test and the consequences of undiagnosed cervical cancer, the low PPV is acceptable.

What are the guidelines for breast cancer screening?

Some controversy exists, but the general guidelines are as follows:

A baseline examination between ages 35 and 39 years [National Cancer Institute (NCI), baseline examination at age 40 years]

Examination every 1–2 years between ages 40 and 49 years

Annual examination after age 50 years

What test is used to screen for breast cancer?

Mammogram

Is the mammogram simple, safe, inexpensive, and acceptable to patient and provider?

In general, yes. However, the test is only relatively inexpensive. Annual mammograms of 0.5 rad carry a small risk of radiation exposure, but the clinical significance of this risk is not known.

What is the sensitivity of a mammogram?

Eighty-five percent

What is the specificity?

Eighty percent

What are the guidelines for colorectal cancer screening?

The ACS and NCI recommend an annual digital rectal examination after age 40 years.

The ACS offers 5 screening options, to begin at age 50:

1. Fecal occult blood sampling every year (FOBS)
2. Flexible sigmoidoscopy every 5 years
3. FOBS every year plus flexible sigmoidoscopy every 5 years
4. Double contrast barium enema every 5 years
5. Colonoscopy every 10 years

All individuals considered high risk (strong family history, familial polyposis, and ulcerative colitis) should have periodic screening with colonoscopy.

What test is used to screen for colorectal cancer?

Fecal occult blood sampling (FOBS; not a stool guaiac in the office). In this test, patients are given six stool guaiac cards. The patient must follow dietary restrictions, such as no meat and vegetables, for 1–2 days prior to the test. The patient then takes consecutive stool samples, places them on the cards, and mails them to the physician.

Is FOBS simple, safe, inexpensive, and acceptable to patient and provider?

The test is safe and relatively inexpensive. However, patients comply poorly with this test, indicating that most patients find the test unacceptable.

What is the sensitivity of FOBS?

Fifty percent

What is the specificity of FOBS?

Unknown; in general, 2% of the test results are positive, and the PPV is 30%. The positive test results also include polyps as well as carcinomas. Of all individuals with positive test results, only 20%–25% have cancer.

What are the guidelines for endometrial cancer screening?

The ACS recommends that women have a pelvic examination at the onset of menopause and that high-risk women have an endometrial biopsy when identified as high risk.

There is currently no indication to biopsy asymptomatic women.

Endometrial cancer is the most common genital cancer in women in the United States.

Which women are considered at high risk for endometrial cancer?

Women with a history of infertility, obesity, failure to ovulate, abnormal uterine bleeding, diabetes, tamoxifen use, or unopposed estrogen use

What test is used to screen for endometrial cancer?

Endometrial biopsy. In this test, a small catheter is placed through the cervical os into the uterine cavity. The endometrium is then aspirated into the catheter for sampling.

What are the guidelines for lung cancer screening?

Although lung cancer is the most lethal cancer in men and women, there is no benefit at this time from screening for lung cancer, even in high-risk populations. Several large studies have shown no benefit in screening chest radiographs or sputum cytologies. The mortality rate from lung cancer is the same in screened populations as in unscreened populations.

39

Preinvasive Neoplastic Disease of the Cervix, Vagina, and Vulva

CERVICAL NEOPLASTIC DISEASE

What are the two histologic regions of the cervix?	Endocervix and ectocervix, based on epithelial type
What is the ectocervix?	The portion of the cervix that is continuous with the vagina
What type of epithelium covers the ectocervix?	Squamous epithelium that is continuous with the squamous epithelium lining the vagina
What is the endocervix?	The portion of the cervix that is adjacent to the external cervical os and extends into the endocervical canal
What type of epithelium covers the endocervix?	Mucin-secreting columnar epithelium that is continuous with the cuboidal cells of the endometrial lining
What is the original squamocolumnar junction (OSCJ)?	The histologic boundary in the fetus that separates the squamous epithelium of the vagina from the columnar epithelium of the endocervix
Where is the OSCJ located?	Its position varies, lying on the ectocervix in 66% of fetuses, within the canal in 30%, and on the vaginal fornices in 4%.
What is the new squamocolumnar junction (NSCJ)?	During a woman's life, the OSCJ moves closer to the endocervical canal by a process called metaplasia; the NSCJ represents the boundary between mature and immature squamous metaplasia.

What is the significance of the NSCJ in the diagnosis of dysplasia?

The NSCJ is the upper limit of squamous intraepithelial neoplasia and the lower limit of any adenocarcinoma in situ for the following reasons:

The NSCJ defines the upper border of any histologically definable dysplasia in women who have not undergone previous therapy.

It does not, however, define the upper limit of squamous metaplasia (ULSM). ULSM extends up into the endocervical canal, above the NSCJ

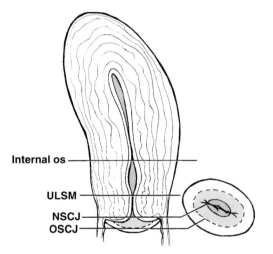

Figure 39-1. OCSJ = old squamocolumnar junction; NSCJ = new squamocolumnar junction; ULSM = upper limit of squamous metaplasia.

What is the transformation zone?

One to three centimeter (cm) area of squamous metaplasia between the old and new squamocolumnar junctions that separates the ectocervix and endocervix.

What is the significance of this zone in cervical cancer?

Location is most susceptible to the development of both preinvasive and invasive cervical neoplastic disease.

Why is this zone susceptible to malignant transformation?

The metaplastic process occurring in this region appears to predispose the area to malignant transformation.

What is metaplasia?

A reversible change in which one type of fully differentiated cell type is replaced by another fully differentiated cell type.

Is metaplasia a malignancy?

No

What is dysplasia?

The abnormal growth or development of organs, tissues, or cells; characterized by an increased mitotic rate and atypical cytologic features (size, shape, organization)
Potentially reversible

What is the relationship of dysplasia to cancer?

Dysplastic changes may be found adjacent to foci of cancer.
Dysplasia may progress to cancer.

What are the different types and frequencies of the various forms of cervical cancer?

Squamous cell neoplasias: 80%–90%
Adenocarcinoma and adenosquamous carcinomas: approximately 20%; incidence of these forms seems to be increasing in a relative sense.
Other types (e.g., melanomas, sarcomas, lymphomas): approximately 1%

What are the causative factors of squamous cell neoplasia?

Cervical squamous cancer and its precursors appear to follow a pattern typical of a sexually transmitted disease. Risk factors are consistent with this pattern and include:
Early age at first coitus (under 20 years)
Multiple sexual partners
Venereal infection, especially HPV infection
Young age at marriage
Young age at first pregnancy
High parity
Divorce
Lower socioeconomic status
Coitus with high-risk males (sexual partner with multiple sexual partners)

	Other factors include cigarette smoking, pelvic radiation, immunodeficiency, and vitamin A and C deficiency.
What is currently thought to be the principal causative agent of cervical squamous cell neoplasia?	Human papilloma virus (HPV)
For what other neoplasias is HPV thought to be the principal causative agent?	Cervical intraepithelial neoplasia (CIN), vaginal intraepithelial neoplasia (VAIN), vulvar intraepithelial neoplasia (VIN), and penile neoplasia HPV is also thought to be the principal causative agent of invasive vulvar and vaginal malignacies.
What percentage of cervical condylomata contain HPV DNA?	Over 90%
What percentage of cervical cancers contain HPV DNA?	Nearly all
Does a type-specific association between HPV subtype and severity of cervical cancer exist?	Yes
How many subtypes of HPV exist?	More than 70
What are the most common subtypes found in genital lesions?	6, 11, 16, 18, 31, and 33
What subtypes are associated with malignant transformation (i.e., commonly seen in highgrade CIN as well as invasive cervical malignancies)?	16, 18, 31, 33, 35, 45, 51, 52, 56, and 58

Of the two main HPV subtypes associated with malignant transformation, which subtype also appears to influence the progressive potential of a precursor lesion?

HPV 18 is reported to be a more progressive subtype than HPV 16 (i.e., it is associated with poor prognostic features and frequently occurs in younger patients with adenocarcinomas and in tumors that tend to recur).

In contrast, HPV 16 DNA has been found in almost all large-cell keratinizing tumors, which tend to recur infrequently.

Is herpesvirus infection a causative factor in genital cancers?

A cause-and-effect relationship with genital cancer has not been proven although it is suspected.

What is the definitive predisposing factor of adenomatous and adenosquamous neoplasia of the cervix?

Transplacental exposure to diethylstilbestrol (DES)

Is HPV associated with adenocarcinomas of the cervix?

Recent data show that many adenocarcinomas are associated with HPV.

What are the predisposing factors of the other types of cervical cancer?

Little is known about predisposing factors for other types of cervical cancer.

List the systems that have been used in the classification of cervical neoplasia.

Papanicolaou system
Cervical intraepithelial system (CIN)
Bethesda system

Describe the Bethesda system.

Table 39.1. Bethesda Cytology Classification System

Bethesda System

Within normal limits

Infection (organism should be specified)

Reactive and reparative changes

Squamous cell abnormalities
Atypical squamous cells of undetermined significance
Low-grade squamous intraepithelial lesion (LSIL)
High-grade squamous intraepithelial lesion (HSIL)
Squamous cell carcinoma

Glandular Abnormalities
Atypical glandular cells of undetermined significance (AGUS)

What are the PAP and CIN systems?	Systems previously used to classify abnormal smears. They are not currently used.
What is the Bethesda system?	The most recent classification system; intended to replace the Papanicolaou system Reports in this system contain: A statement on adequacy of the specimen for interpretation Diagnostic category (normal or other) A descriptive diagnosis Introduced the terms "low-grade" and "high-grade" squamous intraepithelial lesions (LSIL and HSIL). LSIL is more commonly associated with a histology of CINI. HSIL is more commonly associated with a histology of CINII or CINIII.

Is cervical cancer rapidly or slowly progressive?

Slowly progressive

In what Bethesda classes does spontaneous regression occur frequently? Rarely?

Frequently: LSIL
Less frequently: HSIL

What is the estimated duration of disease in women with CIN 3 who progress to invasive cancer?

Three to ten years

What percentage of untreated CIN 3 disease will progress to invasive disease?

Thirty-six percent

What procedure is used to screen for cervical cancer?

Cervical cytology [Papanicolaou (Pap) smear]

How is a Pap smear performed?

Samples of cervical epithelial cells are taken from the ectocervix using a wooden spatula, and samples of endocervical cells are obtained with a cytobrush which is inserted into the external os and rotated.

Since the introduction of Pap smear screening, how has the mortality rate from cervical cancer changed?

Prior to the widespread use of the Pap smear, cervical cancer was the leading cause of cancer death among American women.
Mortality rate has declined by more than 50% to 9 deaths per 100,000 women per year.
Five-year survival after diagnosis of cancer has also increased.

What is the major benefit of the Pap smear?

Its ability to detect preinvasive disease

What are some problems with Pap smear screening?

It is not possible to screen all high-risk patients before they develop invasive disease; many high-risk patients do not have access to screening services.

The Pap smear is not as successful in identifying adenocarcinoma; therefore, the rates of this type of cervical carcinoma have not declined.

With the advent of thinprep PAP smears, the false negative rate is <10%. The false negative rate for invasive cancer may be 10–15%, due to interpretaion in the face of inflammation and necrosis that may accompany the lesion.

Patients do not always obtain follow-up after an abnormal Pap smear.

It is often difficult to evaluate the transformation zone in postmenopausal women because of its location high in the endocervical canal.

What are the current American College of Obstetricians and Gynecologists recommendations for Pap smear screening?

Screening and pelvic examinations should begin at age 18 or at onset of sexual activity, whichever is earlier

Annual screening and pelvic examination until three negative results; thereafter less frequent screening and examinations at discretion of physician

An annual physical and pelvic examination and an annual Pap smear for patients at high or unknown level of risk

What constitutes high risk?

American Cancer Society's criteria are intercourse by age 20 or more than two lifetime sexual partners.

When defining the high-risk patient, it is important to remember that the majority of women are considered high-risk by this definition.

In addition, it is impossible to determine a woman's level of risk without knowing the sexual history of each of her previous partners.

How should a patient with an abnormal Pap smear be managed?

Complete history and physical examination to look for grossly abnormal lesions or discoloration within the vulva, vagina, or perianal region that may identify a likely source of the abnormal cytology; all three areas must be examined because of the prevalence of multicentric disease.

Colposcopy: examination by microscopy
Mandatory in the following abnormalities:
ASCUS, with positive high risk cervical HPV DNA
LSIL
HSIL
AGUS
Carcinoma
When no gross invasive lesion is visible, a colposcopic exam may help identify subclinical disease that may be the source of the abnormal cells.

Why is colposcopy necessary in diagnosis?

Because the lesions of CIN are located in the transformation zone and because early lesions are located primarily on the ectocervix, many of the more subtle lesions can be visualized by colposcopy. This allows for a directed biopsy for histologic diagnosis.

Visualization of what structure constitutes an adequate colposcopic examination?

Visualization of the NSCJ

What is the follow-up if the colposcopic exam is normal after an abnormal Pap smear?

Exfoliation from other sites must be considered (e.g., endometrial, fallopian tube, ovarian, or metastatic breast cancer).

Cellular contamination from a vulvar or urinary tract lesion should also be considered.

If a CIN smear is not explained after examination by an experienced colposcopist, the smear itself should be sent for expert review. If the presence of a high-grade cytologic abnormality is confirmed, diagnostic conization is mandatory.

What are the indications for colposcopically directed biopsy?

Biopsy is used as an adjunct to colposcopy.

Carefully directed punch biopsies taken of the most abnormal appearing areas of epithelium can adequately sample a CIN lesion that is visible in its entirety.

What is the main problem with colposcopically directed biopsy?

Risk of not selecting the most abnormal sites for target biopsy, as the most prominent areas of colposcopic change do not always coincide with the areas of greatest histologic abnormality.

How can this problem be overcome?

Representative biopsy specimens should be taken from all significant acetowhite areas including the most prominent area of epithelial opacity and the most prominent area of vascular atypia.

Any area suspected of occult invasion must also be sampled carefully.

What kind of lesions can endocervical curettage (ECC) identify?

Lesions in the endocervical canal that are invisible to the colposcope

When is ECC used in the diagnosis of cervical cancer?

Experts vary as to when to perform an ECC.

Some advocate mandatory ECC to rule out an extension of a lesion into the endocervix. Others feel that if the entire NSCJ is visualized and a surrounding rim of normal columnar epithelium is seen within the lower canal, ECC can be omitted (in previously untreated patients).

ECC is not performed in pregnant patients because it may result in obstetrical complications.

How is a final outpatient evaluation performed?

All three parameters of the study [PAP cytology, colposcopic examination, and histologic results of colposcopically directed biopsy/ECC] should be reviewed.

All "diagnoses" should be compatible before definitive outpatient therapy is begun (e.g., cytology, colposcopy, and biopsies should indicate similar degrees of CIN).

How are treatment decisions made based on results of all three parameters of study?

If all parameters agree, the area may be treated with close follow-up of mild abnormality. If lession is more severe, it may be treated with ablation or excision.

If significant correlation is lacking, additional evaluation, usually with a cold knife cone (a large cervical biopsy including all of the transformation zone and the canal) is mandatory.

When is conservative (also known as local or superficial ablative) therapy indicated?

Invasive cancer must be excluded.

Patients with squamous lesions are suitable for superficial ablative therapies provided that:

The entire transformation zone can be visualized colposcopically.

The biopsy is consistent with the Pap smear.

The ECC is negative.

Occult invasion after cytologic or colposcopic evaluation is not suspected.

What therapeutic modalities are used in conservative therapy?

Cone biopsy or superficial ablative techniques such as electrocoagulation diathermy, cryosurgery, or CO_2 laser

Is hysterectomy beneficial as a treatment of uncomplicated CIN?

No. It is no longer considered appropriate treatment of uncomplicated CIN.

What is excisional conization?

Surgical excision of a cone of tissue containing the abnormal area of epithelium with a cold knife, a tightly focused beam of superpulsed CO_2 laser energy, or an electrical wire loop.

What are the indications?

Inability to visualize the NSCJ on colposcopy

CIN 2–3 on ECC

Colposcopic suspicion of occult invasion, even if target biopsies show only CIN 3

Significant discrepancies (2 grades) between cytology and histology

Cytologic suspicion of adenocarcinoma in situ

Microinvasion on the punch biopsy

When colposcopic expertise is unavailable

What are the complications?

Complication rate is about 12% and seems to depend on the configuration of the excised cone (i.e., the rate of cervical incompetence increases with larger excisions due to removal of a greater portion of fibromuscular cervix).

Possible complications include hemorrhage, sepsis, infertility, cervical stenosis, and cervical incompetence.

What is loop electrosurgical excision procedure (LEEP)?

Surgical excision of the transformation zone and the distal cervical canal under anesthesia using an electrosurgical wire loop; the loop can also be used for fulguration and electrocoagulation.

What are the complications?	Similar to those of continuous wave laser ablation, including hemorrhage (1%–8%), postoperative pelvic cellulitis or abscess formation, cervical stenosis (1%), cervical deformity, and midtrimester abortion due to cervical incompetence
What is electrocoagulation diathermy (not commonly used in the United States)?	Ablation of abnormal epithelium using high-voltage electricity in two different processes, fulguration and electrocoagulation.
What is fulguration?	An electrode is held just above the surface of the epithelium which produces an arc of electricity from the energy source (electrode) to the ground (the epithelial surface). The heat produced rapidly desiccates the tissue at the site of the spark.
What is electrocoagulation?	Deeper and more widespread tissue destruction is caused by insertion of the electrode below the epithelial surface. Energy is conducted along tissue planes, resulting in heat denaturation and enzymatic degradation of structural proteins within large volumes of tissue.
How is electrocoagulation diathermy different from radial electrocautery?	Electrocautery produces a simple conduction burn at the epithelial surface with a red-hot wire. It does not destroy the epithelium of the cervical crypts, and therefore will not adequately treat cervical dysplasia.
What is cryosurgery?	Application of liquid refrigerants, such as N_2 to the epithelial surface by use of a metal probe. Evaporation of the refrigerant induces hypothermia accompanied by cryonecrosis of the tissue.

What are the benefits of cryosurgery?	It is a cost-effective, well-tolerated means of outpatient treatment of cervical dysplasia.
	Large studies have reported a primary success rate of about 84% in the treatment of CIN 3, however, the treatment of choice for high grade dysplasia is more often excision.
	Anesthesia is not necessary (although premedication with nonsteroidal anti-inflammatory drugs may help relieve discomfort associated with prostaglandin release from dying cells).
What problems are associated with cryosurgery?	Cryonecrosis is not uniform. Adequately treated areas of epithelium are surrounded by a wide margin of sublethal tissue injury.
	Success rate also appears to be dependent on both the extent of the lesion and the volume of tissue that must be destroyed.
How can the cryosurgery treatment failure rate be reduced?	By using a freeze-thaw-refreeze cycle, which increases the reliability of cell death
When is CO_2 laser ablation used?	Due to its short wavelength, the CO_2 laser may be used for superficial ablation of abnormal epithelium as well as for conization.
What are the indications for more radical therapy (i.e., hysterectomy)?	If gynecologic indications exist that would be well-treated by hysterectomy, or if a permanent means of sterilization is desired
	In these circumstances, invasive cancer must be excluded prior to hysterectomy.
Why is follow-up important after conservative therapy?	Cervical epithelial abnormalities may recur

Cervical epithelial abnormalities probably increase the risk of vaginal and vulvar lesions as well.

When should Pap smears be evaluated following conservative therapy? Why?

Pap smears should not be evaluated for 3 months after treatment (especially after cryotherapy) because of the reparative process.

Why is follow-up important after hysterectomy?

Recurrences (on the vaginal mucosa) have occurred up to 10 years after therapy.

PREINVASIVE NEOPLASTIC DISEASE OF THE VAGINA

What is the frequency of vaginal cancer?

Carcinoma of the vagina is rare, accounting for 1%–2% of all gynecologic malignancies.

What is the incidence of vaginal cancer?

Age-adjusted incidence is 0.6 per 100,000.

Between what ages does peak incidence occur?

Between ages 60 and 70

What is the most common type of vaginal cancer?

Squamous cell carcinoma
Multicentric disease (i.e., neoplasia involving several different anatomic sites within the lower genital tract)

What is the cause of vaginal cancer?

Risk factors commonly associated with carcinoma of the cervix and vulva have not shown the same degree of significance in patients who develop vaginal carcinomas.
Long-term pessary use and long-standing uterine procidentia (prolapse of the uterus which causes the cervix to protrude from the vaginal opening) or both may predispose to vaginal cancer by causing chronic local irritation of the vaginal mucosa; however no causal link has been proved.

Whereas the role of a sexually transmitted infectious agent has not been proved in vaginal cancer, the multicentric nature of the disease has led the search for a common agent to which the mucosa of the cervix, vagina, and vulva is exposed, e.g., HPV.

How is vaginal cancer screened for?

Due to the low incidence of vaginal carcinoma, it is not cost-effective to screen all women.

However, most physicians screen with a vaginal Pap as part of periodic check-ups.

What is a predisposing factor to adenocarcinoma of the vagina?

DES exposure *in utero*

What is the incidence of clear cell adenocarcinoma in women exposed to DES?

Estimated to be 1 in 1000 or less

At what stage are most of these adenocarcinomas diagnosed?

Approximately 70% of these vaginal adenocarcinomas are diagnosed at Stage I

What percentage of women with vaginal intraepithelial neoplasia (VAIN) 3 and vulvarintraepithelial neoplasia (VIN) 3 have preexisting or synchronous cervical neoplasia (preinvasive or invasive).

VAIN 3: about 60%
VIN 3: about 30%

What percentage of women with primary vaginal carcinoma have a history of in situ or invasive cervical cancer treated at least 5 years earlier?

Up to 30%

What percentage of women who have vaginal cancer have had a hysterectomy?

Sixty percent

What is benign condyloma acuminatum?

Focal capillary and epithelial proliferation that results in formation of a local papilloma or "wart"

Condylomata are the result of HPV infection.

Condylomata often involve vulva as well as vagina.

What are the most common subtypes of HPV found in benign condylomata, and do these subtypes have neoplastic potential?

HPV types 6 and 11; they have a lower neoplastic potential (excluding verrucous carcinoma), but they have been documented in invasive squamous disease

What HPV subtypes are associated with malignant transformation and in what percent of benign condylomata are they found?

HPV 16 or 18; 7% of histologically benign condylomata

In what percentage of VAIN lesions can HPV DNA be isolated?

Seventy percent

Is the prevalence increasing or decreasing?

Increasing

Is the mean age at diagnosis increasing or decreasing?

Decreasing

What is the malignant potential of VAIN?

Unknown

How is VAIN diagnosed?

By PAP smear
By colposcopy

What are the clinical features of VAIN?	VAIN usually involves the posterior upper third of the vagina. Two clinical patterns can be distinguished: Keratotic plaques, often visible with the naked eye Flat patches of acetowhite epithelium that are often completely invisible before vinegar application
What is the treatment of VAIN?	Often difficult to treat Historically treated by surgical excision or vaginal irradiation; however, current therapy is generally more conservative and consists of laser ablation or topical 5-FU application.
What are the requirements for conservative therapy?	Physician with expert training in colposcopy Directed biopsies consistent with the abnormality seen on the Pap smear No cytologic or colposcopic suspicion of occult invasion Choice of conservative versus radical therapy also depends on the amount of tissue involved and clinical circumstances.

PREINVASIVE NEOPLASTIC DISEASE OF THE VULVA

What is the frequency of vulvar malignancies?	Vulvar cancer is rare, representing about 4% of gynecologic malignancies.
What are the relative frequencies of the various forms of vulvar cancer?	Squamous cell carcinoma: most common intraepithelial lesion of the vulva; accounts for about 90% of all vulvar cancers Malignant melanoma: 2% of vulvar cancers Basal cell carcinomas: 2% of vulvar cancers Vulvar sarcomas: 1%–2%

Lymphomas, plasmacytomas, endodermal sinus tumors, and Paget's disease: extremely rare

What is the cause of vulvar cancer?

The association between cervical neoplasia and vulvar cancer has led to the belief that the common pathogen is HPV.

What is the relationship between vulvar carcinoma in situ and sexually transmitted disease?

Patients with vulvar carcinoma in situ have an increased frequency of sexually transmitted disease.

What is the relationship between vulvar cancer and condylomata acuminata or herpes simplex vulvitis?

At least 5% of vulvar cancers have been estimated to develop within preexisting genital condylomata. Antecedent or concurrent condylomata acuminata or herpes simplex vulvitis is age-associated; patients are usually age 40 or younger.

What is the relationship between vulvar cancer and HSV?

Remains to be determined

What other sexually transmitted diseases are associated with vulvar cancer?

Syphilis (approximately 5% of patients with vulvar cancer have a positive serologic test for syphilis) Lymphogranuloma venereum Granuloma inguinale

What other factors are associated with vulvar cancer?

Obesity
Hypertension
Diabetes mellitus
Arteriosclerosis
Menopause at an early age
Nulliparity
Immunosuppression: Progression from vulvar intraepithelial neoplasia (VIN) to invasive cancer is most often seen in elderly and immunosuppressed patients.

What is the malignant potential of vulvar dystrophies?

Recent studies suggest that the malignant potential of vulvar dystrophies is small.

Adequately treated, a vulvar dystrophy should not significantly predispose a patient to the development of vulvar cancer.

Less than 5% of such patients followed for periods of up to 25 years develop vulvar cancer.

What factors increase the risk of vulvar cancer in patients with vulvar dystrophy?

Cellular atypia on the initial biopsy; occurs in less than 10% of cases

What is vulvar intraepithelial neoplasia (VIN)?

Preinvasive neoplastic disease of the vulva

Is the prevalence of VIN increasing or decreasing?

Substantially increasing; largest increases have been of the multifocal variety, especially in young women.

What are the risk factors for VIN?

Patients with preinvasive and invasive squamous lesions of the cervix and vagina have an increased risk of developing VIN.

Patients with vulvar intraepithelial neoplasia have a 15%–30% chance of having synchronous or metachronous cervical or vaginal squamous neoplasia or both.

Where are VIN lesions typically located?

Hairless areas of the vulva; the skin of the interlabial folds, posterior fourchette, and perineum are most frequently affected.

Twenty-five percent of cases have perianal involvement.

Multifocal disease is common, especially in younger patients.

What are the signs and symptoms of VIN?

Fifty percent of patients are asymptomatic at diagnosis.
Pruritus is the most common symptom.
There is no characteristic appearance of the lesions.
Lesions may be macular or papular in shape.
Discoloration is usual. The color may be white, red, pink, gray, or brown.

What does each color signify?

White: hyperkeratosis and epithelial thickening
Red: hypervascularity and parakeratosis
Gray or brown: melanocyte overactivity and pigment incontinence (premalignant keratinocytes are unable to retain melanin, which is then deposited within macrophages.)

What histologic changes are characteristic of VIN?

Disorganization of the epithelial architecture
Disorders of cytoplasmic and nuclear maturation
Changes usually but not always extend the full thickness of the epithelium.
Giant cells with abnormal nuclei
Multinucleated cells

What histologic type of VIN is most common?

Squamous
Two-thirds of cases have confluent or multicentric lesions.

What procedures are used in diagnosis of VIN?

Toluidine blue
Colposcopy with application of 3% acetic acid
Pap smears of the cervix or vagina to exclude concurrent disease in these areas

What are the mainstay treatments used in VIN?

Ablation
Surgical excision
Methods for excising the lesions include vulvectomy, superficial "skinning" vulvectomy, or wide local excision.

What is the relationship between the amount of tissue removed and recurrence rate?

The amount of tissue removed has not been shown to significantly influence recurrence rate (which is approximately 30% for all three modalities).

Emphasis should be placed on retaining vulvar tissue for both aesthetic and functional reasons.

When is total/radical vulvectomy indicated?

It is not indicated in the management of preinvasive disease.

What is skinning vulvectomy?

Removal of vulvar skin and replacement with a split-thickness skin graft

What are the benefits?

Effective in treating multifocal or extensive disease which may be difficult to treat by excision alone

Subcutaneous tissues of the vulva are preserved, allowing for an increased probability of an excellent functional and cosmetic result.

What are the drawbacks?

Cosmetic and functional results are still unpredictable.

What is wide excision?

Surgical excision of a vulvar lesion and a disease-free margin of approximately 5 millimeters (mm) with primary reapproximation of the skin edges

What are the indications?

Discrete lesions less than 2 cm in diameter and exclusion of invasive disease.

What are the benefits?

It produces excellent, nonmutilating results in the treatment of small foci.

What is CO_2 laser evaporation?

Use of a short wavelength laser to ablate tissue

What are the indications?

It is an acceptable treatment alternative to local excision provided patients are carefully evaluated and undergo biopsy prior to treatment to exclude microinvasive or invasive carcinoma.

What are the benefits?

Treatment is nonmutilating.
It is very effective, particularly for multiple, small lesions.

What are the drawbacks?

Because occult invasion > 1 mm carries a risk of lymph node metastases, there is little room for error.
Unlike excisional techniques, this method does not allow for any histologic evaluation.

What is a drawback of topical therapy with dinitrochlorobenzene or 5FU in the treatment of VIN?

It does not allow for proper histologic evaluation.

What is observation?

Patients are followed closely for a period of 6 months to 1 year.

What are the indications?

Young patients who are pregnant or recovering from recent herpetic vulvitis may be observed closely, as spontaneous regression has been reported in this population.

What is the prognosis for patients with VIN?

Clinical course cannot be predicted on the basis of histopathology or DNA analysis.
Lesions rarely progress.
The rate of invasive vulvar cancer associated with VIN is about 8%, and four-fifths of this number are superficially invasive (< 1 mm).

What is Paget's Disease?

A disease of abnormal differentiation of cells derived from the germinal layer of the epidermis

What is the histologic appearance?

Pathognomonic abnormal cells, called "Paget's cells," are rich in mucopolysaccharide, a diastase-resistant, periodic acid-Schiff (PAS)-positive substance

Histochemical staining can be used to differentiate Paget's disease from what other diseases?

Carcinoma in situ, amelanotic melanoma, and junctional nevi

What is the relationship between Paget's disease and vulvar cancer?

In about 20% of cases, Paget's disease is associated with an underlying adenocarcinoma.

In about 29% of patients, it may herald synchronous or metachronous invasive cancer at other sites.

What is the treatment of Paget's disease?

Because histologically demonstrable disease extends farther than the visible lesion, very wide local excision is required to decrease the likelihood of recurrence.

A wide superficial vulvectomy is often necessary with extensive disease.

What is the treatment of recurrences?

Recurrences are almost always in situ and may be treated by minor local excision or laser therapy if detected early.

40

Breast Cancer

GENERAL

What is the incidence of breast cancer?	One in every 9 women will have breast cancer in her lifetime. Leading cause of cancer death among American women ages 44–55 years Second most common cause of cancer death in women overall after lung cancer
What percentage of women with breast cancer die of the disease?	Fifty percent
What age-group is affected?	Less than 2% of cases occur in women younger than age 30 years. The incidence increases rapidly in the fourth decade. After menopause, the rate of increase slows.
Risk factors?	Age Breast cancer in a first-degree relative: Increases the risk two- to threefold Relative with premenopausal breast cancer: Increase is threefold. With bilateral breast cancer: Increase is 5.5-fold. With premenopausal bilateral breast cancer: Increase is ninefold. Personal history of contralateral breast cancer: Increases the risk twofold Nulliparity Late pregnancy: First full-term pregnancy after age 30 years poses greater risk than nulliparity. Late menopause: Women who reach menopause after age 55 years have twice the risk of women who reach menopause before age 45 years.

Early menarche: Weak risk factor
Ionizing radiation
BRCA1 and 2 mutations
Alcohol - two-fold risk
Atypical hyperplasia: Increases risk fourfold; with positive family history of breast cancer, increases risk ninefold

Is obesity a risk factor?

In postmenopausal women: Weak risk factor
In premenopausal women: Protective

Do oral contraceptive pills increase the risk of breast cancer?

No

Is long-term estrogen only replacement therapy a risk factor?

Controversial
One study found that long-term estrogen replacement therapy increases the risk of breast cancer by 40%. The increased risk may be related to the proliferative effect of estrogen on undiagnosed microscopic breast cancer.

Is long-term combination estrogen-progesterone HRT a risk factor?

A very recent study suggests that there is a small increase in the incidence of breast cancer if taken more than 5 years

DIFFERENTIAL DIAGNOSES

What benign diseases should be included in the differential diagnosis?

Fibrocystic disease
Fibroadenoma
Cystosarcoma phylloides
Intraductal papilloma
Fat necrosis
Mammary duct ectasia
Galactocele
Gynecomastia
Granular cell myoblastoma (rare)
Breast abscess
Mastitis

What is fibrocystic disease of the breast?

Denotes a variety of noninflammatory histopathologic changes in the breast, including epithelial, stromal, and duct proliferation

What is the cause of fibrocystic disease?

Multifactorial, including genetic and hormonal factors (estrogen)

What are the signs and symptoms of fibrocystic disease?

Diffuse breast fullness
Fibronodularity
Cysts may or may not be present.
In general, pain and fullness are noticed immediately before menses; symptoms gradually decrease over 10 to 14 days.

How is the diagnosis of fibrocystic disease confirmed?

Clinically by palpation
Fine-needle aspiration of single cysts
Aspirate should be straw-colored or greenish. Bloody fluid or lesions that do not resolve with aspiration raise suspicion of malignancy.

What is the treatment of fibrocystic disease?

Mild analgesia
Reduction in caffeine intake
Oral contraceptive pills in refractory cases

What is the most common tumor in women younger than 30 years of age?

Fibroadenoma

What is fibroadenoma?

Benign tumor consisting of stromal and epithelial elements

How is the tumor characterized?

Most are solitary, solid, well encapsulated, well circumscribed, rubbery, firm, nontender, lobulated, mobile breast masses 1–4 cm in size.
Hormonally dependent, so may fluctuate in size
Giant fibroadenoma is typically > 5 cm.

What is the treatment of fibroadenoma?

Excisional biopsy for definitive diagnosis and treatment

What is cystosarcoma phylloides?

A rare variant of fibroadenoma that has greater cellularity and pleomorphism and a tendency to recur after simple excision

Some undergo malignant transformation with 10% metastasizing, usually to the lungs

What are the signs and symptoms of cystosarcoma phyllodes?

Large, often teardrop mass with microscopic penetration

Overlying skin may be warm and erythematous.

Mass is not well encapsulated

What is the treatment of cystosarcoma phyllodes?

Smaller lesions: Wide local excision with at least 1-cm margin

Larger, breast-occupying lesions: Simple mastectomy (without axillary node dissection)

What is the most common breast mass after trauma to the breast?

Fat necrosis

Why is fat necrosis easily confused with carcinoma?

The mass of fat necrosis is firm and tender with ill-defined borders and is often surrounded by ecchymosis, skin retraction, and other skin changes.

What is the most common cause of bloody nipple discharge in premenopausal women?

Intraductal papilloma

What is the treatment of intraductal papilloma?

Wedge resection of ductal lesion

What is mammary duct ectasia?

A benign, **painful** mass due to duct dilatation and plasma cell infiltration

What are the signs and symptoms of duct ectasia?

Breast edema, dermal fixation, inflammatory changes; nipple inversion may or may not be present.

What diagnostic/ therapeutic procedures *must* be performed in mammary ectasia?

Multiple biopsies to rule out malignancy and local excision

TYPES OF BREAST CANCER

What is the most common type of breast cancer?

Infiltrating ductal carcinoma
Represents 70%–80% of all breast cancers

What are the two types of noninvasive breast cancer?

Ductal carcinoma in situ (DCIS)
Lobular carcinoma in situ (LCIS)

Which type is commonly characterized by multicentricity and a significant risk of progressing to invasive cancer?

DCIS; 25%–30% of patients progress to invasive breast cancer.

What percentage of patients with LCIS have bilateral disease?

25% to 40%

What percentage of patients with LCIS will have recurrent LCIS in the ipsilateral or contralateral breast?

25% to 40%

What are some types of invasive carcinoma that have a low risk of metastasis?

Colloid carcinoma, medullary carcinoma, tubular carcinoma, comedocarcinoma, and papillary carcinoma

Which type is known to enlarge rapidly because of hemorrhage and necrosis?

Medullary carcinoma, which represents 3%–5% of all breast cancers, is typically a mobile, deeply set encapsulated tumor that is otherwise slow growing.

Which of these breast cancers has the best 5-year survival rate?

Papillary carcinoma has the lowest frequency of axillary nodal spread. It is typically bulky and centrally located. It is usually seen in younger patients and is not derived from intraductal papilloma.

Which of the moderately metastasizing carcinomas is characterized by numerous microcalcifications?

Infiltrating ductal carcinoma has microcalcifications and significant fibrosis, whereas infiltrating lobular carcinoma extensively infiltrates and does not have microcalcifications.

What is inflammatory carcinoma?

A rare, highly aggressive form of carcinoma of any histologic type that causes skin changes such as erythema and peau d'orange and other local inflammatory changes

Represents 1.5%–3% of all breast cancers

Poor prognosis, with a 5-year survival rate of 3%–5%

Seventy-five percent of patients present with palpable axillary metastasis.

What is Paget's disease of the nipple?

DCIS or infiltrating ductal carcinoma involving the epidermis causing inflammatory, eczematous dermatitis of the nipple and areola

Represents 1%–3% of all breast cancers

One-third of patients present with axillary node metastasis.

Usually a favorable prognosis secondary to early diagnosis

DIAGNOSIS OF BREAST CANCER

What are typical presenting signs and symptoms of breast cancer?

Palpable breast mass that is firm, ill defined, not freely mobile, and usually nontender

Unilateral bloody nipple discharge

Nipple retraction, flattening, or thickening

Skin changes, including dimpling, peau d'orange, crusting

Palpable lymph nodes

Diffuse breast pain (rare)

Constitutional symptoms such as weight loss, anorexia, bone pain (advanced disease)

Abnormal mammogram

Where are most breast cancers located?

Upper outer quadrant (tail of Spence)

What is peau d'orange?

Swollen, pitted skin overlying carcinoma of the breast; resembles orange peel

Caused by stromal infiltration and edema due to lymphatic obstruction

What are the common sites for metastasis?

Bone, lungs, liver, and brain

What procedures are used for breast cancer screening?

Breast self-examination monthly, preferably 1 week after menses (sensible, but without proven benefit)

Physical examination:
Every 3 years for women ages 20–40 years and annually for women age 40 years or older

Known breast lesions should not be followed for more than two menstrual cycles without a diagnosis.

Mammogram:
The recommended schedule for screening mammogram is continually being reevaluated and revised.

Some current guidelines include first screening mammogram at age 40 years, every 2 years until age 50, and yearly after age 50 years.

What size mass can a mammogram detect?

Masses ≥ 0.5 cm

What are the false-negative and false-positive rates of mammography?

False-negative rate: 5%–15%
False-positive rate: < 5%

Why is it more difficult to evaluate young women by mammography?

The breasts of young women contain more fibrous tissue than those of older women.

What findings on mammography require further evaluation?

Spiculated, stellate, clustered microcalcifications (< 1 mm)

What diagnostic tests are helpful in evaluating a breast mass?

Ultrasound can differentiate between cystic and solid masses.

Fine-needle aspiration biopsy
Hemocult-positive fluid should be examined cytologically.
Cysts that do not resolve with two aspirations should be evaluated with needle or excisional biopsy.

Needle biopsy for superficial, fairly well circumscribed lesions > 1 cm; establishes diagnosis in 80% of patients

Open biopsy: definitive diagnostic method
Excisional biopsy (i.e., total removal) for benign tumors and for lesions < 3 cm
Incisional biopsy (or needle biopsy) for suspect lesions ≥ 3 cm immediately before planned mastectomy

Estrogen/progesterone receptor studies and flow cytometry of tissue biopsy samples can aid in formulating treatment plan in some cases.

STAGING AND TREATMENT OF BREAST CANCER

What tests are necessary for staging and treatment planning of breast cancer?

Essential: Examination, bilateral mammogram, complete blood count, chemistry panel including liver function tests, chest radiograph
Selected studies based on results of tests: Radionuclide bone scan, liver computed tomography scan

What classification is used in breast cancer staging?

TNM classification: T (primary **t**umor), N (regional **n**odes), M (**m**etastasis)

What are the TNM stages of breast cancer?

Tumor size
   Tx: Cannot assess
   T0: No evidence of primary tumor
   Tis: In situ
   T1: $\leq$ 2 cm
   T2: > 2 cm but < 5 cm
   T3: > 5 cm
   T4: Extension onto chest wall/skin
Regional node status
   Nx: Cannot assess
   N0: No regional lymph node spread
   N1: Mobile ipsilateral axillary nodes
   N2: Fixed ipsilateral axillary nodes
   N3: Ipsilateral internal mammary
      nodes
Metastasis
   Mx: Cannot assess
   M0: No distant metastasis
   M1: Distant metastasis; includes
      ipsilateral supraclavicular lymph
      nodes

What are the available treatment options for breast cancer?

Surgical:
   Lumpectomy with axillary dissection
      and radiation
   Simple mastectomy
   Modified radical mastectomy
   Systemic treatment:
   Radiation therapy
   Chemotherapy
   Hormonal treatment: Tamoxifen, an
      antiestrogen; oophorectomy in
      premenopausal women; and
      adrenalectomy or hypophysectomy
      (rarely)

What is the difference between simple mastectomy and modified radical mastectomy?

Modified radical mastectomy includes axillary node dissection.

What are the complications of mastectomy/axillary dissection?

Injury to the thoracodorsal nerve to the
   latissimus dorsi
Injury to the long thoracic nerve to the
   serratus anterior, causing "winging of
   the scapula"

Lymphedema of the ipsilateral upper
extremity
Loss of sensation due to injury of
intercostobrachial nerves
Injury to the medial and lateral thoracic
nerves to the pectoralis muscles

**For what pathologic type is
radiation therapy most
effective?**

Local chest wall lesions, regional lymph
node metastasis, and bony and brain
metastasis

**What are the side effects
of tamoxifen?**

Mild nausea
Hot flashes, particularly in
premenopausal women
Transient thrombocytopenia or
leukopenia

**For each of the following
stages of breast cancer, list
the current recommended
treatment options and
prognosis.**
    **Clinically local disease,
    stage I–II**

Treatment options:
    Lumpectomy ± axillary dissection ±
    radiation therapy
    Modified radical mastectomy
    Add adjuvant chemotherapy for
    positive lymph nodes
Prognosis:
    Overall 5-year survival rate for stage I
    is 85%.
    Overall 5-year survival rate for stage II
    is 66%.

    **Clinically advanced local
    disease, stage III**

Treatment: Simple mastectomy +
    radiation therapy + chemotherapy
Prognosis: Overall 5-year survival rate
    for stage III is 41%.

    **Systemic disease, Stage
    IV**

Treatment: Systemic therapy
Prognosis: Overall 5-year survival rate
    for stage IV is 10%.

41

Cervical Cancer

GENERAL

What is the incidence of cervical cancer?

Approximately 15,000 new cases occur per year.

Second most common gynecologic malignancy following uterine malignancies

What are the signs and symptoms of cervical cancer?

The most common symptom is vaginal bleeding, which may be postcoital, postmenopausal, or intermenstrual. Later in the disease, vaginal discharge, pelvic pain, or back pain secondary to ureteral obstruction may develop. Ten percent to twenty percent of patients complain of pain radiating to the back or legs.

How is cervical cancer diagnosed?

Cervical biopsy provides definitive diagnosis and is easily performed if the patient has a visible cervical tumor.

If an abnormal PAP smear or routine examination raises suspicion of cervical cancer, colposcopically directed biopsy may be helpful.

What colposcopic findings are suggestive of cervical cancer?

Abnormally branched, looped, or punctate blood vessels (secondary to neovascularization of the tumor and distortion of the blood vessels by the growing mass)

Abnormal appearance of the surface of the cervix

What procedures are used in the staging of cervical cancer?

Cervical cancer is clinically staged, based on careful pelvic examination and general physical examination with particular attention to inguinal and supraclavicular lymph nodes.

Other procedures that may be used for clinical staging include chest x-ray, intravenous pyelogram, barium enema, cystoscopy, proctoscopy, and cervical conization and examination under anesthesia.

What procedures are useful in treatment planning, but not in staging?

Computed tomography (CT) scan, magnetic resonance imaging (MRI), ultrasound, and lymphangiogram

What are the stages of cervical cancer?

Stage 0: Carcinoma in situ

Stage I: Carcinoma is limited to the cervix.

Ia: Microscopic diagnosis only

Ia1: Minimal invasion ≤ 3 mm

Ia2: Lesions not exceeding 5 mm in depth from the surface epithelium or 7 mm in horizontal spread

Ib_1: Lesions ≤ 4 cm, limited to cervix

Ib_2: Lesion > 4 cm, limited to cervix

Stage II: Carcinoma extends beyond the cervix, but has not extended to the pelvic sidewall or to the lower third of the vagina.

IIa: No obvious parametrial involvement

IIb: Obvious parametrial involvement

Stage III: Carcinoma extends to the pelvic sidewall or lower third of the vagina or there is evidence of hydronephrosis.

IIIa: No extension to the pelvic sidewall but the lower third of the vagina is involved

IIIb: Pelvic sidewall involvement or hydronephrosis

Stage IV: Carcinoma extends outside the true pelvis or clinically involves the mucosa of the bladder or rectum.

IVa: Spread to adjacent organs
IVb: Distant spread

What are the histologic types of cervical cancer and their frequency?

Squamous cell carcinoma: 80%
Undifferentiated: 10%
Adenocarcinoma: 5%
Sarcoma: 3%
Primary melanoma, small cell, lymphoma: rare

SQUAMOUS CELL CARCINOMA

Describe the demographics of squamous cell carcinoma.

Mean age is 50 to 55 years with a bimodal distribution (peaks occur at 35 to 39 years and at 60 to 64 years).

What are the risk factors for squamous cell carcinoma?

Early age at first coitus, multiple sexual partners, human papillomavirus (HPV) infection, smoking, multiparity

What are the treatment options for squamous cell carcinoma?

Radiation therapy with concurrent chemosensitization can be used for **all** stages of cervical cancer. Surgery, however, is limited to stages I and IIa disease.
Chemotherapy alone is occasionally an option.

What is the treatment of stage Ia1?

No involvement of lymphovascular space: cervical conization, if patient wants to preserve fertility, or a type I hysterectomy
Nonsurgical candidates: intracavitary radiotherapy

What is the treatment of stage Ia2?

No involvement of lymphovascular space; invasion less than 3 mm: type I hysterectomy or cervical conization
Involvement of lymphovascular space; invasion less than 3 mm: type I or type II hysterectomy with a pelvic node dissection

Invasion of 3 to 5 mm: type II
hysterectomy with a pelvic node
dissection

Intracavitary radiotherapy is an option.

**What is the treatment of
stages Ib and IIa?**

Surgery and radiotherapy with
concurrent chemotherapy offer the
same cure rates for these stages.

Surgery:

Surgical candidates have lesions less than
4 to 5 centimeters (cm).

Type III or radical hysterectomy with
pelvic node dissection and para-aortic
node sampling

Radiotherapy:

4500 cGy external beam with weekly
cisplatin chemosensitization and
intracavitary radiation

External beam radiotherapy with
chemosensitization may be followed
with type I hysterectomy in patients
whose lesions respond poorly to
radiation.

**What is the treatment of
stages IIb through IVa?**

Radiotherapy using external beam and
weekly cisplatin chemosensitization and
intracavitary radiation

**What is the treatment of
stage IVb?**

Chemotherapy is the primary treatment
modality for metastatic disease. The
most effective chemotherapeutic agent
is cisplatin.

Radiotherapy may be used to control
local disease and relieve bleeding,
edema, or pain.

**What are the complications
of surgery?**

Immediate postoperative complications:
hemorrhage, ureterovaginal or
vesicovaginal fistulas, fever, sepsis,
pulmonary embolus, and wound
infection

Long-term complications: lymphocyst
formation, bladder dysfunction,

ureteral strictures, and fistula formation, GI dysfunction

What are the complications of radiotherapy?

Acute: nausea, diarrhea, and superficial skin damage

Long-term: fistula formation involving the bladder, bowel, and vagina; vaginal stenosis and sexual dysfunction; rectal bleeding from radiation proctitis; and ureteral stenosis

What is the treatment of recurrent disease?

Generally, patients who were initially treated surgically are candidates for radiotherapy, and patients initially treated with radiotherapy may be candidates for surgical excision of recurrent disease.

Surgical options include local excision or pelvic exenteration [anterior, posterior, or total].

What is the overall 5-year survival rate for squamous cell carcinoma?

Sixty percent

What is the 5-year survival rate for each stage of squamous cell carcinoma?

Stage I: 85% to 90%
Stage II: 60% to 80%
Stage III: 30%
Stage IV: 10%

UNDIFFERENTIATED CARCINOMAS

Describe the demographics of undifferentiated carcinomas.

The patient demographics are not like those of squamous cell carcinoma; however, these carcinomas tend to occur in a similar age-group.

What are the risk factors for undifferentiated carcinomas?

No specific risk factors

What is the treatment?	The treatment of each stage is the same as the treatment of each stage of squamous cell carcinoma.
What is the prognosis?	The numbers are too small to assign percentages; however, overall prognosis is worse than that of squamous cell carcinomas because of the more aggressive or poorly differentiated histopathologic component of these carcinomas.

ADENOCARCINOMAS

Describe the demographics of adenocarcinomas.	The frequency of this type of cancer is increasing; however, this increase may be due to improvement in the early detection of squamous cell carcinomas. The average age is 56 years. Eighty percent of patients have stage I or II disease at the time of diagnosis.
What are the risk factors?	Same as squamous cell carcinomas
In general, what are the treatment options for adenocarcinoma?	Generally, the treatment is the same as that of squamous cell carcinoma. These tumors may occasionally be "bulkier" than squamous cell carcinomas. Therefore, radiotherapy may be advocated, even with early stage disease, because it is technically difficult to achieve negative margins with surgery. In some cases, radiation and chemosensitization plus type I hysterectomy is proposed for bulky stage I and stage II tumors.
What is the prognosis?	Adenocarcinoma and squamous cell carcinoma have similar patterns of lymphatic dissemination; however, adenocarcinoma is more aggressive in

both lymphatic spread and local extension. Therefore, the survival rates are lower in adenocarcinoma compared with squamous cell carcinoma.

What is the overall 5-year survival rate for adenocarcinoma?

Fifty percent

What is the 5-year survival rate for each stage of adenocarcinoma?

Stage I: 70% to 75%
Stage II: 30% to 40%
Stage III: 20% to 30%
Stage IV: < 15%

42

Ovarian Neoplasms

GENERAL

What is the incidence of ovarian cancer in the United States?

About 1 in 70 women will develop ovarian cancer.

Incidence begins to rise around the fifth decade of life and is highest in postmenopausal women.

Ovarian cancer is the leading cause of death from gynecologic cancer in the United States.

How are ovarian neoplasms classified?

According to the tissue type from which they originate:

Coelomic epithelium

Sex cord–ovarian stroma

Germ cell

Nonspecialized stroma

Metastatic tumors

EPITHELIAL OVARIAN NEOPLASMS

GENERAL FEATURES AND GENETICS

What is the embryologic origin of epithelial neoplasms?

Arise from coelomic epithelium (i.e., the mesothelium), which covers and is incorporated into the ovary during embryonic development

This epithelium also gives rise to peritoneum and the paramesonephric (müllerian duct), which explains the histologic similarities between lesions of ovaries, peritoneum, and urogenital tract.

In what age group do most epithelial ovarian cancers occur?

Greater than 80% of epithelial ovarian cancers occur in postmenopausal women, with a peak incidence at age 62.

Approximately 30% of ovarian epithelial neoplasms in postmenopausal women are malignant, compared with only 7% in premenopausal women.

Is there a hereditary pattern of development for ovarian cancers?

Hereditary or familial cases are seen, but account for < 5% of all ovarian malignancies.

What is a feature that distinguishes hereditary cases of epithelial ovarian cancers?

Tend to present about 10 years earlier than nonfamilial cases

How can patients at risk for hereditary epithelial ovarian cancer be identified?

A specific genetic marker is not available.

A pedigree analysis is useful and may reveal an autosomal dominant pattern of transmission.

How are patients with familial risk of ovarian cancer managed?

Management is controversial because of the lack of reliable screening methods. In general, women who have a significant family history of ovarian cancer and wish to preserve their fertility should be followed by transvaginal ultrasonography every 6 months.

Women who no longer wish to maintain their fertility should be offered prophylactic bilateral salpingo-oophorectomy; they should be informed that peritoneal carcinomas occasionally occur after this operation.

What specific inheritance patterns for ovarian cancer have been identified?

Site-specific familial ovarian cancer

Patients with two first-degree relatives with epithelial ovarian cancer: risk of developing ovarian cancer is as high as 50%, representing an autosomal dominant mode of transmission.

Patients with a single first-degree relative with epithelial ovarian cancer: risk is increased three- to ten-fold over those without a family history.

Breast/ovarian familial cancer syndrome

May exist if there is familial history of epithelial ovarian and breast cancers.
Recently, this syndrome has been associated with the BRCA1 gene, a locus on the 17q chromosome.

Lynch II syndrome

Syndrome of multiple adenocarcinomas involving familial colon cancer (Lynch I syndrome) and ovarian, endometrial, breast, and other cancers
Women with this syndrome appear to have at least three times the risk of the general population for development of epithelial ovarian cancer.

What are the signs and symptoms of ovarian cancer?

Majority of patients are either asymptomatic or present with symptoms that are nonspecific and usually ignored
Early stage disease: urinary symptoms and/or constipation (secondary to a growing pelvic mass), irregular menses, and pelvic pain or pressure
Advanced disease: abdominal distention, bloating, constipation, anorexia, nausea, and early satiety secondary to ascites and intestinal spread

What is the most important sign that should raise suspicion of ovarian cancer?

Presence of a pelvic mass on physical examination

What is the role of screening in the diagnosis of this disease?

Currently, no tests are available that are specific and sensitive enough to serve as a valuable screening tool for ovarian cancer.

How is ovarian cancer diagnosed?

An ovarian mass requires definitive diagnosis, which usually entails exploratory laparotomy/laparoscopy.

In premenopausal patients, observation with pelvic ultrasound and hormonal suppression with oral contraceptives to check for regression of the mass before proceeding with laparotomy are reasonable.

Ultrasound may be helpful in characterizing the nature of the mass. Young women with sonographic findings suggestive of a benign process may be followed. Persistent masses require definitive diagnosis by tissue sample.

What are the differential diagnoses for an ovarian mass?

Gynecologic causes:
Functional cysts of the ovaries
Pelvic inflammatory disease (PID)
Endometriosis
Massive edema of the ovary (secondary to torsion)
Pedunculated uterine leiomyomas
Ectopic pregnancy
Nongynecologic causes:
Inflammatory or neoplastic colonic mass
Lymphoma
Metastasis from distant primary tumors (e.g., breast)

What is the role of tumor markers in the diagnosis and treatment of epithelial cancers?

CA 125
Elevated in about 80% of patients with epithelial ovarian cancers, but it is not specific
Positive values are highly predictive of recurrence of disease; however, negative values are not sensitive in predicting the absence of disease.
Carcinoembryonic antigen (CEA)
Elevated in the majority of patients with mucinous ovarian cancer
However, it is neither sensitive nor specific enough to be useful in patient screening.

How do epithelial ovarian cancers spread?

Primarily by "surface implantation" throughout the peritoneal cavity, lymphatic dissemination involving pelvic and para-aortic nodes, and less commonly, hematogenous dissemination

Describe the general staging system for ovarian cancers.

Ovarian cancer is surgically staged:

Stage I: growth limited to the ovaries

Stage II: growth involving one or both ovaries with pelvic extension

Stage III: tumor involving one or both ovaries with peritoneal implants outside the pelvis, positive retroperitoneal or inguinal nodes, or superficial liver metastasis

Stage IV: growth involving one or both ovaries with distant metastasis; includes pleural effusion with positive cytology and parenchymal liver metastasis

What histologic features are used to determine the grade of an ovarian tumor?

Pattern of differentiation, extent of cellular anaplasia, and proportion of undifferentiated cells are used for grading lesions on a scale of 1 (few changes from normal morphology) to 3 (poorly differentiated and rapidly dividing).

Name the different histologic types of epithelial ovarian neoplasms.

Serous

Mucinous

Endometrioid

Clear cell

Brenner

Mixed epithelial

Undifferentiated

What classification system is used to describe the likelihood of metastasis of epithelial neoplasms?

Each histologic type (except for undifferentiated) is further subclassified as:

A: benign

B: low malignant potential (LMP), also called borderline

C: malignant based on the extent of proliferation, nuclear features, mitotic activity, and stromal invasion

TYPES OF EPITHELIAL NEOPLASMS

Serous neoplasms

What is the most common type of epithelial neoplasm?

Serous histology is seen in both the majority of benign and malignant epithelial ovarian tumors (75% of all epithelial cancers).

What percentage of serous neoplasms are benign? Malignant? LMP?

Benign: 70%
LMP: 5% to 10%
Malignant: 20% to 25%

How frequently do bilateral serous tumors occur?

Overall, serous tumors are bilateral 10% of the time. Malignant tumors are more frequently bilateral (35%–50%).

What are psammoma bodies and what is their significance?

Concentric calcifications that occur occasionally in benign serous neoplasms and frequently in serous cystadenocarcinomas

Mucinous neoplasms

What percentage of mucinous tumors are benign?

Eighty percent

What is the bilateral occurrence rate of malignant mucinous tumors?

Ten percent to twenty percent

What is pseudomyxoma peritonei?

Secretion of large amounts of gelatinous mucinous material into the peritoneal cavity by the neoplastic epithelium

Most commonly associated with appendiceal adenocarcinomas; well-differentiated colorectal adenocarcinomas; and less frequently, ovarian mucinous adenocarcinomas

Endometrioid neoplasms

What are some examples of LMP endometrioid epithelial neoplasms?

LMP tumors can have various morphologic presentations (e.g., tumors with a prominent fibrous component are sometimes referred to as "adenofibromas")

What histologic features alter the prognosis of malignant endometrioid tumors?

Good prognosis if histology shows benign squamous metaplasia
Poor prognosis if histology shows mixed adenosquamous carcinoma

What is the relationship between ovarian endometrioid lesions and similar lesions in the endometrium?

Ovarian endometrioid tumors are associated with similar lesions in the endometrium.

What is the management of cases with associated ovarian and endometrial tumors?

It is important to differentiate multifocal disease (i.e., separate primaries) from disease that has metastasized from the uterus because of the much better prognosis associated with the former.

Clear cell neoplasms

Which type of epithelial ovarian tumor is most frequently associated with hypercalcemia and hyperpyrexia?

Clear cell tumors

What histologic features are characteristic of clear cell tumors?

Clear cells with vacuolated or clear cytoplasm
Hobnail cells in which the nuclei are projected to an apical cytoplasm

Sometimes associated with focal areas of endometriosis or endometrioid carcinoma

Brenner tumors

Do Brenner tumors tend to be benign or malignant?

Less than 2% of these tumors are malignant.

What are the gross and histologic features of Brenner tumors?

Gross features: resemble ovarian fibromas due to their solid consistency and white or yellow-white color

Histologic features:

Stromal proliferation around nests of epithelial cells resembling transitional epithelium of the urinary tract

These tumors are associated with mucinous cystadenomas or dermoid cysts in the same or contralateral ovary.

TREATMENT OF EPITHELIAL NEOPLASMS

What are the main principles in the treatment of ovarian cancers?

Three concepts:

1. Importance of meticulous and extensive surgical staging in disease that on inspection appears to be limited to the ovaries
2. Importance of "adequate" cytoreduction [macroscopic disease should be reduced to ≤ 1 cm]
3. Importance of platinum-based combination chemotherapy in all stages

What is the treatment of choice of stage Ia and Ib (tumor limited to one or both ovaries with no

If no evidence of spread beyond the ovary: abdominal hysterectomy and bilateral salpingo-oophorectomy (TAH-BSO)

evidence of extra-ovarian spread), grade 1 lesions?

The uterus and the contralateral ovary may be preserved if patient wants to preserve fertility.

What is the treatment of stages Ia and Ib, grades 2 and 3, and stage Ic?

No single optimal treatment exists; however, surgery alone is not sufficient.

Options:

Chemotherapy with a single agent (e.g., cisplatin, carboplatin, or taxol)

Combination chemotherapy (cisplatin and taxol or cyclophosphamide with or without adriamycin)

Radiation (intraperitoneal ^{32}P or whole abdominal radiation)

What is the treatment of stages II, III, and IV lesions?

Surgery followed by chemotherapy/ radiation

Initial surgery: maximal removal of disease including metastases (cytoreductive or debulking procedure)

Upon the completion of surgery plus chemotherapy/radiation, patients with no clinical evidence of disease and negative tumor markers may undergo a reassessment laparotomy or a "second look surgery." If disease is still present, second-line or salvage therapy may be recommended.

What clinical factors negatively affect the prognosis?

Advanced age, residual tumor after primary surgery, volume of ascites

What is the 5-year survival rate for ovarian cancers?

Great variability exists in survival of patients with same-stage ovarian cancer because survival is highly dependent on tumor grade, sensitivity to chemotherapeutic agents, success of debulking procedure, and many other factors. Thus, the 5-year survival rate is not a practical concept in ovarian cancer.

In general, for properly staged patients,
5-year survival rates are:
Stages I and II: 80% to 100%
Stage IIIa: 30% to 40%
Stage IIIb: 20%
Stage IIIc and IV: 5%

NONEPITHELIAL OVARIAN NEOPLASMS

What is the prevalence of nonepithelial ovarian cancers?

Nonepithelial ovarian cancers comprise only 10% of all ovarian cancers.

What are the three main types of nonepithelial tumors?

1. Germ cell tumors
2. Sex cord–stromal tumors
3. Tumors metastatic to the ovary

How are these tumors staged?

They are surgically staged in the same manner as epithelial cancers.

GERM CELL TUMORS

Germ cell tumors comprise what percentage of all ovarian neoplasms?

Neoplasms: 20%
Of ovarian malignancies?
Malignancies: < 5% (in western countries)

What percentage of germ cell neoplasms are malignant?

About 33% (one-third)

In what age group are most germ cell tumors seen?

Second and third decade of life

What is the embryologic origin of germ cell neoplasms?

Arise from primitive germ cells and may occur within, or more commonly, outside the gonads
Extragonadal involvement may occur from the pineal gland to the retroperitoneum. This widespread involvement is due to the embryonic migration of germ cells from the

caudal portion of the yolk sac to the posterior mesentery before they are incorporated into the developing gonads. These cells are often multipotent cells and may present as embryonic, extraembryonic, or mixed structures.

Name the main histologic types of germ cell neoplasms.

Dysgerminoma (also called germinoma)
Teratoma
Endodermal sinus tumor (EST)
Embryonal carcinoma
Polyembryoma
Choriocarcinoma
Gonadoblastoma
Mixed germ cell tumors

What are the benign types of germ cell neoplasms?

Gonadoblastomas and mature cystic teratomas

Name the secretory markers for different pure malignant germ cell tumors.

Placental alkaline phosphatase (PLAP) and lactate dehydrogenase (LDH) are commonly produced by dysgerminomas.
Human chorionic gonadotropin (hCG) and alpha fetoprotein (AFP) are secreted by many different tumors (see Table 42-1).
Mixed germ cell tumors may secrete more than one marker.

Table 42–1.

Tumor type	hCG produced	AFP produced
Dysgerminoma	no	no
Embryonal carcinoma	yes	yes
Teratoma	no	no
Endodermal sinus tumor	no	yes
Choriocarcinoma	yes	no

What are the signs and symptoms of germ cell tumors?

Subacute pelvic pain (secondary to characteristic rapid growth rate of these tumors)

Bladder and rectal symptoms

Menstrual irregularities (may be confused with pregnancy)

Torsion or rupture of the adnexa may be confused with appendicitis.

What is the diagnostic workup for germ cell tumors?

In the presence of a pelvic mass on physical examination, preliminary evaluation includes ultrasound and serum hCG, AFP, PLAP, and LDH measurements. Chest x-ray is important because germ cell tumors can metastasize to lungs or mediastinum.

When and why is karyotyping indicated?

A karyotype should be obtained on all premenarchal girls with germ cell tumors because of the association between these lesions and gonadal dysgenesis.

Which germ cell tumors tend to be associated with gonadal dysgenesis?

Gonadoblastomas, dysgerminomas, and ESTs

When should surgical exploration be considered?

Premenarchal patients: adnexal mass ≥ 2 cm

Postmenarchal premenopausal patient: adnexal mass > 8 cm

DYSGERMINOMAS

What percentage of germ cell tumors are dysgerminomas?

Thirty percent to forty percent

In what age-group are most dysgerminomas seen?

Between ages 10 and 30

What percentage of ovarian malignancies associated with pregnancy are dysgerminomas?

Twenty percent to thirty percent

What is the association between dysgerminomas and gonadal dysgenesis?

Five percent of dysgerminomas are discovered in phenotypic females with abnormal gonads, hence the need for karyotyping.

How common is the involvement of the contralateral ovary?

Dysgerminomas are the only malignant germ cell tumor with a **significant rate of bilateral occurrence** (about 10%–15%)

What is the treatment of dysgerminomas?

Unilateral oophorectomy in order to preserve fertility

Surgery may be followed with chemotherapy; contralateral ovary, fallopian tube, and the uterus can therefore be preserved even in the presence of metastatic disease because the tumor is sensitive to chemotherapy.

What is the treatment if karyotyping reveals a Y chromosome?

Bilateral gonadectomy

Should the contralateral ovary be biopsied?

Yes, because not all bilateral lesions have obvious ovarian enlargement

When is chemotherapy used in treatment?

For advanced or incompletely resected tumors

What chemotherapy regimen is prescribed in these cases?

Combination chemotherapy using bleomycin, etoposide, and cisplatin (BEP)

Can radiation be used in the treatment of dysgerminomas?

Although dysgerminomas are very sensitive to radiation, loss of fertility limits its use to recurrent or chemoresistant cases.

What is the prognosis after treatment of dysgerminomas?	Cure rates of 85% to 90%, even for patients with advanced disease, with the use of BEP chemotherapy

TERATOMAS

What are teratomas?	Tumors composed of totipotent cells capable of differentiating into derivatives of more than a single germ layer
In what age-group are most teratomas seen?	First two decades of life
How are teratomas classified?	Classified as mature or immature based on histologic appearance of nervous tissue elements of the tumor and the malignant behavior observed in immature teratomas
What is the prevalence of immature teratomas?	Represent < 1% of all teratomas
What is the incidence of bilateral presentation in teratomas?	Bilateral incidence of mature teratomas is 15% to 20%. Immature teratomas are almost always unilateral, although metastasis to the contralateral ovary may occur.
Do mature teratomas transform into immature teratomas?	Mature and immature teratomas are thought to represent related but separate neoplastic processes, and the mature form does not transform into the immature form. Malignant degeneration of mature cystic teratomas is thought to occur in only 1% to 2% of cases; in this situation, the most frequent malignancy developed is squamous carcinoma.
What is Rokitansky's protuberance and what is its significance?	Definition: protuberance on the inner wall of the cyst containing a wide variety of tissue present in the tumor

Significance: must be sectioned
thoroughly because it often contains
populations of immature cells
important to the accurate grading of
the lesion

What are the possible complications of mature cystic teratomas?

Other than malignant transformation,
they include torsion, rupture and
hemorrhage, infection, and gliomatosis
peritonei.

Rupture is uncommon, but becomes
more common in pregnant patients
and may occur during labor.

What is gliomatosis peritonei?

Implantation of benign, mature glia in
the peritoneal cavity; may occur
following the rupture of a mature cystic
teratoma

What are the three specialized forms of teratoma?

Dermoid cyst: consists entirely of skin
and appendages (i.e., ectodermal
derivatives).

Struma ovarii: consists primarily of
thyroid tissue

Carcinoid: composed of gut
neuroendocrine cells which secrete
serotonin and/or other
catecholamines

What is the treatment of mature teratomas?

Ovarian cystectomy with preservation of
remaining normal ovarian tissue, if
possible

What is the treatment of immature teratomas?

Premenopausal patients who want to
preserve fertility: unilateral
oophorectomy if the tumor is limited
to a single ovary

Postmenopausal patients: TAH-BSO

Chemotherapy (VAC) for all patients
except those with stage Ia grade 1
tumors; chemotherapy is also
indicated if ascites is present,
regardless of the tumor grade.

What is the most important prognostic factor for survival following treatment of teratomas?

Grade of the lesion

What other factors influence survival?

Patients with incompletely resected tumors prior to chemotherapy have a lower probability of cure compared to those with complete tumor resection.

What are the 5-year survival rates for patients with grades 1, 2, and 3 lesions?

Grade 1: 82%
Grade 2: 62%
Grade 3: 40%

ENDODERMAL SINUS TUMORS

What is the epidemiology of endodermal sinus tumors (ESTs)?

Also known as yolk sac tumor
   Represents the second most common germ cell malignancy
This aggressive malignancy tends to occur in young females (median age is 18) and is almost always unilateral.

What are Schiller-Duval bodies?

Cystic spaces lined by a flattened endothelium that contain a tuft with a vascular core resembling a glomerulus; they are characteristic of EST histology.

Is there a useful marker for ESTs?

Most lesions secrete AFP.
However, AFP is not useful as a screening tool but can be used to monitor response to therapy and recurrence.

What is the treatment of ESTs?

Surgical exploration and unilateral salpingo-oophorectomy
Gross metastases should be removed, but thorough debulking is not indicated because all patients must receive chemotherapy.

Chemotherapy currently consists of cisplatin-containing combination regimens.

EMBRYONAL CARCINOMA

How common are embryonal carcinomas?	Rare tumor of young females (median age is 14)
What feature of embryonal carcinoma distinguishes it from choriocarcinoma?	Histologic absence of trophoblastic cells
What are the characteristic tumor markers for embryonal carcinoma?	Frequently secrete hCG and AFP May secrete estrogen May lead to precocious pseudopuberty or irregular bleeding at presentation
What is the treatment of embryonal carcinoma?	Same as that of endodermal sinus tumors (i.e., unilateral oophorectomy followed by cisplatin-based combination chemotherapy)

CHORIOCARCINOMA OF THE OVARY

What is choriocarcinoma of the ovary?	A tumor composed of trophoblastic tissue
How frequently does choriocarcinoma occur in nonpregnant patients?	Purely nongestational occurrence in the ovary is extremely rare. These patients tend to be younger than 20 years old, and the majority have metastases at the time of presentation.
What tumor markers are associated with this disease?	hCG secretion is common. AFP elevation indicates an endodermal sinus component.
What is the treatment of choriocarcinoma?	Combination chemotherapy has been employed in these rare cases using methotrexate, actinomycin D, and

cyclophosphamide (same as treatment of gestational trophoblastic disease), or alternatively, BEP

What is the prognosis after treatment?

Poor

POLYEMBRYOMA

In what age group do polyembryomas occur?

Very young patients

How common is this tumor?

Extremely rare

What is the characteristic histology of this tumor?

The tumor is composed of embryoid bodies that reflect the histology of early embryonic differentiation (ectoderm, endoderm, mesoderm).

What tumor markers are associated with this tumor?

Elevated hCG, AFP

Can polyembryoma be associated with precocious puberty?

Yes

GONADOBLASTOMA

What is gonadoblastoma?

Benign neoplasm composed of a mixture of germ cells and sex cord derivatives; found in patients with gonadal dysgenesis

Are gonadoblastomas ever malignant?

No; however, they are associated with the development of malignant germ cell tumors in up to 50% of cases.

What is the characteristic genetic abnormality seen in gonadoblastomas?

The karyotype commonly reveals a Y chromosome or a fragment of it.

What is the significance of the presence of a Y chromosome in a female patient?	Prompt bilateral gonadectomy is required because of the risk of malignancy. The exception is patients with androgen insensitivity syndrome in whom this procedure can be delayed until age 30 (before this age, the risk of developing cancer is not significant).

MIXED GERM CELL TUMORS

What are mixed germ cell tumors composed of?	Contain two or more of the above tumor elements
What is the incidence of dysgerminoma, EST, immature teratoma, and choriocarcinoma in mixed germ cell tumors?	Dysgerminoma: 80% EST: 70% Immature teratoma: 53% Choriocarcinoma: 20%
What factors determine the prognosis in these tumors?	Tumor size and the relative amounts of the most malignant component

SEX CORD–STROMAL TUMORS

How common are sex cord–stromal tumors?	Account for 5% of all ovarian malignancies
What is the origin of these neoplasms?	Derived from sex cords and ovarian mesenchyme
What differentiation patterns are seen in these tumors?	Because the primitive stromal cells can differentiate into either male or female, these tumors can have predominantly male or female characteristics.
What are the three general groups of sex cord–stromal tumors?	1. Granulosa–stromal (including granulosa and thecoma–fibroma tumors)

2. Androblastomas (Sertoli-Leydig cell tumors)
3. Gynandroblastomas

GRANULOSA–STROMAL CELL TUMORS

What is a granulosa–stromal cell tumor?

Tumor defined by the presence of granulosa cells, with or without thecal elements

In what age-groups are these tumors usually seen?

Occur in women of all ages

What are the signs and symptoms?

Granulosa-stromal cell tumors typically secrete estrogen. Depending on the reproductive age of the patient, signs and symptoms include sexual pseudoprecocity, menstrual irregularity, secondary amenorrhea, endometrial hyperplasia, or even endometrial carcinoma.

Why aren't granulosa and theca cell tumors classified separately?

A strict division between granulosa and theca cell tumors is not useful because of frequent histologic coexistence and similar endocrinologic effects.

What is the gross appearance of these tumors?

Vary in size, tend to be yellow or gray in color, and have a smooth lobulated surface

What are Call-Exner bodies?

Arrangement of granulosa cells in small clusters around a central cavity; present in granulosa–stromal cell tumors

What is the metastasis/recurrence pattern seen in these tumors?

Usually stage I at diagnosis, but may recur 5 to 30 years later.
Hematogenous spread to lungs, liver, or brain is also possible and may occur years after the initial diagnosis.

What factors should be taken into account when planning treatment of granulosa–stromal cell tumors?	Age of patient, desire to preserve fertility, and extent of disease determined by surgical staging
What is the treatment if fertility is not an issue?	TAH/BSO Primary therapy with chemotherapy and radiation reserved for recurrent or metastatic disease
What is the treatment if fertility preservation is desired?	For stage Ia disease, unilateral salpingo-oophorectomy followed by a dilatation and curettage of the uterus because of the possibility of coexistent endometrial carcinoma
What is the prognosis following treatment?	Granulosa tumors have a prolonged natural history with possibility of late recurrence. Ten-year survival is about 90%; drops to a rate of approximately 75% after 20 years.

SERTOLI-LEYDIG CELL TUMORS

How common is this malignancy and in what age group does it usually occur?	Quite rare (0.5% of all ovarian cancers) Occur most frequently in the third and fourth decades of life
What are the signs and symptoms?	Virilization secondary to androgen production is seen in about 85% of cases. Signs of virilization include acne, hirsutism, breast atrophy, oligomenorrhea or amenorrhea, receding hairline, and a deepening of the voice.
What laboratory abnormalities may be associated with Sertoli-Leydig tumors?	Plasma testosterone and androstenedione levels may be elevated. Rarely, these tumors may produce estrogen (gynandroblastomas) and may

thus cause signs and symptoms typical of granulosa-theca cell tumors.

What is the treatment? Because bilateral lesions are rare (< 1%), the usual treatment is unilateral salpingo-oophorectomy with evaluation of the contralateral ovary.

What is the prognosis following treatment? Five-year survival rate is about 70% to 90%, and recurrences are uncommon.

TUMORS METASTATIC TO THE OVARY

What percentage of ovarian tumors are metastases from distant primaries? Approximately 5%

What primary tumors tend to metastasize to the ovaries? Tumors of the female genital tract, breast, or gastrointestinal (GI) tract
About 25% of women who die of metastatic breast cancer have evidence of ovarian involvement (usually bilateral) at autopsy.

What is a Krukenberg tumor? Cells characterized by a mucin-filled "signet ring" histologic appearance that have metastasized to the ovary, usually from the GI tract
The primary tumor most frequently originates from the stomach, and less commonly, from the colon, biliary tract, or the breast.
These tumors tend to occur bilaterally and usually present at an advanced stage of the primary disease. Most patients die of their primary tumor within a year.

What other malignancies tend to involve the ovaries?

Leukemias and lymphomas; involvement tends to be bilateral.

What hematologic malignancies most commonly involve the ovaries?

Burkitt's lymphoma: most common
Advanced-stage Hodgkin disease: About 5% of patients have some involvement of the ovaries.

What is the treatment of metastatic tumors to the ovaries?

Therapy consists of treating the primary disease.

43

Endometrial Carcinoma

What is endometrial carcinoma?

An adenocarcinoma involving the lining of the uterus

What is the incidence of endometrial cancer in the United States?

The most common malignancy of the female genital tract in the United States

Approximately 36,000 new cases and 5900 deaths occur each year.

What is a possible cause of endometrial cancer?

Exact cause is unknown; however, a positive correlation exists between exposure to unopposed estrogen and development of endometrial cancer.

What are examples of hyperestrogenic states associated with development of endometrial cancer?

Estrogen replacement therapy, obesity, anovulatory cycles (polycystic ovary disease), and estrogen-secreting tumors (such as granulosa-theca cell tumors)

What factors tend to be protective against endometrial cancer?

States of decreased estrogen or increased progestin levels (e.g., oral contraceptives)

What is the typical profile of a patient with endometrial carcinoma?

Patients tend to be obese, postmenopausal women of low parity.

What are the signs and symptoms of endometrial carcinoma?

Postmenopausal bleeding, perimenopausal intermenstrual bleeding, or premenopausal abnormal uterine bleeding, particularly in the presence of anovulation.

How is endometrial carcinoma diagnosed?

All patients presenting with the previously mentioned signs and symptoms should undergo an endometrial biopsy.

Because of a 10% false-negative rate, a negative endometrial biopsy in a symptomatic patient should be followed by fractional curettage under anesthesia.

Describe the current staging system for endometrial carcinoma.

Endometrial carcinoma is surgically staged (as recommended by the International Federation of Gynecologists and Obstetricians).

Stage I: tumor limited to the uterine corpus

Ia–limited to the endometrium

Ib–invasion of less than half of the myometrium

Ic–invasion of greater than half of the myometrium

Stage II: cervical involvement

IIa–endocervical glandular involvement only

IIb–cervical stromal invasion

Stage III: local spread

IIIa–invasion of the serosa, adnexa, or both, with or without positive peritoneal cytology

IIIb–vaginal metastasis

IIIc–metastasis to pelvic nodes, para-aortic nodes, or both

Stage IV: distant spread

IVa–invasion of bladder/bowel mucosa

IVb–distant metastasis, including intra-abdominal or inguinal nodes

How does this cancer spread?

Direct extension is the most common route.

Can also spread via the following routes:

Transtubal dissemination, leading to widespread peritoneal metastasis

Lymphatic spread to pelvic and para-aortic nodes

Hematogenous spread (usually to lungs)

What tumor features represent important prognostic factors?

Advanced tumor grade and increased depth of myometrial invasion are associated with increased risk of hematogenous and lymphatic spread, local vault recurrence, adnexal metastasis, and positive peritoneal cytology.

What are the histologic subtypes of endometrial carcinoma?

Approximately 90% are endometrioid. Remaining 10% to 15% consist of papillary serous, adenosquamous, clear cell, malignant mixed mesodermal tumors, sarcomas, undifferentiated and, rarely, squamous cell carcinomas. The uncommon subtypes are associated with a poorer prognosis.

How does the presence or absence of hormone receptors affect survival?

Presence of estrogen receptors (ER) and progesterone receptors (PR) is associated with increased survival, even in patients with lymph node metastasis.

What is endometrial hyperplasia and what is its relationship to endometrial cancer?

All endometrial hyperplasia was once thought to represent the benign end of a continuum of morphologic severity eventually resulting in carcinoma in situ, but this concept has been recently challenged. Endometrial hyperplasia with atypia is thought to be premalignant.

What are the risks of progression to carcinoma for endometrial hyperplasia and hyperplasia with atypia?

Simple hyperplasia 1%
Complex hyperplasia 3%
Simple hyperplasia with atypia 9%
Complex hyperplasia with atypia 30%

What is the treatment of stage I endometrial cancer?

Total abdominal hysterectomy and bilateral salpingo-oophorectomy (TAH-BSO)
Some authorities treat microscopic cervical involvement (unofficially designated as stage II occult disease) in the same manner as stage I disease.

What is the treatment of stage II disease?

Two options:
1. TAH-BSO with bilateral pelvic lymphadenectomy
2. Combined preoperative radiation (external pelvic irradiation and intracavitary radium or cesium), followed in 6 weeks by surgery.

What risks are associated with the second option?

Ten percent risk of associated severe gastrointestinal/urologic complications

What is the treatment of stage III disease?

Treatment is individualized and is aimed at surgical eradication of all macroscopic tumor, including any enlarged pelvic or para-aortic nodes, to improve the prognosis.

What is the treatment of stage IV disease?

Management, because patients with stage IV disease respond poorly to treatment

Treatment is individualized and usually involves surgery (palliative), radiation therapy, and progestins. Pelvic exenteration may be considered if disease extension is limited to bladder or rectum.

What are the 5-year survival rates for each stage of endometrial carcinoma?

Stage I: 70% to 95%
Stage II: 60% to 85%
Stage III: 40%
Stage IV: < 10%

44   Gestational Trophoblastic Disease

GENERAL

What is trophoblast?

The extraembryonic ectoderm surrounding the blastocyst

What is gestational trophoblastic disease (GTD)?

Tumors originating from trophoblastic tissue

These tumors may spread either locally or distantly metastasize.

How are the types of GTD classified?

Benign GTD
1. Complete hydatidiform mole
2. Partial hydatidiform mole

Malignant GTD
1. Invasive mole
2. Gestational choriocarcinoma
3. Placental site trophobastic tumor

The three types of malignant GTD can be metastatic or nonmetastatic.

How are these types differentiated?

On the basis of histopathologic and cytogenetic findings

However, the clinical features are more important in determining prognosis.

What are the tumor markers for GTD?

With the exception of placental site trophoblastic tumor, which is marked by human placental lactogen (HPL), the primary tumor marker is human chorionic gonadotropin (hCG).

In general, what is the diagnostic evaluation for all forms of GTD?

Complete history and physical examination

Ultrasound

Measurement of serum hCG level

Hepatic, renal, and thyroid function tests

What is the diagnostic evaluation for metastatic disease?

Chest x-ray

Ultrasound or computed tomography scan of the abdomen and pelvis

Measurement of the hCG level in cerebrospinal fluid (hCG levels are elevated in central nervous system metastatic disease)

When should a diagnostic evaluation for metastatic disease occur?

If hCG levels either plateau or continue to rise

List the common metastatic sites of GTD and their relative incidence.

Lung: 80%
Vagina: 30%
Pelvis: 20%
Brain: 10%
Liver: 10%
Bowel, kidney, spleen: < 5%
Other: 10%

How is GTD staged?

Stage I: limited to the uterus

Stage II: extends outside the uterus, limited to the genital structures

Stage III: extends to the lungs

Stage IV: all other metastatic sites

What factors indicate a good prognosis?

Less than 4 months since the pregnancy
hCG level < 40,000 mIU/ml
No liver or brain metastasis
No prior chemotherapy

What factors indicate a poor prognosis?

More than 4 months since the pregnancy
hCG level > 40,000 mIU/ml
Evidence of liver or brain metastasis
History of prior chemotherapy
Following a term pregnancy

What is the overall cure rate for GTD?

Ninety-two percent

What are the cure rates for each stage of GTD?

Stage I: 100%
Stage II: 88%
Stage III: 90%
Stage IV: 40%

What is the cure rate for low-risk disease (good prognosis)?

Ninety-seven percent

What is the cure rate for high-risk disease (poor prognosis)?

Sixty-four percent

What is the effect of GTD on subsequent pregnancies?

Patients with complete molar pregnancy have no increased risk of antenatal or intrapartum complications in later pregnancies.

Partial mole: Available data are limited but reassuring.

Choriocarcinoma: with successful treatment with chemotherapy, no increased risk of complications in later pregnancies

The frequency of congenital anomalies is not increased despite the teratogenic and mutagenic potential of the chemotherapeutic agents.

Risk of molar pregnancy in subsequent pregnancies:

Patients with molar disease are at an increased risk of developing molar pregnancy in later conceptions. The incidence is 0.6%–2.0%.

After two episodes of GTD, the risk of repeat disease rises to 28%.

HYDATIDIFORM MOLE

What is the definition of hydatidiform mole?

A proliferative disorder of the trophoblast cells that occurs in conjunction with pregnancy

What is the incidence?

In the US, the incidence is 1/1000 pregnancies. The incidence is 1/100 in Asian countries.

What percentage of patients will develop malignant sequelae?

Approximately 20% of patients with complete moles and 10% of patients with partial moles

Do these tumors metastasize?

No, unless persistent disease develops

What are the risk factors?

Maternal age:
    Increased risk in women over age 35
    Risk is five times greater in women over age 40.
    Risk may be increased in teenagers.
Previous molar pregnancy: Women with a previous mole have 10 times the risk of having a subsequent mole, regardless of partner.
Paternal age: increased risk if father is over age 45

What are the cytogenetic features of a hydatidiform mole?

Maternal genome regulates the growth and development of the embryonic tissue, while the paternal component regulates tissue proliferation.
In general, a haploid normal sperm fertilizes an ovum; the sperm then duplicates its own chromosomes, producing a 46XX karyotype. Maternal chromosomes may be either inactive or absent.
46XY complete moles result from fertilization of an empty ovum by two separate sperm, one contributing the X, the other the Y.

What are the differences between complete and partial moles?

Table 44–1.

	Complete	Partial
Fetal or embryonic tissue	Absent	Present
Hydatidiform swelling of villi	Diffuse	Focal
Trophoblastic hyperplasia	Diffuse	Focal
Trophoblastic stromal inclusions	Absent	Present
Karyotype	46XX (90%)	69XXY, 69XXY (66%)
	46XY (10%)	diploid (33%)
	diploid (33%)	
% of total hydatidiform moles	95%	5%
% that develop to persistent disease	20%	5%

What are the signs and symptoms of complete and partial moles?

Table 44–2.

	Complete (%)	Partial (%)
Vaginal bleeding	97	73
Excessive uterine size	51	4
Prominent ovarian theca lutein cysts	50	0
B-hCG > 100,000	50	6
Pre-eclampsia	27	3
Hyperemesis	26	0
Hyperthyroidism	7	0
Trophoblastic emboli	2	0

Vaginal bleeding is the presenting symptom in over 90% of moles.
Pre-eclampsia in the first half of pregnancy is virtually diagnostic of mole.
Hyperthyroidism is secondary to the high level of hCG, which behaves like TSH.

What is the treatment of hydatidiform mole?	The preferred method of treatment is evacuation of the uterus by suction and curettage. Hysterectomy is an alternative in selected patients.
What % of patients will be cured after uterine evacuation?	80%
What is invasive hydatidiform mole?	Features are those of hydatidiform mole, but edematous chorionic villi persist with invasion into the myometrium and continue to produce hCG. Rarely metastasize
What is the treatment of invasive hydatidiform mole?	First-line therapy is methotrexate (MTX). Since MTX is secreted by the kidney, urine creatinine levels must be normal before each treatment. Patients whose levels of hCG plateau or rise during therapy should be switched to alternative therapy. Alternative therapy: actinomycin-D or etoposide Early hysterectomy shortens the duration and amount of chemotherapy needed to produce remission.
What is the follow-up for hydatidiform mole?	Weekly measurement of serum hCG levels until levels are normal for 6 consecutive months. If levels plateau or rise during the 6-month interval, patient should be evaluated for metastasis. Virtually all episodes of malignant sequelae occur within 6 months of evacuation. Patient must use effective contraception for the entire interval of hormonal follow-up.

GESTATIONAL CHORIOCARCINOMA

What is choriocarcinoma?

Malignant form of trophoblastic disease, generally referred to as gestational trophoblastic neoplasm and always preceded by a pregnancy

Characterized by proliferation of cytotrophoblasts and syncytiotrophoblasts, but in contrast to invasive hydatidiform mole, no villi are present

What percentage of patients develop metastatic disease?

Approximately 50%

What is the incidence of gestational choriocarcinoma?

Rare, but can follow any type of pregnancy:
  Forty percent follow hydatidiform moles
  Thirty percent follow spontaneous abortions
  Twenty-four percent follow term deliveries

Difficult to assess exact incidence of choriocarcinoma because of its rarity and the difficulty in distinguishing between an invasive mole and nonmetastatic choriocarcinoma.

In North America and Europe, the rate is 1 in 20,000 to 1 in 40,000 pregnancies.

Slightly higher risk in Asia

What are the risk factors for choriocarcinoma?

History of hydatidiform mole
  3 percent of women with a molar pregnancy will develop choriocarcinoma.
  Approximately 50% of patients with choriocarcinoma have a history of a mole; the other 50% have had either a spontaneous abortion or a term delivery.

Maternal Age
  Increased risk after the age of 35
  Women over age 40 have a 5% to
    15% greater risk than younger
    women.
  ABO blood group incompatibility:
    More cases than statistically
    expected occur in women with
    blood type A.
  Oral contraceptive pill (OCP) use:
    Long-term OCP use has been
    associated with an increased risk.

What are the features and histologic findings?

No chorionic villi
Cytotrophoblasts and
  syncytiotrophoblasts

What are the signs and symptoms?

Same as those for hydatidiform mole

What is the treatment of choriocarcinoma?

Low risk (good prognosis)
  MTX or actinomycin-D
  Hysterectomy in conjunction with
    chemotherapy
High risk (poor prognosis)
  Triple therapy (MTX, actinomycin-D,
    cyclophosphamide, vincristine)
  Hysterectomy does not appear to
    improve the outcome in patients
    with high-risk metastatic disease.
  ± Radiation therapy to brain and liver
    to control metastatic disease

What is the follow-up for choriocarcinoma?

Weekly measurements of serum hCG
  levels until levels are normal for 3
  consecutive months
Monthly measurements of serum hCG
  levels until levels are normal for 12 to
  24 consecutive months depending on
  the stage of the disease
Again, effective contraception is a
  MUST.

PLACENTAL SITE TROPHOBLASTIC TUMOR

What is placental site trophoblastic tumor?

Consists primarily of intermediate trophoblasts

Usually limited to the uterus but may metastasize late in the course of disease

What is the incidence of placental site trophoblastic tumor?

Rarest form of GTD

What are the risk factors?

All are subsequent to a pregnancy; 5% of patients may have a history of a spontaneous abortion.

What are the features and histologic findings?

Histologically composed of only one cell type (intermediate trophoblast)

Can follow any type of pregnancy

What features of placental site trophoblastic tumor differentiate it from other GTDs?

Differs from choriocarcinoma primarily because of absence of syncytioblasts and cytotrophoblasts

Unlike other forms of GTD, hCG production is variable or may be absent and does not correlate with the extent of the disease. Measurement of HPL may be more reliable than hCG.

What are the signs and symptoms?

One-third of patients present with amenorrhea, positive β-hCG, and uterine enlargement.

Patients may present with menometrorrhagia.

What is the treatment of placental site trophoblastic tumor?

Often can be treated with dilation and curettage, but if it persists, it is fairly resistant to chemotherapy. Therefore, early hysterectomy is recommended.

45

Vulvar Cancer

GENERAL

Vulvar cancer comprises what percentage of all malignancies of the female genital tract?

Four percent

What are the etiologic factors?

A specific factor has not been identified.
The relationship of vulvar cancer to vulvar intraepithelial neoplasia, human papillomavirus (HPV), multiple sexual partners, and smoking is controversial.

In younger women with vulvar cancer, what percentage have evidence of HPV infection?

About 85% in warty squamous carcinomas and 40% in keratinizing squamous carcinomas

What are the signs and symptoms?

The usual presenting symptom is a palpable mass on the vulva. Most of the lesions occur on the labia majora, although vulvar cancer may occur anywhere on the external genitalia.
Many women present with vulvar itching.
Other presenting symptoms include bleeding and an abnormal discharge.

How is vulvar cancer diagnosed?

Definitive diagnosis is made by biopsy.

How is vulvar cancer staged?

Vulvar carcinomas are surgically staged because of the importance of evaluating the regional lymph nodes.
Stage 0: Carcinoma in situ, including Paget's disease
Stage I: Tumor confined to the vulva, < 2 cm in diameter, negative nodes
Stage II: Tumor confined to the vulva, > 2 cm in diameter, negative nodes

Stage III: Tumor of any diameter with the following:

Spread to urethra, vagina, anus; and/or

Unilateral regional lymph node metastases

Stage IV: Tumor of any diameter with any of the following:

Infiltration of the bladder or rectal or urethral mucosa

Fixed to the bone, or bilateral regional lymph node metastases

Distant metastases

What are the histologic types of primary vulvar cancer and their frequency?

Primary vulvar cancer comprises 92% of vulvar cancers.

Squamous cell carcinoma: 92%

Melanoma: 2–4%

Bartholin gland carcinoma: 1%

Basal cell carcinoma: 2%

Sarcoma: 1%–2%

Lymphoma, endodermal sinus: Rare

What percentage of vulvar cancers are metastases from other primary tumors?

Eight percent

What primary cancers typically metastasize to the vulva?

Cancers of the cervix, endometrium, kidney, and urethra

SQUAMOUS CELL CARCINOMA

What is the mean age of patients with squamous cell carcinoma of the vulva?

Age 65 years

What are the signs and symptoms?

A mass usually located on the labia majora. However, the labia minora, clitoris, and perineum may be involved. In 10% of cases, the location of the primary lesion cannot be determined because of the presence of multiple lesions at the time of presentation.

Pruritus, bleeding, or discharge

How does squamous cell carcinoma of the vulva spread?

By direct extension to adjacent tissues

By lymph nodes, primarily to the inguinal lymph nodes, then to the femoral lymph nodes and the external iliac lymph nodes (pelvic lymph nodes)

By circulation (hematogenous spread), primarily to the lung, liver, and bone; hematogenous spread usually occurs late in disease and is uncommon without lymphatic involvement.

Spread to how many lymph nodes increases the risk of distant metastatic disease?

More than three

What is the incidence of lymphatic spread?

Thirty percent

What factors influence the likelihood of lymphatic spread?

The size of the lesion and the depth of invasion

What is the treatment of stage I disease?

Before any treatment, the cervix, vagina, and vulva should be examined colposcopically.

Surgery:

Is the mainstay treatment: either wide local excision of the lesion or a radical vulvectomy

Wide local excision for vulvar cancer involves an incision carried down to the underlying fascia and a 1-cm negative surgical margin.

A radical vulvectomy involves excising both labia majora and the mons pubis to the depth of the underlying fascia.

A 1-cm negative surgical margin is predictive of excellent local control.

Wide local excision is the most appropriate treatment for lateral or posterior lesions, whereas radiotherapy may be preferred for anterior or periclitoral lesions.

Small vulvar lesions respond well to radiotherapy.

Groin lymph node dissection:

Must be considered, even in patients suspected of having only stage I disease, if there is >1 mm stromal invasion

The only patients without significant risk of lymph node metastases are those with < 1 mm of invasion.

Recurrent disease in the undissected groin carries a high mortality rate.

For unilateral lesions, the groin dissection only needs to be performed on the ipsilateral side.

If the lesion is midline, a bilateral groin dissection should be performed secondary to the increased risk for contralateral lymph node involvement.

What is the difference between early and late stage III disease?

Early stage III disease involves a lesion of any size with spread to adjacent organs. However, there is no unilateral lymph node metastasis, as there is with advanced stage III cancer.

What is the treatment of stage II and early stage III disease?

Surgery:

Radical vulvectomy and either ipsilateral or bilateral groin lymphadenectomy depending on the location of the lesion

Partial resection of other involved areas, such as the urethra, if necessary

Radiation therapy with concomitant chemosensitization: Preoperative radiation therapy may decrease the size of the primary lesion and thus allow a less extensive surgery.

What is the lymph node dissection that should be performed in stage II and early stage III disease if one positive lymph node is found?

No additional treatment is needed, and a contralateral lymph node dissection is not necessary.

Two or more positive nodes?

Contralateral dissection; patient should be considered for postoperative radiation to the groin and pelvis.

When is a pelvic lymph node dissection necessary?

There is a < 10% incidence of pelvic lymph node involvement; therefore, a pelvic lymph node dissection does not need to be performed unless:

More than three positive unilateral groin nodes are found; same-side pelvic nodes should be evaluated.

There are positive bilateral groin nodes.

What is the treatment of advanced stage III and stage IV disease?

Radical vulvectomy and bilateral groin dissection

Postoperative radiation therapy to the pelvis and groin if more than two groin nodes are positive

Preoperative radiation with or without chemotherapy can be considered as primary treatment in very advanced lesions (in poor surgical candidates, this may be the only option).

Pelvic exenteration may be necessary if bladder or rectal mucosa is involved.

What is the treatment of recurrent disease?

If the primary lesion is > 4 cm, there is a significant risk for recurrence. Treatment is further surgical resection or radiotherapy if the patient was not previously radiated to maximal dosage.

Systemic recurrences (lung, bone) are treated with chemotherapy; the most commonly used agents are cisplatin, cyclophosphamide, methotrexate, bleomycin, or mitomycin C. Systemic recurrences are associated with poor prognosis.

What are the complications from treatment?

Radical vulvectomy and groin dissection are associated with wound infection and breakdown in 40%–50% of patients secondary to the inability adequately to mobilize healthy skin to close the defect.

Sixty to 70% of patients will have chronic leg edema.

Mortality rate from radical vulvectomy is 2%, usually as a result of a pulmonary embolism or myocardial infarction.

Seromas occur in 10%–15% of patients and can be treated by aspiration if the patient is symptomatic.

Femoral nerve injury may occur, resulting in sensory loss to the anterior thigh; often resolves spontaneously.

Chronic cellulitis occurs on the side of the lymph node dissection in approximately 10% of patients.

Rare: Femoral hernias and fistula formation

What is the overall 5-year survival rate?

Seventy percent

What are the 5-year survival rates for each stage?

Stage I: 98%
Stage II: 85%
Stage III: 74%
Stage IV: 31%

What is the most important predictor of recurrence in squamous cell carcinoma of the vulva?

Number of involved groin nodes

What are the rates of recurrence based on this factor?	Less than three positive nodes: 12% rate of recurrence to the vulva, groin, pelvis, or systemically More than three positive nodes: 66% rate of local or systemic recurrence
What is another predictor of recurrence in squamous cell carcinoma of the vulva?	Location of positive lymph nodes
What are the 2-year survival rates based on the location of the positive lymph nodes?	Unilateral groin nodes: 70%–80% Bilateral regional nodes: 50% Bulky regional nodes: 30% Pelvic nodes: 10%

MELANOMA

What is the incidence of primary vulvar melanomas?	Rare
In what age group and race do these cancers commonly occur?	Postmenopausal white women
Where on the vulva do the melanomas commonly arise?	May arise either de novo or from a previously existing nevus Occur primarily on the labia minora or the clitoris
What are the signs and symptoms?	Patients usually present with a mass, bleeding, or pruritus.
What staging criteria are used for primary vulvar melanomas?	Traditional staging for vulvar cancer does not apply, because the prognosis for melanomas depends on the depth of invasion. Clark, Chung, or Breslow staging criteria are used. Breslow is most commonly used for vulvar melanoma. It measures the thickness of the lesion from the surface to the deepest point of invasion.

What are the Breslow stages for primary vulvar melanomas?

Stage I: < 0.76 mm
Stage II: 0.76–1.50 mm
Stage III: 1.51–2.25 mm
Stage IV: 2.26–3.0 mm
Stage V: > 3 mm

What is the treatment of lesions with < 1 mm of invasion?

Wide local excision

What is the treatment of lesions with > 1 mm of invasion?

Radical excision and groin dissection. If the lesion is located laterally, an ipsilateral dissection is needed. If the lesion is located medially, a bilateral dissection is indicated.
If the groin lymph nodes are involved, there is no benefit from a pelvic lymph dissection secondary to the poor prognosis.
No role for radiation therapy
Poor results with chemotherapy or immunotherapy

What is the overall 5-year survival rate?

20% to 30%

What is the 5-year survival rate for lesions with < 1 mm of invasion?

One hundred percent

BARTHOLIN GLAND CARCINOMA

Where are the Bartholin glands located?

In the labia majora

What is the most commonly occurring type of cancer of the Bartholin glands?

Multiple histologic types occur because of the various cell types that comprise a gland; the most commonly occurring type is adenocarcinoma.

What is the treatment?

Wide local excision of the primary tumor or a hemivulvectomy with ipsilateral groin lymph node dissection.
If the ipsilateral groin nodes are positive, the patient may benefit from a contralateral lymph node dissection and pelvic radiation therapy.

What is the overall 5-year survival rate?

Similar to that for a primary squamous cell carcinoma of the vulva

BASAL CELL CARCINOMA

In what age-group and race do basal cell carcinomas commonly occur?

Primarily postmenopausal white women

Where are these cancers commonly located?

On the labia majora

What is the treatment?

Three percent to five percent contain a squamous cell component and should be treated as a primary squamous cell to the vulva.
Primary treatment is wide local excision.

What is the prognosis?

Overall, good. There are too few cases to assign percentages.

Is metastatic disease to the lymph nodes common or rare?

Rare

What is the rate of local recurrence?

Twenty percent

VULVAR SARCOMA

What are the most common histologic subtypes of vulvar sarcoma?

Multiple; the most common are leiomyosarcoma and rhabdomyosarcoma.

Where does leiomyosarcoma commonly occur and what is the most common presentation?

In the labia majora and usually presents as a large, painful lesion

What is the treatment of vulvar leiomyosarcoma?

Wide local excision because lymph node involvement is rare

What is the overall 5-year survival rate for vulvar leiomyosarcoma?

Thirty percent

Rhabdomyosarcoma is the most common vulvar sarcoma of what age group?

Children

In what percentage of vulvar rhabdomyosarcomas is the pelvis involved?

Twenty percent

What is the treatment of vulvar rhabdomyosarcomas?

Similar to that for rhabdomyosarcoma in other pelvic organs (see Chap. 44)

Involves a combination of surgical resection, chemotherapy, and radiation therapy

What is the overall 5-year survival rate for vulvar rhabdomyosarcoma?

20% to 30%

46

Fallopian Tube Carcinoma

GENERAL

Primary fallopian tube carcinoma comprises what percentage of all primary cancers of the female genital tract?

0.3%

Fallopian tube carcinoma is similar to what other female genital tract cancer?

Epithelial ovarian carcinomas; diagnosis, treatment, and prognosis are therefore similar.

What primary cancers commonly metastasize to the fallopian tubes?

Ovarian, uterine, breast, and gastrointestinal tract

In what age group does fallopian tube carcinoma primarily occur?

Fifth to sixth decades of life

What are the signs and symptoms?

Classic triad of symptoms occurs in 15% of patients:
　Profuse, watery vaginal discharge
　Pelvic pain
　Pelvic mass
Fifty percent of patients present with vaginal bleeding or vaginal discharge.
Sixty percent of patients have a pelvic mass at the time of presentation.
Ten percent of patients have abnormal cells detected on a routine Papanicolaou smear.

How is fallopian tube carcinoma staged?

Staging is based on that used for ovarian carcinoma.
Stage I: Confined to the fallopian tubes, with or without malignant ascites

Stage II: Extends beyond the fallopian tubes but confined to the pelvic organs, with or without malignant ascites

Stage III: Confined to the abdominal cavity

Stage IV: Distant metastases

What are the histologic types of fallopian tube carcinoma and their frequency?

Epithelial serous: > 90%

Sarcoma: Rare

EPITHELIAL SEROUS CARCINOMA OF THE FALLOPIAN TUBES

What are the signs and symptoms?

Classic triad of pelvic pain, pelvic mass, and a watery discharge

What is the percentage of patients who present at each stage?

Stage I: 20%–25%
Stage II: 20%–25%
Stage III: 40%–50%
Stage IV: 5%

What is the treatment?

Overall, identical to that for ovarian carcinomas

The mainstay of treatment is exploratory laparotomy to resect the bulk of the tumor and adequately stage the disease. Adequate staging includes lymph node evaluation, biopsies of suspect areas, and cytologic evaluation of the peritoneal fluid.

The chemotherapeutic regimens are similar to those for ovarian cancer. First line agents are taxo- and carboplatin.

What is the overall 5-year survival rate?

Forty percent

What is the 5-year survival rate for each stage?	Stage I: 65% Stage II: 50%–60% Stages III–IV: 10%–20%

SARCOMA OF THE FALLOPIAN TUBES

What is the most common sarcoma of the fallopian tubes?	Primary mixed müllerian mesodermal tumor (MMMT)
Is MMMT common or rare?	Very rare
What is the common stage at presentation?	Advanced stage III–IV disease
Treatment?	Attempted resection of disease as described previously, with adjuvant chemotherapy. Radiation therapy has limited usefulness.
What is the overall 5-year survival rate?	Zero percent

47

Vaginal Cancer

GENERAL

Primary vaginal cancer comprises what percentage of all malignancies of the female genital tract?	1% to 2%
What percentage of vaginal cancers are metastases from other primary cancer?	80% to 90%
What cancers *usually* metastasize to the vagina?	Cervical or vulvar
What other cancers can metastasize to the vagina?	Uterine, gestational neoplasms, and (by direct extension) rectal and bladder
What are the signs and symptoms?	Fifty percent to seventy-five percent of patients present with painless vaginal bleeding, either postcoital or postmenopausal. Vaginal discharge is common. Five percent present with pelvic pain. Five percent to ten percent of patients are asymptomatic.
How is vaginal cancer diagnosed?	Diagnosis is often difficult if the lesion is small or endophytic or if the lesion is covered by the blades of the speculum. The speculum should be manipulated so that the anterior and posterior vaginal walls are well visualized. Definitive diagnosis: Biopsy
What findings are suspect for vaginal cancer?	An abnormal Papanicolaou smear and normal cervical colposcopy

How is vaginal cancer staged?	Clinically staged (similar to cervical cancer) based on physical examination, cystoscopy, proctoscopy, and chest radiography:
	Stage 0: Carcinoma in situ
	Stage I: Limited to vaginal mucosa
	Stage II: Submucosal tissue involvement but no extension to the pelvic sidewall
	Stage III: Extension to the pelvic sidewall
	Stage IV: Extension beyond the pelvis or involvement of the bladder or rectal mucosa
	IVa: Extension to adjacent organs
	IVb: Spread to distant organs
What are the histologic types of primary vaginal cancer and their frequencies?	Squamous cell carcinoma: 84%
	Adenocarcinoma: 9%
	Sarcoma: 3%
	Melanoma: 2%
	Miscellaneous (e.g., lymphoma, small cell): 2%

SQUAMOUS CELL CARCINOMA

What is the mean age of patients with squamous cell carcinoma?	Age 50–60 years
Where is squamous cell carcinoma usually located?	Upper posterior wall of the vagina
From what metastatic cancers is squamous cell carcinoma of the vagina difficult to differentiate?	Metastases from the cervix or vulva
Is squamous cell carcinoma associated with human papillomavirus?	Yes
What percentage of patients have a history of severe cervical dysplasia or cervical cancer?	Thirty percent
	May be secondary to the treatment for cervical cancer, especially if previously treated with radiation therapy.

If diagnosed more than 5 years after the cervical cancer, it is most likely a second primary lesion.

What percentage of patients present at each stage?

Stage I: 25%
Stage II: 34%
Stage III: 25%
Stage IV: 16%

How does squamous cell carcinoma spread?

Direct spread or invasion
Lymphatic spread, primarily to the inguinal and the pelvic lymph nodes
Hematogenous spread

What is the treatment of squamous cell carcinoma?

Overall, radiation is preferred.
Surgical treatment is indicated in a few circumstances:
Stage I disease in the upper vagina
In young patients, to preserve ovarian function
Patients with advanced local disease may undergo pelvic exenteration.
Radiation failures

What are the treatment options for carcinoma in situ?

Surgical excision to rule out invasive cancer
Laser ablation
Interstitial radiation
Radioactive implants placed in the vagina to provide local radiation dose to the affected area
Topical chemotherapy with 5-fluorouracil

What are the treatment options for stage I disease?

Radical hysterectomy with pelvic lymphadenectomy and partial vaginectomy
Interstitial radiation

What are the treatment options for stages II, III, and IV disease?

External and interstitial radiation

What are the complications from treatment?	Complications occur in 10%–15% of patients and include radiation cystitis, fistula formation, vaginal stenosis, and proctitis.
What is the overall 5-year survival rate?	Forty-two percent
What are the 5-year survival rates for each stage?	Stage I: 70% Stage II: 46% Stage III: 30%–40% Stage IV: 10%–15%

ADENOCARCINOMA

What is the frequency of primary adenocarcinoma of the vagina?	Rare
In what age group does this cancer primarily occur?	Except for clear cell adenocarcinoma, primarily in postmenopausal women Most clear cell adenocarcinomas occur in women 17–20 years of age.
What is the relationship between diethylstilbestrol (DES) exposure and clear cell adenocarcinomas?	Sixty-five percent of women with clear cell adenocarcinoma have documented evidence of DES exposure. Ten percent have exposure to a "unknown" drug. Twenty-five percent were not exposed to DES.
What is the estimated risk of clear cell carcinoma in DES-exposed women?	One in 1000
Where are adenocarcinomas primarily located?	In the exocervix or the upper third of the vagina
At what stage do most patients present?	Seventy percent present with stage I disease.

What is the treatment?	Similar to that for squamous cell carcinoma
	Stage I disease: Surgery is the primary treatment.
	Advanced stages: Radiation therapy is the primary treatment.
What is 5-year overall survival rate?	Seventy-eight percent
What are the 5-year survival rates for each stage?	Stage I: 87%
	Stage II: 76%
	Stage III: 30%

EMBRYONAL RHABDOMYOSARCOMA

What are the two types of embryonal rhabdomyosarcoma?	Solid and cystic.
	The cystic form is referred to as sarcoma botryoides, and is the most common vaginal tumor in infants and children.
In what age group do most embryonal rhabdomyosarcomas commonly occur?	Ninety percent occur in children younger than 5 years of age.
Where in women of reproductive age are embryonal rhabdomyosarcomas primarily located?	The cervix
Where in postmenopausal women are embryonal rhabdomyosarcomas primarily located?	The uterus
At what stage do most patients present with embryonal rhabdomyosarcoma?	Usually at an advanced stage

What is the treatment?
Previously treated with exenteration, which was ineffective and associated with a high complication rate
Currently, treatment involves a combination of surgical resection, chemotherapy, and radiation therapy.

What is the overall 5-year survival rate?
20% to 30%

MELANOMA

What is the mean age of patients with melanoma?
Age 60 years

In what race do melanomas almost always occur?
White

What are the signs and symptoms?
Most patients present with vaginal bleeding, discharge, or a mass.

Where are melanomas primarily located?
Most commonly arise in the distal vagina and may or may not be pigmented.

At what stage do most patients with melanoma present?
Melanoma is too rare to assign percentages.

What is the treatment?
Surgery has been the primary treatment, including radical exenteration, although local control is difficult to achieve with surgery alone.
Radiation therapy may be helpful in selected patients.

What is the overall 5-year survival rate?
Less than 10%

48

General Gynecologic Oncology

RADIATION THERAPY

What is radiation therapy?

Use of x-rays and gamma rays to treat cancer

How does radiation therapy kill cancer cells?

Cells are sensitive to the effects of radiation during the G2 phase of mitosis. The radiation kills cells by breaking DNA strands, either directly or by producing free radicals.

What is the relationship between tumor size and depth and the dose of radiation required to cause cell death?

As a tumor increases in size and depth, an increasing dose of radiation needs to be applied to cause cell death.

How is radiation therapy administered?

External beam: X-ray beam therapy in which electromagnetic energy is directed to the target tissue from an "external" source

Brachytherapy: Gamma-ray therapy in which the source is placed into the patient's body

In interstitial therapy, the source (e.g., cesium needles) is placed directly into the area of the tumor.

In intracavitary therapy, the source is placed indirectly in the area of the tumor (e.g., vaginal colpostats and uterine tandems).

Radioisotopes: Radiation therapy in which a radioisotope in solution (e.g., gold in solution) is placed in the peritoneal cavity to deliver radiation directly to the surface of the tumor

What is the inverse square law?

The dose of radiation delivered to the tissue is the inverse square of the distance from the source to the tissues.

What is the conventional unit of radiation used in radiation oncology?

Centigray (cGy)
One cGy is equal to 1 rad.

What are the dosage limitations for normal tissues?

Ovary: 1000 cGy
Kidney: 2500 cGY
Liver: 5000 cGY
Intestine: 6000 cGY
Bladder: 6500 cGY

What are the complications?

Both tumor cells and normal cells absorb radiation; surrounding tissues also undergo cell damage.

Acute complications: Nausea and diarrhea secondary to mucosal damage leading to mucosal irritation and sloughing; "sun burn" secondary to radiation absorption by the skin

Chronic complications: Radiation causes microvascular damage and fibrosis, leading to poor tissue oxygenation and repair.

Genitourinary tract: Fistulas between the bladder and surrounding organs, ureteral strictures, hemorrhagic cystitis

Gastrointestinal tract: Fistulas and strictures that may require surgical resection and repair

Vaginal stenosis, fistula tract formation

Ovarian failure with subsequent anovulation; hormone replacement should be considered in premenopausal women.

CHEMOTHERAPY

What is chemotherapy?

Use of drugs that exert a cytotoxic effect on cells

What are cycle-specific drugs?

Act only during a specific phase of cell division and therefore depend on cellular proliferation

What are cycle-nonspecific drugs?

Act during all phases and therefore depend less on cellular proliferation

What are the mechanisms of cytotoxicity of chemotherapeutic agents? Give examples of drugs for each mechanism.

DNA synthesis inhibitors [e.g., 5-fluorouracil (5-FU), methotrexate, bleomycin]

Mitotic inhibitors (e.g., vincristine, vinblastine, taxol)

Alkylating agents [e.g., ifosfamide, cyclophosphamide, doxorubicin (Adriamycin), cisplatin, carboplatin]

How are dosages calculated?

Most dosages are determined in clinical trials. Dosages are then individualized to the patient based on renal and hepatic function, body surface area, and side effects such as myelosuppression, nephrotoxicity, and neurotoxicity.

What is the mechanism of action of 5-FU?

Interferes with DNA synthesis by disrupting the DNA chain. It is a DNA synthesis inhibitor and cycle specific, and acts during the G2 phase of the cell cycle.

When is 5-FU used?

Primarily to treat cervical cancer and for vulvar and vaginal dysplasia

How is 5-FU excreted?

Renal

What are its toxicities?

Myelosuppression, nausea, vomiting, alopecia

What is the mechanism of action of methotrexate?

Interferes with DNA synthesis by interfering with folate reduction. It is a DNA synthesis inhibitor and cycle-specific, and acts during the G2 phase of the cell cycle.

When is methotrexate used?

Primarily to treat gestational trophoblastic disease

How is it excreted?

Renal

What are its toxicities?

Myelosuppression, mucositis, liver and kidney damage, alopecia

What is the mechanism of action of bleomycin?

Bleomycin is an antibiotic that forms free radicals that cause breaks in the DNA strand during mitosis. It is a DNA synthesis inhibitor and cycle-specific, and acts during the G2 phase of the cell cycle.

When is bleomycin used?

To treat squamous cell carcinoma of the vagina and vulva and ovarian germ cell tumors

How is it excreted?

Renal

What are its toxicities?

Interstitial pneumonitis, alopecia, and pulmonary fibrosis
Total dose must be limited to 400 mg secondary to an increased risk of pulmonary fibrosis.
Patients should be followed by chest x-ray and diffusion capacity of carbon monoxide.

What is the mechanism of action of vincristine?

Vincristine interferes with microtubule function during mitosis. It is a mitotic inhibitor and cycle-specific.

When is vincristine used?

To treat gestational trophoblastic disease and ovarian germ cell tumors

How is it excreted?

Renal

What are its toxicities?

Myelosuppression, neurotoxicity, alopecia

What is the mechanism of action of vinblastine?

Interferes with spindle formation during mitosis. It is a mitotic inhibitor and cycle-specific.

When is vinblastine used?

For the same conditions as vincristine

How is it excreted?

Renal

What are its toxicities?

Nausea, vomiting, myelosuppression, stomatitis, alopecia, and neurotoxicity

What is the mechanism of action of Taxol?

It is an alkaloid derived from the yew tree and acts by interfering with spindle cell function during mitosis. It is a mitotic inhibitor and cycle-specific.

When is Taxol used?

Primarily to treat ovarian cancer, but also used as second-line therapy for uterine and cervical carcinomas

How is it excreted?

Hepatic

What are its toxicities?

Myelosuppression, allergic reactions including anaphylaxis with cardiopulmonary collapse, seizures, nausea, vomiting, alopecia, neurotoxicity

What is the mechanism of action of ifosfamide?

Interferes with DNA linkage. It is an alkylating agent and cycle-nonspecific.

When is ifosfamide used?

To treat cervical and ovarian cancers, all sarcomas

How is it excreted?

Renal

What are its toxicities?

Myelosuppression, nausea, vomiting, alopecia, hemorrhagic cystitis, nephrotoxicity

What is the mechanism of action of cyclophosphamide?

Interferes with DNA linkage. It is an alkylating agent and cycle-nonspecific.

When is cyclophosphamide used?

Used primarily to treat ovarian and endometrial carcinoma

How is it excreted?

Renal

What are its toxicities?

Myelosuppression, nausea, vomiting, alopecia, hemorrhagic cystitis

What is the mechanism of action of doxorubicin?

Doxorubicin is an antibiotic that interferes with DNA and RNA synthesis by forming free radicals. It is an alkylating agent and cycle-nonspecific.

When is doxorubicin used?

To treat uterine and ovarian cancer

How is it excreted?

Hepatic

What are its toxicities?

Myelosuppression, nausea, vomiting, cardiomyopathy
Cardiomyopathy is dose-related; usually begins with 500 mg/m^2

What is the mechanism of action of carboplatin?

Carboplatin cross-links DNA. It is an alkylating agent and cycle-nonspecific.

When is carboplatin used?

To treat ovarian carcinoma

How is it excreted?

Renal

What are its toxicities?

Thrombocytopenia, nausea, vomiting, nephropathy, peripheral neuropathy

What is the mechanism of action of cisplatin?

Cross-links DNA; it is an alkylating agent and cycle-nonspecific.

When is cisplatin used?

To treat ovarian carcinoma and cervical cancer

How is it excreted?

Renal

What are its toxicities?

Decreased white blood cell count, ototoxicity, nephrotoxicity, peripheral neuropathy

SURGICAL PROCEDURES

What is a type I hysterectomy?
Surgical removal of the uterine corpus and cervix

What is a type II hysterectomy?
Surgical removal of the uterine corpus, cervix, and medial half of the cardinal ligaments

What is a type III hysterectomy?
Surgical removal of the uterine corpus, cervix, cardinal ligaments, uterosacral ligaments, and upper third of the vagina with pelvic lymph node dissection. Also known as a radical hysterectomy.

What is a type IV hysterectomy?
Type III hysterectomy with removal of periureteral tissues and three-fourths of the vagina

What is a type V hysterectomy?
Type IV hysterectomy with removal of the distal ureters and bladder; similar to an anterior exenteration

What is an anterior exenteration?
Removal of the uterine corpus, cervix, bladder, and vagina

What is a posterior exenteration?
Removal of the uterine corpus, cervix, rectum, and vagina

What is a total pelvic exenteration?
Removal of the uterine corpus, cervix, bladder, rectum, and vagina

49

Urinary Incontinence

INTRODUCTION

What is urinary incontinence?

The objective, involuntary loss of urine; presents a social and/or hygienic problem for the patient

Note: Urinary incontinence is a symptom, not a diagnosis, and therefore requires careful, thorough evaluation.

How common is it?

Reports among women less than 65 years of age range from 15% to 30%. In patients older than 65 years, the estimated prevalence is 30%.

ETIOLOGIES

What are some causes of urinary incontinence (especially in elderly patients)?

Anatomic abnormalities
Urinary infection
Drugs
General atrophy
Neurologic impairment

What is the most common form of urinary incontinence among women?

Stress incontinence (SUI) occurs during periods of increased intra-abdominal pressure (e.g., coughing, sneezing, exercise).

What is the pathophysiology of SUI?

In general, there is loss of anatomic support of the urethra, bladder, and/or urethrovesical junction, which allows the proximal urethra to be located outside the abdominal pressure zone. Thus, any increase in intra-abdominal pressure is transmitted to the bladder without a simultaneous rise in urethral pressure, so urine is involuntarily lost.

What factors contribute to the development of stress incontinence?

Denervation injuries from labor, childbirth, or pelvic surgeries
Previous bladder surgeries
Advanced age
Hypoestrogenism

What is intrinsic urethral sphincter deficiency?

Specific type of SUI, which may or may not coexist with an anatomic abnormality of the urethra
Usually results from previous bladder surgery or severe denervation injury
Urethra is rigid ("pipe stem")

How is the condition diagnosed?

Urodynamic evaluation

What is the treatment?

Pubovesical sling or collagen injections

What is urge incontinence?

Involuntary loss of urine associated with an abrupt and strong desire to void
Also known as **detrusor instability** because of overactivity of the detrusor muscle
In the presence of detrusor overactivity and a neurologic lesion (e.g., Parkinson's disease), the term **detrusor hyperreflexia** is commonly used.

How does the detrusor muscle normally serve to maintain urinary continence?

Normal micturition is under voluntary and involuntary control. The detrusor muscle is the smooth muscle wall of the bladder and normally contracts reflexively after voluntary relaxation of the pelvic floor and urethral musculature.

What is mixed urinary incontinence?

Urinary incontinence due to both detrusor instability and genuine stress incontinence

What are some other causes of urinary incontinence?	Urethral diverticulum Congenital abnormalities (e.g., ectopic ureter) Urinary fistula Bladder cancer

What drugs can cause incontinence?	Diuretics:
	  Methyldopa
	  Prazosin
	Antihistamines:
	  Phenothiazines
	  Diazepam

What is overflow incontinence?	Results from underactivity of the detrusor muscle, most commonly from a neurogenic (e.g., diabetic) or postoperative bladder Bladder fails to empty adequately, resulting in a large postvoid residual (PVR), usually > 300 ml Leakage can thus be precipitated by small increases in intra-abdominal pressure because the bladder is always full.

EVALUATION

What are the pertinent questions to ask when taking the patient's history?	"Do you leak when coughing, sneezing, laughing, or with exercise?" (suggests SUI) "Do you leak before you reach the toilet with a strong urge to void?" (suggests urge incontinence) "How many voids per day?" (frequency suggests infection or overflow) "Nocturia or incontinence with intercourse?" (suggests urge incontinence) "Do you wear pads? How disabling is the problem?" "How often do you have leaking?" "History of UTIs?" "Painful urination?" (suggests obstruction, cancer, infection)

"Hematuria?" (suggests cancer, infection)

"Difficulty initiating voiding?" (suggests obstruction, loss of bladder support, neurologic impairment)

"Straining with urination?" (suggests obstruction)

"Feeling of incomplete emptying?" (suggests obstruction, loss of bladder support)

Note: Some patients may benefit from keeping a voiding diary.

What should be looked for on physical examination?

Atrophy
Vaginal infection
Urethral diverticulum
Cystocele
Descent of bladder

What is the Q-tip test?

A Q-tip lubricated with viscous lidocaine is placed in the urethra at the urethrovesical junction.

To check for hypermobility of the urethra (a condition often associated with stress incontinence), have the patient Valsalva. If the Q-tip deviates more than about 30°, the test is positive.

What tests can be performed in the office to assess urinary incontinence?

Urinalysis with culture should always be performed.
Urine cytology for women with unexplained hematuria

What are office cystometrics?

After the patient empties her bladder, postvoid residual is checked.

A sterile catheter is then placed in the bladder, which is filled with increments of 50 to 100 cc sterile water.

Patient is asked to relay her first filling sensation, first urge to void, and maximum bladder capacity.

What does a detrusor contraction look like?

A rise in the meniscus of fluid in the catheter suggests a detrusor contraction.

What is a stress test?

After maximal filling, the patient is asked to cough.

If she **immediately** leaks urine, the test is positive.

If leakage occurs several seconds after provocation, the patient may have a component of detrusor instability.

It is essential to check in both the supine and the standing position.

Who should be referred for more sophisticated urodynamic testing?

Approximately 10% to 15% of patients will require multichannel urodynamic testing for diagnosis. Such studies might be useful for patients with:

Mixed urge and stress symptoms

Prior bladder surgeries

Suggestive history, but negative office evaluation

Also used to rule out intrinsic sphincter deficiency, which may predict surgical failure

What are the benefits of cystoscopy?

Can diagnose fistulae, foreign bodies, tumors, or aberrant ureters

What is the purpose of multichannel urodynamic tests?

Specialized catheters simultaneously record urethral, vesical, and intra-abdominal pressures, and precisely diagnose detrusor instability and/or stress incontinence.

TREATMENT

What are the treatment options for urinary incontinence?

Behavioral modification
Pharmacologic treatment
Surgical management

What are some behavioral techniques used to treat urinary incontinence?

Encouraging patient to avoid excess fluid and/or caffeine intake
Regularly scheduled voiding

Biofeedback techniques

Clean, intermittent self-catheterization

Vaginal pessaries, if pelvic organ prolapse is also present

What are some pharmacologic agents used to treat urinary incontinence?

Antispasmodics (e.g., oxybutynin)

Tricyclic antidepressants (e.g., imipramine)

α-adrenergic agents (e.g., phenylpropanolamine)

Is hormone replacement recommended?

In postmenopausal women, estrogen replacement (topical or oral) has some benefit in treating stress or urge incontinence.

What is the Burch procedure?

Abdominal retropubic urethropexy operation

Uses suture to suspend the paravaginal fascia (which supports/surrounds the urethra) to the abdominal side of the pubic bone

Point of attachment is Cooper's ligament, better known as the iliopectineal line

Success rate is 75% to 90%

What complications are associated with the Burch procedure?

An enterocele (occurs in 7% to 15% of patients)

What is the Marshall-Marchetti-Krantz procedure?

Abdominal retropubic urethropexy operation

Uses suture to suspend the paravaginal fascia to the abdominal side of the pubic bone

Point of attachment is the cartilage in the symphysis pubis

Success rate is 75% to 90%

What complication is associated with the MMK procedure?

Osteitis pubis, a painful inflammatory condition (occurs in up to 5% of patients)

What is a Pereyra procedure?

Type of vaginal suspension for SUI

What is the advantage of a Pereyra procedure?

Vaginal approach

What is the disadvantage of this procedure?

Potential bladder injury and smaller objective cure rate (40%–70%)

What is a suburethral sling procedure?

Reserved for patients at most risk for operative failure (those with intrinsic sphincter deficiency, severe obesity, prior surgical failures, or a scarred, fibrotic urethra)

Restores continence by elevating the urethrovesical junction and mechanically compressing the urethra against the pubic symphysis

Autologous graft material, usually a thin strip of rectus fascia, is tunneled under the urethra and sewn to the abdominal wall

What are the possible complications of a suburethral sling procedure?

Postoperative voiding dysfunction, especially urinary retention

What are some other surgical techniques?

Periurethral collagen injections

Insertion of an artificial urinary sphincter

Index